A Researcher's Guide to Usir
Electronic Health Records

In an age when electronic health records (EHRs) are an increasingly important source of data, this essential textbook provides both practical and theoretical guidance to researchers conducting epidemiological or clinical analysis through EHRs.

Split into three parts, the book covers the research journey from start to finish. Part 1 focuses on the challenges inherent when working with EHRs, from access to data management, and raising issues such as completeness and accuracy which impact the validity of any research project. Part 2 examines the core research process itself, with chapters on research design, sampling, and analysis, as well as emerging methodological techniques. Part 3 demonstrates how EHR research can be made meaningful, from presentation to publication, and includes how findings can be applied to real-world issues of public health.

Supported by case studies throughout, and applicable across a range of research software programs (including R, SPSS, and SAS), this is the ideal text for students and researchers engaging with EHRs across epidemiological and clinical research.

Neal D. Goldstein, PhD, MBI, is an Associate Professor of Epidemiology at the Drexel University Dornsife School of Public Health. He can be reached through his website: www.goldsteinepi.com.

A Researcher's Guide to Using Electronic Health Records

From Planning to Presentation

Second Edition

Neal D. Goldstein

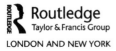
Routledge
Taylor & Francis Group

LONDON AND NEW YORK

Cover image credit: © Getty Images

Second edition published 2023
by Routledge
4 Park Square, Milton Park, Abingdon, Oxon, OX14 4RN

and by Routledge
605 Third Avenue, New York, NY 10158

Routledge is an imprint of the Taylor & Francis Group, an informa business

First edition published by Routledge 2017

British Library Cataloguing-in-Publication Data
A catalogue record for this book is available from the British Library

ISBN: 978-1-032-19372-4 (hbk)
ISBN: 978-1-032-16959-0 (pbk)
ISBN: 978-1-003-25887-2 (ebk)

DOI: 10.4324/9781003258872

Typeset in Bembo
by KnowledgeWorks Global Ltd.

To Joanna and Reid

Contents

Figures

Tables

Boxes

About the author

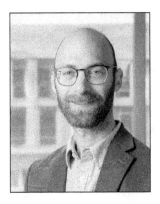

Neal D. Goldstein, PhD, MBI is an Associate Professor of Epidemiology at the Drexel University Dornsife School of Public Health. With a background in biomedical informatics, he focuses on computational approaches in complex data settings, especially electronic health records and disease surveillance, to understand infectious disease transmission. This has been demonstrated through his work with bloodborne pathogens, COVID-19, vaccine-preventable diseases, and healthcare-associated infections. Dr. Goldstein is well-published, his work has been profiled in national and local media outlets, and he has been featured in countless interviews. More information can be found on the book website, https://www.goldsteinepi.com/books/ehr/, including errata, data, source codes, and more.

Preface to the Second Edition

It should come as no surprise that EHRs are near ubiquitous in clinical practices in the U.S. and abroad. Likewise, we have witnessed the "big data" movement in healthcare, where massive and high-dimensional data sets are commonplace in research. Given the accessibility of EHR data to clinicians, researchers, and data scientists, individuals are engaging in EHR-based research at an unprecedented rate that will only continue to increase. When the first edition of this book was released in 2017, there was a lack of books devoted to epidemiological research of EHRs, and even as this second edition comes to the press, this problem persists. However, scholarly output using EHR data has exploded, most often in the form of academic journal articles, making this second edition timelier than ever.

Following the first edition, I received numerous letters from colleagues and readers of the book requesting a fuller treatment of EHR research. This sentiment was echoed in an ongoing EHR workshop I annually host. The first edition focused mostly on data management aspects of EHRs as the basis for valid epidemiological analysis, and in fact, this was reflected in the lofty and verbose title *Improving Population Health Using Electronic Health Records: Methods for Data Management and Epidemiological Analysis*. This second edition covers the entire spectrum of using EHRs for health research, no longer just data management. These additions include understanding the architecture of the EHR, clinical workflow, and the healthcare system; designing EHR-based research and asking appropriate research questions; obtaining data from the EHR; cleaning the data and other data management steps; conducting an epidemiological analysis with specific focus on challenges and solutions for working with EHR data; and advanced and emerging methodologic techniques. Case studies are included that reinforce the concepts presented throughout the book, and may be used for discussion in a classroom setting.

While all readers may not be hands-on in each one of these steps in this continuum, it is nevertheless important to understand what is required at each step, which ultimately improves the validity of the research. Underscoring the entire book is the notion of EHR data literacy, which carries through the spirit of both the first and second editions. This second edition also moves beyond entry-level and incorporates material for intermediate and advanced EHR-based epidemiological investigations, while at the same time maintain the approachability of the original edition that so many readers appreciated.

I am indebted to those who provided feedback on the first edition as well as drafts of the second edition. I would especially like to thank my clinical colleagues who have contributed their time and expertise in the series of interviews that provided invaluable perspectives on the use of EHRs for clinical and research needs. My ambitious hope is this second edition will become a definitive reference on EHR research in epidemiology, perhaps motivating dedicated graduate courses in the analysis of electronic health records. I welcome feedback, positive or negative, on this edition, and can be contacted through the book website: https://www.goldsteinepi.com/books/ehr/.

Neal D. Goldstein
December 2022
Philadelphia, PA

Introduction

1 The Rise of Electronic Health Records

The collection of health information on a large-scale basis may not be new, but the availability of tools and techniques to analyze electronic health record (EHR) data enables efficient and effective health research. Today's personal computers are capable of astounding feats that a mere generation ago would have necessitated not only large, air-conditioned rooms, but also capital investments that all but a few of the largest corporations could afford. No longer is technology the limiting factor in clinical and public health research; it is the interconnection of disparate systems and the expertise of cross-discipline researchers that represents the current shortcoming.

With the goal of improving health outcomes via epidemiological analysis of EHR data, researchers need to be cognizant of the entire spectrum of data acquisition, management, analysis, and interpretation. Due to the variety of stakeholders in the process (Figure 1.1), research tends to be disjointed, with individuals of varied experiences and expertise handling discrete components in isolation. For example, the clinician has experience in the ascertainment and interpretation of health information, whereas a statistician is an expert in analytic methodology. Without communication between the two individuals, a statistician may misunderstand the data in the EHR, whereas a clinician may misinterpret the results from the study. This is not ideal; the research process is a continuum, dependent on previous steps, and the goal of improving health can only be realized through seamless transition in the workflow.

Another way to visualize the relationship between clinical practice, health informatics and information technology, and the researcher is through a "zone" model as described by Verheij et al. (2018). Figure 1.2 depicts the processes and actors involved in the secondary analysis of EHR data. One can see how the roles of care delivery, data management, and research become compartmentalized and any data "hand off" may result in the contamination of data. Indeed, based on this workflow, the authors identified 13 potential sources of "bias" that can occur in the EHR research workflow. The validity of EHR data and epidemiological research is a unifying theme in this book.

What follows in this book are two overarching aims: one didactic and one pragmatic. Didactically, the book aims to improve the reader's comprehension of the EHR research continuum as well as the data encountered therein.

DOI: 10.4324/9781003258872-2

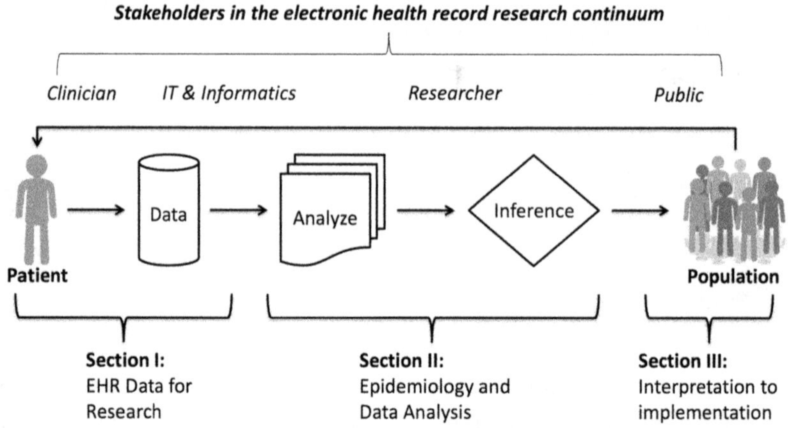

Stakeholders in the electronic health record research continuum
Clinician
IT & Informatics
Researcher
Public
Data
Analyze
Inference
Patient
Population
Section I:
EHR Data for Research
Section II:
Epidemiology and Data Analysis
Section III:
Interpretation to implementation

Figure 1.1 From patient to results: the electronic health record research process and its stakeholders.

Care zone
Database zone
Research zone
Delivery of care
Clinical practice
Recording in EHR
EHR system
Extraction from EHR
Translation into database
Database manager
Prepare dataset for researcher
Research methods
Researcher
Outcome and interpretation

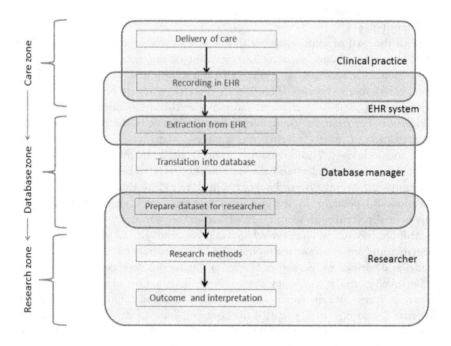

Figure 1.2 A zone model of stakeholders in electronic health record research.

Pragmatically, the book provides concrete guidance for the researcher working with EHR data, from preparing the data, to performing the analysis, and finally interpreting and disseminating the results. For example, extracting and linking EHR data has traditionally been viewed as a role for information technology (IT) or informatics, with minimal appreciation by the researcher for the underlying data architecture. Yet, by examining this architecture, the researcher can be better prepared to analyze the data properly, minimizing the chance for errors due to miscommunication or misunderstanding of what a data point represents (Figure 1.2).

Evolution of the modern EHR

A key driver of large-scale health research has been the adoption of EHRs by hospital systems, as well as an increasing number of small practices, and the connection of these systems together through health information exchanges (HIEs). Modern-day EHRs are not simply electronic copies of patients' medical charts: they represent a suite of applications and tools that enable the electronic management of health. However, initially, EHRs were mere data repositories – termed clinical data repositories – and in some crude cases represented scanned versions of paper medical charts. Early adopters of "medical computing" included notable institutions like Massachusetts General Hospital in the late 1960s with the Computer Stored Ambulatory Record (Oregon Health & Science University, 2015a), Indiana University Medical Center in the early 1970s with the Regenstrief Medical Record System (Oregon Health & Science University, 2015b), and the Veterans Health Administration with the Veterans Health Information Systems and Technology Architecture in the late 1970s (Oregon Health & Science University, 2015c). These systems provided electronic health data capture and retrieval, as well as primitive decision support services. Concurrent with these efforts were a variety of other small- and large-scale practices both nationally and internationally (Oregon Health & Science University, 2015d).

One of the primary drivers toward widespread use of EHRs came from the Health Information Technology for Economic and Clinical Health (HITECH) Act portion of the 2009 American Reinvestment & Recovery Act, which demanded the evolution of these systems to their current incarnation of interconnected health tools that exist first and foremost to improve health outcomes (U.S. Department of Health & Human Services, 2021a). Although some providers balked at the notion of implementing EHRs, mainly from expense and early inefficiency, by 2014 nearly 75% of US-based providers had implemented them (Jamoom, Yang & Hing, 2016). Independent and smaller private practices have traditionally lagged behind EHR adoption compared to integrated practices (Everson, Richards & Buntin, 2019), and as such represent the healthcare settings least likely to have EHRs. Yet the trend toward ubiquity will only continue as independent practices consolidate or are pressured from competition and patient expectations for services offered in the EHR (e.g., virtual visits, electronic prescriptions, digital imaging, automated referrals, and so on). Combined with the "meaningful use" incentives for adopting EHRs as put forth in the HITECH act, requirements of Medicare and Medicaid, and a newer generation of clinicians raised with EHRs, reverting to a paper-based system is a near impossibility.

Population health research was a natural extension of HITECH, and specific sections of the act called for "improved population health outcomes" and "more robust research data on health systems" also as part of meaningful use (U.S. Department of Health & Human Services, 2021b). As EHRs largely necessitate coded data entry, research from these data is greatly improved, both in terms of accuracy and efficiency. Even among noncoded free-text data, as warranted to capture specific nuance or subtlety common in certain medical domains like behavioral health, natural language parsing makes it possible to transform free-text data to coded data (discussed further in Chapter 12).

The interconnection of the various EHRs was the logical next step. Again, spurred on by the HITECH act, a joint health record was needed that acknowledged patients interact with a variety of providers, and many of these providers stored data in "silos," inaccessible by other providers. By connecting data silos together in health information networks, also known as HIEs, providers now have a longitudinal view of patient outcomes over time (Oregon Health & Science University, 2015e). The data linkage and management have been done for them, and therefore a much richer set of data are available to track patient outcomes. Unfortunately for the researcher, access to a complete longitudinal view of a patient's health may still be out of reach, especially in areas where patients have choice as to where to seek care. The legislation that enabled statewide HIEs may specifically prohibit their use for research purposes: readers will need to consult with their respective state's HIE-enabling legislation to assess what is permissible.

In short, the current state of EHRs is the result of evolution over 50 years, and researchers are likely to encounter a variety of systems and vendors in practice. A best-of-breed or hybrid model has been used by many organizations, which is intended to select the most appropriate EHR product given specific departmental or functional requirements at that time. On the other hand, some organizations have favored a single vendor, unified system that enables efficient data sharing and consistent user experience, while potentially sacrificing features or cost. As of July 2017, among providers participating in the Medicare EHR Incentive Program, the top five most common EHR vendors in outpatient medicine were Epic Systems Corporation, Allscripts, eClinicalWorks, NextGen Healthcare, and GE Healthcare (Office of the National Coordinator for Health Information Technology, 2017a) and the top five most common EHR vendors in inpatient medicine were Epic Systems Corporation, Cerner Corporation, Medical Information Technology (MEDITECH), McKesson, and MEDHOST (Office of the National Coordinator for Health Information Technology, 2017b).

Using electronic health records for research

A paper written during the nascent stages of EHR adoption identified the merits of paper-based charts, including familiarity, portability, flexibility, and readability (Hersh, 1995). Since space was at a premium, the information recorded in a paper chart tended to be concise with only the most (subjectively) relevant details recorded. Yet for the researcher, paper records for large-scale health research were next to useless because they were often inaccessible to anyone outside of the practice, may lack readability and interpretability, and may not reflect a population sample (discussed further in Chapters 6, 7, and 9). With electronic data linkage, EHRs can address the shortcomings of paper records. EHRs allow for efficiency of scale in data capture – since space is no longer a limited factor – and standardized coding. The public health value in aggregating medical data in real-time and large-scale ways has already been demonstrated, for example, through identification of lead poisoning of children in Flint, Michigan (Hanna-Attisha et al., 2016), or real-time surveillance for COVID-19 in the United States (Burke et al., 2021). Public health surveillance using EHRs is discussed in detail in Chapter 14. Yet researchers must recognize that *more data do not equal better research*, and there are many common elements of sound epidemiologic research inherent in paper- and EHR-based research, including proper study design, appropriate measurement of data, and correct analytic techniques, all of which are accompanied by potential for bias that may jeopardize findings.

The secondary uses of EHR data for research have rapidly increased over the past few decades. Indeed, a simple PubMed search for "electronic medical record" (a term historically more used than EHR) reveals nearly 80,000 citations through December 31, 2021, and shows a remarkable growth in citation numbers in the current millennium (Figure 1.3). Such data are used for a variety of reasons: administrative reporting, certification and accreditation, quality and safety monitoring, public health, and, of course, research and analysis (Safran et al., 2007). EHR data may inform our understanding of the prevalence of morbidities, be used to associate putative "exposures" with health outcomes (for purposes of estimating relative or absolute risks), or further our understanding of how the healthcare environment itself may contribute to diseases. One contemporary use of EHR data that has attracted much attention is measuring and describing a community's health based on patients captured within a healthcare system, supplementing metrics obtained from traditional public health surveillance programs (Kruse et al., 2018). In fact, the use of EHR data for research has resulted in entire books dedicated to this topic, including the first edition of this book (Goldstein, 2017), as well as others (MIT Critical Data, 2016). The reader is also referred to these review articles that summarize the challenges and opportunities of EHR-based research (Casey et al., 2016; Cowie et al., 2017; Gianfrancesco & Goldstein, 2021; Raman et al., 2018; Shortreed et al., 2019).

This book is grounded in EHRs as a data source for health research, although the methods discussed are broadly applicable to other health data sources that present similar challenges when working with high dimensional data. For example,

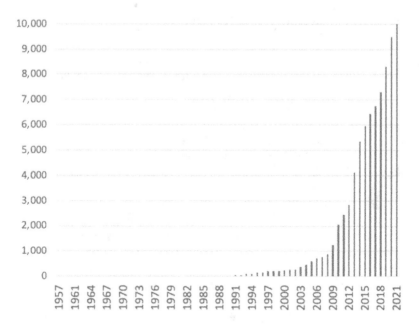

Figure 1.3 Citations in PubMed matching the search term "electronic medical record" through December 31, 2021.

large electronic registries, such as immunization information systems, notifiable disease systems, cancer registries, claims databases, and so on, provide population-level data useful to researchers and are often under the charter of local or regional health departments (except billing and insurance which may be from private entities). Although registries are not explicitly discussed, they can be thought of as special cases of EHRs: the patient has a specific encounter with a provider that leads to data generated in an electronic system and is a process dependent on the provider encounter. There are also many types of EHR research possible: observational studies, safety surveillance, clinical research, as well as regular activities (see Table 1 in Cowie et al., 2017, for specific examples). The specific type of research will be qualified if needed; again, the goal is for a generic representation of health research from the EHR.

EHRs and "big data"

Big data is an abstract concept, but it is not a new concept. The term gained popularity in the early 2000s. Data tend to become "big" when they have certain properties, and depending on the scope of the EHR, may or may not fulfill the theoretical definition. An academic medical center may contain millions of records capturing thousands of data points while a small private practice may only have a thousand patient panel with significantly fewer variables. Although this book is not intended to offer a new definition of big data, or explore its theoretical underpinnings, there is a need to ground big data in theory, so as researchers we can be consistent in its definition.

The META Group, now part of the Garner Group (Stamford, CT), offered one of the original definitions in 2001 centered around three "V"s of big data, namely data volume, velocity, and variety (Laney, 2012). The definition has since been adopted by many and altered to incorporate additional "V"s. In the definition's original form, the three "V"s are:

1 *Volume.* In combination with data becoming cheap, it is also a commodity necessary for business, including the business of healthcare. Therefore, the volume of data has increased, and will continue to increase, substantially over time.
2 *Velocity.* The pace at which data are acquired has also increased markedly. In addition to more data being captured, it is being captured quicker.
3 *Variety.* Data are heterogeneous, from primary care provider office notes to medical images to laboratory reports and so on. Data will become increasingly heterogeneous as more systems are incorporated together. Big data repositories must be able to capture a wide variety of data formats and adapt to emerging and yet-to-be-identified types.

This definition was appropriate in 2001, when it was proposed, and has held up since. EHRs certainly fulfill the three "V"s of big data, and in fact, have fulfilled the definition well before its existence. A question arises, what should one do with the increasing volume of disparate health data?

This question seeks to define the architecture of big data repositories, such as a clinical data warehouse, and it is the answer to this question that will have some purists deviating from the architecture proposed in this book. Herein, we propose a simplified architecture of a research database, with an eye toward the most efficient pathway to valid epidemiological analysis, that is likely to satisfy most EHR-based research projects. Yet there are alternative approaches; Chapter 4 discusses the strengths and weaknesses of these alternative approaches. Importantly and regardless of the data architecture, the methods presented in this book will help to ensure valid research.

The intended audience of this text further necessitates a practical, rather than a theoretical framework for big data. The primary readers of this book include the researcher who is new to EHRs; the clinician who needs a concise how-to guide for obtaining data and conducting a study; the IT or informatics professional who seeks to understand the needs of health researchers; the healthcare administrator who has been tasked with assessing health metrics from the EHR; and the public health worker using EHRs for surveillance purposes. *The text is written toward these readers who may have limited resources, and therefore wish to take on multiple roles in the research process.* Besides this primary audience, the text will also prove useful for anyone who interacts with health data, as a better understanding of its use beyond clinical care could only improve data quality and therefore research quality. All levels of experience will benefit from this book, from trainees to seasoned professionals.

Stakeholders in the research process

Perhaps one of the biggest barriers to effective EHR research involves the complexity of the healthcare system. There are a variety of stakeholders in the research process, and each has their own agenda (Figure 1.1). Beginning from the initial encounter into the system, the patient is concerned with an acute or chronic health problem or preventive maintenance. He or she may not even be aware that the data generated as part of that encounter ultimately may get used in research despite the Health Insurance Portability and Accountability Act's Privacy Rule that contains explicit provisions for research from patient data collected during the encounter. From the patient's perspective, the interest is getting well (or staying well) with the expectation that the provider seen has the best treatments available. From the clinician's perspective, their interest also reflects the patient's interest: how can an illness be cured or prevented, or sequelae mitigated. The clinician, whether a physician, nurse, medical assistant, or other healthcare professionals, acts as the gatekeeper to the system. Their knowledge of therapeutics or prophylactics is drawn from experience, literature, and colleagues. Therefore, the physician likely represents the first opportunity for health research, often in the form of a clinical question: "Will this intervention benefit my patient?" Unfortunately, the clinician may lack time, expertise, and data to answer this question, instead relying on existing, and possibly outdated, literature. The data generated from each patient encounter is entered by the clinician or ancillary staff into the EHR.

At this point, the IT or informatics group assumes responsibility for the integrity and accessibility of the health data entered by the provider. IT and their more recent colleagues informaticists, who are trained in both IT and healthcare, maintain the information systems and therefore have the most comprehensive knowledge of the availability and structure of the data. The clinician interested in conducting research therefore needs to effectively communicate with IT to receive the correct data in order to answer the research question at hand. The importance of this step cannot be overstated as it will influence success or failure of the research project. The informaticist serves as the liaison between groups but is likely a luxury only the larger institutions have on staff. In addition, the IT group may have their own policies and procedures in place that can, occasionally and unfortunately, inhibit the research process; as such, one of the goals of this work is to empower the clinician in the research process, making the research data request as efficient as possible and minimizing the burden on IT.

Assuming data are available to answer the original research question, a new stakeholder enters the process: the health researcher. Their background has them well suited to design and analyze the study yet are often dependent on the successful handoff of data. This handoff of data, channeled through IT, originates with the clinician assessing which patient characteristics are most meaningful to study. Working hand in hand with the researcher can further elucidate these characteristics. Finally, after the analysis is completed and the results generated, the findings need to be effectively communicated to all stakeholders in the process, as well as the community at large. In fact, this may be the most crucial point in the research process: findings, whether positive, negative, or equivocal need to be relayed clearly and concisely to others for incorporation into the greater body of scientific knowledge. The entire process becomes a continuum as the community becomes influenced by the outcomes of research and shapes the scope and nature of the patients re-entering the system. Last, but certainly not least, overseeing this entire process is the institutional review board routinely made up of all identified stakeholders, ensuring the research is ethical, lawful, and necessary.

As can be seen in Figures 1.1 and 1.2, this is a process that is highly dependent on each previous step, and initial errors, such as an ambiguous data request, can be further magnified as the research progresses, akin to the telephone game played by children, jeopardizing the results of the research. Furthermore, each stakeholder in the process has a highly specialized skillset. Efficiency in the process can be gained by having researchers cross-trained in the core disciplines (Goldstein, LeVasseur & McClure, 2020); for example, clinicians who obtain epidemiology training, IT personnel who obtain clinical training, and health researchers who obtain IT training. Besides formal training, shadowing individuals provides a valuable appreciation of the healthcare environment, job functions, and workflow of the varied stakeholders. Shadowing can also provide an understanding of the meaning of health data: from how it is collected, to entered and stored in the EHR, to recalled for later use.

Depending on the stakeholders involved, the goals of EHR research may clash. For example, a clinician may want to know how a therapy or intervention will benefit their patient; an epidemiologist may want to know a population average effect rather than a single patient effect; and a hospital administrator may want to know how a quality improvement initiative has changed rates over time. Often our end goal is to establish causality: how some factor or intervention relates to some health state. Yet, as will be discussed in Chapter 11, causality is not always an attainable and practical goal; further, it may not matter for most interventions.

The need for a cohesive view of research

Given the complexity of the data and variety of stakeholders in the healthcare system, the traditional paradigm of research as its own standalone process needs to change. Collaborations are a given in scientific inquiry and should be viewed as crucial to success for a given line of research. Without a clear understanding of disease process, or any health state for that matter, and direction for the research, the right data will not be retrieved from the underlying electronic database. Once an initial research question is formed and testable hypothesis are constructed, the correct stakeholders need to be identified, as they may be the best suited to assess the feasibility of the research.

The remainder of this book serves as a researcher's guide to using EHRs, assuming a research question and data are available. The approach to the subject matter is divided into three distinct sections: understanding the data (Section I), conducting the research (Section II), and interpretation and application of the findings (Section III).

Section I introduces the fundamentals of EHR research and moves into challenges in accessing the data including data extraction and linkage issues. This is a crucial step in the research continuum, and unfortunately is only viewed as a "black box"; that is, a request for data is made and data are provided that may or may not be correct. This may result in a dataset missing data on some key factors while containing information extraneous to research. This section concludes by describing several caveats of EHR data, so the researcher understands the extent and limitation of what is captured in the EHR.

Section II presents the core epidemiology and statistics, introducing essential study designs and statistical techniques needed to analyze *secondary* data, in other words, data retrieved from the EHR originally captured for nonresearch purposes. In addition, this section discusses common threats to validity of EHR research and introduces the quantitative bias analysis to describe the extent that bias may impact study findings. Advanced and emerging epidemiological and statistical methods round out this section.

Section III details preferred methods for presenting results and provides many concrete examples to reinforce these methods. Public health applications of EHR research are also considered as is using the EHR for surveillance purposes. To conclude the book, a variety of case studies are provided to further cement the concepts presented in the text.

For readers wishing to skip ahead or use this book in a piece-meal fashion, Chapter 2 presents a flowchart of the book, and Appendix 1 includes a research planner with specific page numbers and sections most relevant to specific points in the research process. Additional information can be found on the book website, https://www.goldsteinepi.com/books/ehr/, including errata, data, source codes, and more.

References

Burke PC, Shirley RB, Faiman M, Boose EW, Jones RW, Merlino A, Gordon SM, Fraser TG. Surveillance for probable COVID-19 using structured data in the electronic medical record. Infect Control Hosp Epidemiol. 2021 Jun;42(6):781–783.

Casey JA, Schwartz BS, Stewart WF, Adler NE. Using electronic health records for population health research: A review of methods and applications. Annu Rev Public Health. 2016;37:61–81.

Cowie MR, Blomster JI, Curtis LH, Duclaux S, Ford I, Fritz F, Goldman S, Janmohamed S, Kreuzer J, Leenay M, Michel A, Ong S, Pell JP, Southworth MR, Stough WG, Thoenes M, Zannad F, Zalewski A. Electronic health records to facilitate clinical research. Clin Res Cardiol. 2017 Jan;106(1):1–9.

Everson J, Richards MR, Buntin MB. Horizontal and vertical integration's role in meaningful use attestation over time. Health Serv Res. 2019 Oct;54(5):1075–1083.

Gianfrancesco MA, Goldstein ND. A narrative review on the validity of electronic health record-based research in epidemiology. BMC Med Res Methodol. 2021 Oct 27;21(1):234.

Goldstein ND. Improving Population Health Using Electronic Health Records: Methods for Data Management and Epidemiological Analysis. Boca Raton, FL: CRC Press, 2017.

Goldstein ND, LeVasseur MT, McClure LA. On the convergence of epidemiology, biostatistics, and data science. Harvard Data Science Review. 2020; 2(2). doi: 10.1162/99608f92.9f0215e6.

Hanna-Attisha M, LaChance J, Sadler RC, Champney Schnepp A. Elevated blood lead levels in children associated with the Flint drinking water crisis: A spatial analysis of risk and public health response. Am J Public Health. 2016 Feb;106(2):283–290.

Hersh WR. The electronic medical record: Promises and problems. J Am Soc Inf Sci. 1995 Dec;46(10):772–776.

Jamoom EW, Yang N, Hing E. Adoption of certified electronic health record systems and electronic information sharing in physician offices: United States, 2013 and 2014. NCHS Data Brief. 2016 Jan;(236):1–8.

Kruse CS, Stein A, Thomas H, Kaur H. The use of electronic health records to support population health: A systematic review of the literature. J Med Syst. 2018 Sep 29;42(11):214.

Laney D. Deja VVVu: Others Claiming Gartner's Construct for Big Data. Gartner Blog Network/CTOvision.com. https://ctovision.com/deja-vvvu-others-claiming-gartners-construct-for-big-data/ (accessed December 1, 2020), 2012.

MIT Critical Data. Secondary Analysis of Electronic Health Records. Cambridge, MA: Springer, 2016.

Office of the National Coordinator for Health Information Technology. 'Certified Health IT Developers and Editions Reported by Health Care Professionals Participating in the Medicare EHR Incentive Program,' Health IT Quick-Stat #30. https://www.healthit.gov/data/quickstats/health-care-professional-health-it-developers (accessed December 6, 2021), 2017a.

Office of the National Coordinator for Health Information Technology. 'Certified Health IT Developers and Editions Reported by Hospitals Participating in the Medicare EHR Incentive Program,' Health IT Quick-Stat #29. https://www.healthit.gov/data/quickstats/hospital-health-it-developers (accessed December 6, 2021), 2017b.

Oregon Health & Science University. Clinfowiki: Computer Stored Ambulatory Record (COSTAR). http://www.clinfowiki.org/wiki/index.php/Computer_Stored_Ambulatory_Record_(COSTAR) (accessed December 1, 2020), 2015a.

Oregon Health & Science University. Clinfowiki: Regenstrief Medical Record System (RMRS). http://www.clinfowiki.org/wiki/index.php/RMRS (accessed December 1, 2020), 2015b.

Oregon Health & Science University. Clinfowiki: Veterans Health Information Systems and Technology Architecture (VistA). http://www.clinfowiki.org/wiki/index.php/Vista (accessed December 1, 2020), 2015c.

Oregon Health & Science University. Clinfowiki: Historically Important Electronic Medical Record Systems. http://www.clinfowiki.org/wiki/index.php/Historically_Important_Electronic_Medical_Record_Systems (accessed December 1, 2020), 2015d.

Oregon Health & Science University. Clinfowiki: Health Information Exchange. http://www.clinfowiki.org/wiki/index.php/Health_Information_Exchange (accessed December 1, 2020), 2015e.

Raman SR, Curtis LH, Temple R, Andersson T, Ezekowitz J, Ford I, James S, Marsolo K, Mirhaji P, Rocca M, Rothman RL, Sethuraman B, Stockbridge N, Terry S, Wasserman SM, Peterson ED, Hernandez AF. Leveraging electronic health records for clinical research. Am Heart J. 2018 Aug;202:13–19.

Safran C, Bloomrosen M, Hammond WE, Labkoff S, Markel-Fox S, Tang PC, Detmer DE, Expert Panel. Toward a national framework for the secondary use of health data: an American Medical Informatics Association White Paper. J Am Med Inform Assoc. 2007 Jan–Feb;14(1):1–9.

Shortreed SM, Cook AJ, Coley RY, Bobb JF, Nelson JC. Challenges and opportunities for using big health care data to advance medical science and public health. Am J Epidemiol. 2019 May 1;188(5):851–861.

U.S. Department of Health & Human Services. Health IT Legislation. https://www.healthit.gov/topic/laws-regulation-and-policy/health-it-legislation (accessed December 1, 2020), 2021a.

U.S. Department of Health & Human Services. Meaningful Use. https://www.healthit.gov/topic/meaningful-use-and-macra/meaningful-use (accessed December 1, 2020), 2021b.

Verheij RA, Curcin V, Delaney BC, McGilchrist MM. Possible sources of bias in primary care electronic health record data use and reuse. J Med Internet Res. 2018 May 29;20(5):e185.

2 Concepts in Electronic Health Record Research

Unless you are employed as a full-time researcher, research is often conducted as time permits. This book can be used in a similar fashion, and while the reader will obtain the greatest amount of knowledge from an exhaustive study, it can nonetheless be used in a piece-meal approach recognizing that there are many time constraints during the day. Figure 2.1 is a flowchart of the book and depicts how each chapter contributes toward the goal of conducting research from the EHR. The beginning of each chapter includes an abstract that provides a synopsis of the content, and each chapter can be read as a stand-alone entity. Readers are encouraged to review the list of references at the conclusion of each chapter for additional readings relevant to the topic area. Additional information can also be found on the book website, https://www.goldsteinepi.com/books/ehr/, including errata, data, source codes, and more.

The balance of this chapter defines concepts and terms used throughout the book, depicts sample EHR data, and enumerates hardware and software requirements for conducting secondary data research from the EHR. These concepts and requirements are not presented as a mere glossary, but rather a didactic discussion with supporting examples. No specific vendor is endorsed in this text, nor should any mention of a specific vendor be taken as such.

Concepts and terminology

One of the biggest challenges when interfacing with clinicians, information technology (IT) personnel, researchers, policy planners, hospital administrators, and the public is lack of a common language. Clinicians use language specific to biology and medicine, IT personnel use terminology specific to math and engineering, while administrators speak in terms of economics and business. The most effective communicators take complicated processes and translate them into lay terms that a general audience can understand by using common, everyday language in lieu of technical jargon.

Healthcare concepts

Broadly speaking, we can define two types of patient *encounters* with the healthcare system: outpatient (or ambulatory) and inpatient. *Outpatient* medicine focuses on acute or chronic conditions that can be managed in the community

DOI: 10.4324/9781003258872-3

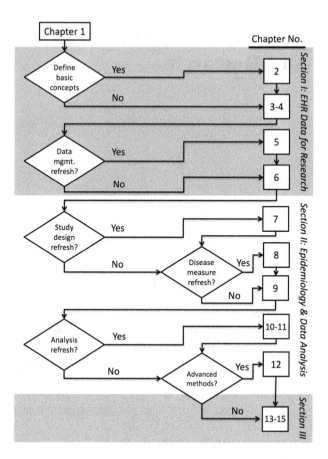

Figure 2.1 A flowchart of the book.

setting. Such settings include clinic offices, urgent, or acute care facilities, physical therapy, and many laboratories and imaging centers. Relevant to research, the encounters generated in outpatient medicine tend to occur across disparate EHRs based on patient (self-)referral patterns. On the other hand, *inpatient* medicine focuses on serious or complex problems requiring management with a team of providers and occur in an institutionalized setting. Such settings include hospitals, rehabilitation centers, nursing homes, and other long-term care facilities. These types of encounters tend to generate data within a single EHR. Inpatient EHR data are longitudinal for the duration of the admission but cross-sectional in nature in terms of the patient's overall life, whereas outpatient data may capture multiple encounters across many years (Figure 2.2). As medicine has evolved, so too has the types of encounters. No longer are encounters strictly face-to-face interactions: for example, they may be virtual or telehealth visits, electronic or phone messaging, or app-based services. These nuanced

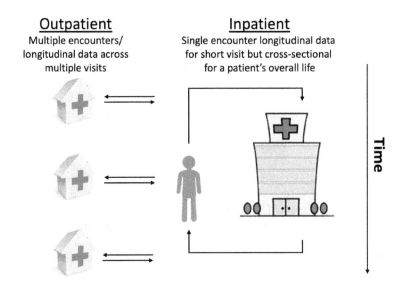

Outpatient
Multiple encounters/
longitudinal data across
multiple visits

Inpatient
Single encounter longitudinal data
for short visit but cross-sectional
for a patient's overall life

Figure 2.2 The relationship between inpatient and outpatient encounters.

encounter types may be of relevance to the research question, but not clearly identified in the EHR.

EHRs represent a population of individuals that have sought care at a specific healthcare location identified by its *catchment* area, also known as the referral network or service area. Yet it is important to keep in mind that at larger academic medical centers or institutions well-known for a particular medical specialty, the catchment may not reflect the local geography. Therefore, the population observed in a hospital's EHR may not be representative of the surrounding area. Further complicating this is possibility of *informed presence bias* where patients in the EHR may be systematically different from those who are not in the EHR. These concepts are discussed in detail in Chapters 6, 7, and 9 of the book.

EHR data typically occur in a hierarchy. At the top level is the patient, usually indexed by a medical record number, and containing information that is less likely to change on a visit-to-visit basis (e.g., patient's name, sex and gender, race, ethnicity, date of birth, and address, to name a few). At the next level, patients will have one or more encounters, usually indexed by a billing or financial identifier, that document specific health findings relevant for that healthcare visit. However, not all encounters may generate a billable event nor be documented in the EHR. Within a given encounter and at the next level of the hierarchy will be documentation on a patient's reason for visit and include their history, physical examination results, medications, plan, and so on, depending on the structure of the EHR. Also depending on the EHR, the problem list may be independent from the encounter and exist at the patient-level, complicating longitudinal analyses. Nevertheless, all levels generate documentation potentially useful for the researcher. Pollard et al. (2016) provide a helpful categorization of EHR data and note common issues to consider for each type: demographics, laboratory, medical imaging, physiologic measurements, medications, diagnosis and procedural codes, and caregiver and procedure notes. Ehrenstein, Kharrazi, and Lehmann (2019) built upon this list of traditional EHR data by describing nontraditional EHR data, such as healthcare utilization, biosamples and genetic information, surveys, and clinical workflow, which is covered in further detail in Chapter 4.

Researchers must be aware of the practice of documentation in the EHR and limitations of these data. *Documentation does not exist for the benefit of the researcher*: it is there for reasons related to patient care and reimbursement. There is also a tension between clinical documentation and billing: sometimes clinical notes occur for billing reasons, and sometimes absence of a billing need will result in absence of clinical documentation. There are differences in documentation by providers, provider role, and institutions (Sohn et al., 2018) as well as differences driven by patient-level factors, such as race (Tahir, 2022). All physicians do not document the same, and physicians, nurses, medical assistants, and other allied healthcare workers all document different aspects of patient care in different fashions in the EHR. The use of medical scribes or patient-entered data is not uncommon and may further impact data accuracy. Indeed, operationalizing a *clinical phenotype*, or health state of a patient, is a central challenge in EHR research (Pendergrass & Crawford, 2019; Richesson et al., 2013). As mentioned earlier, the EHR is a limited view of a patient, dependent upon their encounters or lack thereof, and as a result, ascertaining someone's true health status is difficult. In practice, most phenotypes are operationalized on combinations of billing and diagnostic codes, free text notes, and other ancillary details (Wei & Denny, 2015). The challenge of identifying a diagnosis from the EHR is covered in Chapter 6.

Terminology and data standards

Part of the challenge in those new to EHR research is the language used in healthcare and this section provides a high-level overview of U.S.-centric data standards that researchers are likely to encounter.

There are a variety of *vocabularies* used in the modern healthcare environment. Clinical documentation may occur using the Systematized Nomenclature of Medicine Clinical Terminology (SNOMED-CT) vocabulary and the World Health Organization's International Classification of Diseases (ICD) vocabulary. SNOMED-CT is more comprehensive for clinical documentation, whereas ICD is used primarily for billing or reporting. Insurance payments in the inpatient and outpatient worlds may be coded using the Diagnosis-Related Group (DRG) and the Ambulatory Payment Classification, respectively. DRGs are a Centers for Medicare and Medicaid Services requirement for payment and quality care that most private insurers also require. A full inpatient admission (not observation) receives a DRG code toward discharge for reimbursement purposes that incorporates severity of illness and final diagnosis. In terms of laboratory orders and procedures, the American Medical Association's Current Procedural

Terminology captures laboratory orders, surgical procedures, and medical studies, and the Logical Observation Identifiers Names and Codes standardizes how laboratory orders are transmitted and reported. In certain instances, a laboratory order will be coded as a procedure if a calculation is involved. The U.S. National Library of Medicine Unified Medical Language System (UMLS) integrates terminology from many of these vocabularies in an ontology mapper, and their Interactive Map-Assisted Generation of ICD Codes (i-MAGIC) maps between SNOMED and ICD. The U.S. Food and Drug Administration produces the National Drug Code, used to categorize over-the-counter and prescription medicines, and RxNorm (part of the UMLS) assists with mapping medicines from multiple vocabularies.

Despite standard vocabulary, some places will also have their own coding, and there is also geographic variation in coding. Whenever possible, researchers should request data by the code itself rather than the (human readable) name or interpretation (Table 2.1). An additional complication occurs when EHR-based studies span multiple years and a standard has changed, such as the transition from ICD-9 to ICD-10 in the 2010s. This would require identifying codes from both vocabularies at the outset, or possibly mapping from the older vocabulary to the newer one using one of many freely available tools.

For those who may dive deeper into the architecture of the EHR, they should be familiar with information exchange and data sharing standards, most notably the World Health Organization's Health Level 7 (HL7). This standard is used for reporting clinical and administrative data between healthcare systems. As of this writing, there are two widely used implementations of HL7, version 2.x and version 3.x, and translators exist to convert messages between versions. HL7's clinical document architecture is the standard that governs how clinical documents are encapsulated (Dolin et al., 2001), and in version 3.x, they are implemented in the eXtensible Markup Language (XML), thus making them human readable and easily parsable. The newer HL7 Fast Healthcare Interoperability Resources standard is increasingly being used for more efficient transfer of

Table 2.1 The relationship between clinical documentation and coding vocabularies

Problem list	ICD-9 Mapping	ICD-10 Mapping	SNOMED mapping
Right knee pain	**719.46** Pain in joint, lower leg	**M25.569** Pain in unspecified knee	**30989003** Knee pain
Severe aortic stenosis	**424.1** Aortic valve disorders	**I35.0** Nonrheumatic aortic (valve) stenosis	**60573004** Aortic valve stenosis
Family history of cerebral palsy	**V17.2** Family history of other neurological diseases	**Z82.0** Family history of epilepsy and other diseases of the nervous system	**275940001** Family history: Brain disorder + **128188000** Cerebral palsy

Whenever possible request the code as opposed to the meaning.
ICD, International Classification of Disease; SNOMED, Systematized Nomenclature of Medicine.

health information across networks using modern Internet technology standards (Rae-Dupree, 2020). Aside from HL7, there are other data sharing standards in use in healthcare, such as Digital Imaging and Communications in Medicine.

Technology concepts

Regardless of the EHR vendor and platform, the underlying technology is likely a *database*. A database is a both a technology and an abstract concept and, at its core, is a way of representing data using a certain structure that allows for organization. Just like most kitchen cabinets are sorted to have, say, glassware in one cabinet, plates in another, utensils in a drawer, and so forth, a database has *tables* that contain data with similar features. For example, suppose you are designing a system for collecting immunization data. You may have one table that stores the patient demographics, a second with the vaccine administered, and a third table with provider details, vis-à-vis Figure 2.3. These tables are linked together by a *unique identifier*, an essential variable that matches data from one table to another. The **patient demographics** table is linked to the **vaccine administered** table by the "Patient ID" variable, and the **vaccine administered** table is linked to the **provider details** table by the "Vaccination ID" variable.

Every time a provider submits vaccination events, known as *records* or *observations*, for a given patient (*subject*), they are entered in the appropriate database table, along with the corresponding unique identifier. The data become organized in a logical fashion that facilitates data import, export, linkage, and analysis. Contained within each table are one or more *variables* that represent the individual data. Within the **vaccine administered** table, there may be variables corresponding to vaccine antigen, manufacturer, date administered, route of administration, dose in milliliters, vaccine lot number, and so on. From a research perspective, we may be interested in the antigen and date the vaccine was administered – but not interested in manufacturer, route of administration, dose, or lot number – and therefore we only need to request – or export if the database is accessible – those two variables. Most EHRs, whether local or cloud based, will

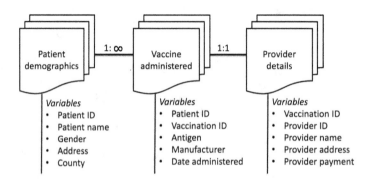

Figure 2.3 An immunization database.

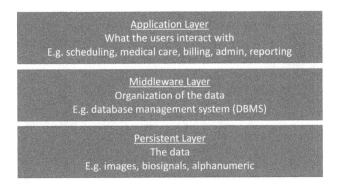

Figure 2.4 Generalized architecture of the EHR.

run a specific database technology, such as SQL Server (Microsoft Corporation, Redmond, WA), Db2 (International Business Machines Corporation, Armonk, NY), MySQL (Oracle Corporation, Redwood City, CA), MariaDB (MariaDB Foundation), or PostgresSQL (PostgreSQL Global Development Group).

Irrespective of the technology, the researcher will need to retrieve specific variables from one or more underlying database tables. Fortunately for the researcher, accessing data is a core function of any database management system; unfortunately for the researcher, the underlying structure of the tables and variables may not be optimal for research purposes. A generalized view of the architecture of the EHR is shown in Figure 2.4. Almost all users interact with the "application layer," as this is the safest view of the data. For example, assembling research data via chart review occurs within this layer. Trusted users may receive access to the "middleware layer," which allows for efficiency in data abstraction and confidence in data integrity. The "persistent layer" contains the actual data and should never be accessed. There is also redundancy built into the EHR databases: there is a primary instance of the database that contains the truth and one or more secondary instances that are virtual copies. This ensures both availability of the data, efficiency of access, and safeguards of data protection. Some institutions also have a "sandbox," which is a periodic snapshot of data that allows developers to test alterations to the EHR without compromising real patient data.

Occasionally, the data are not in a pure database as described above, but the result of an export of the original data, deemed *exported* data. Data can be exported from the original database or from third-party software, such as a statistical package or spreadsheet application. When the data are exported, they may be in a *proprietary* format, readable by only one vendor's products, or in a nonproprietary format, readable by many vendor's products. Further, the data may be in a machine-readable format, also known as binary format, or human readable format, such as a text file. Regardless of the nature of the export, the structure of the data will likely be reflective of the database structure described above: namely, one or more tables of variables containing multiple observations.

Table 2.2 Hypothetical data types for an example database table

Variable	Data type
Antigen	Coded text
Manufacturer	Free text
Date administered	Date/Time
Route of administration	Coded text
Dose in milliliters	Numeric

Researchers should avoid proprietary formats, as this limits the ability to share data with others and potentially inhibits collaboration. Rather this book advocates for a universal human readable format: the *comma separated value* (CSV) file. A CSV file will contain one or more observations comprised of one or more variables for a given table. As such, multiple tables in a database will need to be represented as multiple CSV files, or a single CSV file joined together. Unlike a database, the data type of the variables may be lost in a CSV file export, a potential and important limitation. By *data types* we simply mean the type of data that each variable represents. Continuing with the **vaccine administered** table from previously, the data types for the following variables can be assumed (Table 2.2).

Knowing the data type is important for data consistency and manipulation, and valid statistical inference, which are dealt with in later chapters. *Coded data* (also referred to as discrete data or structured data) types are used when the architect of the database wanted to force the user to adhere to a predetermined format or choice. While coded data are great for research and reporting, they are less well suited for capturing nuance and subtlety, common in some medical specialties including psychiatry. Conversely, *free text* (or unstructured data) allows the user to enter any value, often without constraints, and is quite capable of capturing nuance. On the other hand, free text is a challenge to mine for specific values and requires advanced techniques including natural language processing, discussed in Chapters 4 and 12. A *data dictionary*, if available, describes the underlying data, and may include items such as the variable name, data type, and interpretation of coded values.

Suffice for now to understand that EHR data comprise many *observations* (for many *subjects*) stored in a *database* composed of one or more *tables* containing *variables* that are represented by specific *data types*. Depending on the type of data, the number of observations and subjects may be equivalent. For example, if each patient has only a single vaccine (or, as another example, each patient visited a provider only one time), the number of observations will equal the number of subjects. However, when a single subject has multiple records, in our example multiple vaccinations, or were seen by the provider multiple times, the number of observations exceeds the number of subjects. A special case of this latter situation is the repeated measures, or longitudinal study, discussed further in section II of the book. Figure 2.5 represents a generalized view of the **vaccine administered** table viewed within the immunization database and

Single database table

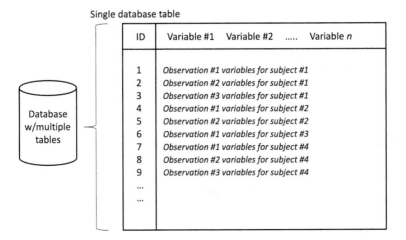

Figure 2.5 A hypothetical table within a database showing multiple observations per subject.

depicts nine total observations corresponding to unique immunization events for four subjects: subject #1 has received three separate vaccinations, subject #2 has received two vaccinations, and so forth.

Once the raw data are exported from the EHR or imported from a secondary source, they will be referred to as the research database. A *research database* is a generalized set of variables and all observations that can be used to explore various research questions under a specific domain, such as vaccine uptake in an outpatient clinic or neonatal outcomes in an intensive care unit. Contrast the research database with the *clinical data warehouse* or *clinical data repository*. A clinical data warehouse is a centralized and unified view of patients and their data in the EHR. While the research database is a snapshot view of patients and their data for a group of related research questions, the clinical data warehouse is an enterprise-wide view that has many uses including clinical, research, and administrative. Meanwhile a *clinical data mart* is a simplified data warehouse intended for a single use, such as research, and is similar to the research database. Development of a research database is the goal of the section I of this book and the research database itself may be stored as a database file, a REDCap website (REDCap Consortium, Vanderbilt University), within the statistical software itself, or using other computer applications.

The research database (or, if available, the clinical data warehouse) drives creation of the *analytic dataset,* a subset of variables and/or observations specific to the research question at hand. Under the proposed paradigm, each separate analysis can have its own analytic dataset extracted from the master research database. Although creating separate analytic datasets requires additional investment of time upfront, the researcher has ensured that the research data are appropriate, clean, and most importantly, reproducible. If sampling was used to create the research database, the research database may be equivalent to the

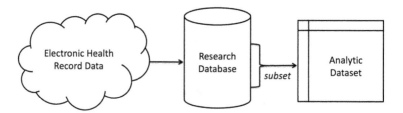

Figure 2.6 Relationship of the EHR to the research database and analytic dataset.

analytic dataset (see Chapter 7). Figure 2.6 depicts the relationship of EHR data to the research database and subsequent analytic dataset.

Epidemiological concepts

Epidemiology has traditionally been defined as a "study of the distribution and determinants of health-related states or events in specified populations and the application of this study to control health problems" (Thacker, 2006). A primary goal of epidemiologic research is to understand the nature of disease in a population, for example the well-known relationship between smoking and lung cancer. It is inherently a quantitative science and a core aspect to the "study of the distribution and determinants" is study design, variable measurement, and analysis.

When designing an epidemiological study, the researcher identifies a population and assembles a sample of individuals. A *population* is a collection of individuals with one or more defining characteristics, such as geographic location. While it may be intuitively desirable to study an entire population, often this is not feasible or even necessary due to practical study constraints; therefore, a *sample* of the population is recruited into a study. In most cases, the sample should be representative of the underlying population; a population-based sample is subset of people specifically drawn for this purpose. When the sample is drawn in such a way that it is not representative, we say the sample may be *biased*. When drawing a sample from a population, the investigator has several choices as to the most appropriate strategy to use, keeping in mind that occasionally practical constraints determine the sampling methodology to use. The specific research aims, as well as practical limitations, will often dictate demographic characteristics of the population, and are then specified as *inclusion* and *exclusion criteria* when forming the study sample.

Epidemiology is not limited to a single type of study. For example, there are epidemiologists who engage purely in *descriptive* studies, seeking to measure the occurrence of a health phenomenon in the population for the purpose of disease control or resource allocation. Classic epidemiologic fieldwork and public health surveillance efforts often fall under this type of work. There are epidemiologists who work with *experimental* and *quasi-experimental* studies with the goal of ascertaining how some sort of intervention, whether pharmacologic or not, impacts health. There are epidemiologists who work with *observational* studies, where there is no experimental manipulation of an intervention, but they still seek to identify associations present in the data. EHR-based studies most frequently would fall under observational work, and more specifically are considered a *secondary analysis* as the EHR data were not originally collected for the purposes of the research aims. Epidemiologists engage in other types of work too, but we will limit our discussion of epidemiological concepts to those most relevant to EHR research.

Epidemiologists may engage in predicative or causal work from the EHR. In a predictive analysis, the researcher is interested in statistical associations between one or more putative risk or protective factors (i.e., *exposures*) and some disease or health state (i.e., *outcome*). The goal here is to identify risk or generate hypotheses, but not to model cause and effect *per se*. For example, a study examining characteristics of an inpatient admission and risk for developing a healthcare associated infection could be considered a predictive analysis. The results may be used to alert clinicians as to when someone is at high risk of infection.

In an *etiologic* analysis, the researcher is interested in the causal association between an *exposure* and *outcome*, including disease or condition. A hypothetical research aim could examine the relationship between large household size – the exposure – and an infectious disease outbreak – the outcome. If the exposure is associated with the outcome, the question becomes, is it causally related to the outcome? Causal inference is the goal of many traditional epidemiologic analyses and implies whether the inference made from a study can be assumed valid and generalizable to some target population. *Statistical inference is not the same as causal inference*, and causal inference incorporates both philosophical and technical frameworks. Saying an exposure truly affects an outcome is not only about study validity, but also about a multitude of assumptions governing the observed relationship, discussed further in section II of this book. Turning to the hypothetical example, while the study may demonstrate that larger households are more likely to have infectious disease outbreaks, this may not have been a direct result of large household size, but rather that larger households were less likely to have fully immunized families. In this case, we say that results were *confounded* by immunization status.

Another hypothetical etiologic analysis may look at the association between an "exposure" of kidney disease and an outcome of infection. In addition to potential confounders of this relationship, such as age, the investigator may wish to consider potential mediators and effect modifiers. A *mediator* is an intermediate factor between the exposure and outcome. If the analysis demonstrates that kidney disease was strongly related to infection, a mediating variable could conceivably be immune dysfunction, in that kidney disease leads to a compromised immune system that leads to infection. An *effect modifier*, on the other hand, will affect (or modify) the relationship between kidney disease and infection. A genetic mutation may strengthen the relationship between kidney disease and infection, while lack of a genetic mutation may not affect the relationship. It is important to correctly identify mediators and moderators in an epidemiologic study, as failure to do so may *bias* the results, such as by modeling a mediator as a confounder. The distinction

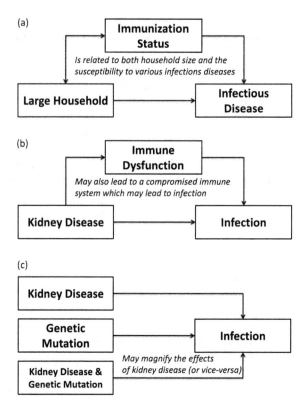

Figure 2.7(a–c) Causal diagrams depicting confounding (a), mediation (b), and effect modification (c). Failure to correctly identify the mechanism may bias the study
results.

between confounders, mediators, and modifiers are more readily depicted using
causal or conceptual diagrams (Figure 2.7a–c, respectively). Causal diagrams are a
wonderful method for uncovering the hypothesized pathway where an exposure
affects an outcome and are discussed in detail within the context of confounding
in Chapter 9.

The specific type of epidemiological analysis is dictated by the study design,
both of which are discussed in detail in section II. A variety of epidemiology textbooks are available and can supplement this brief introduction.

Statistical concepts

The reader is assumed to have a base understanding of biostatistics; if not, there are
a host of introductory statistical textbooks on the market. This section is intended
only as a review of the core terminology, with specific focus on practical definitions rather than theoretical definitions of concepts, which occasionally differ.

The output from a statistical *analysis* may include a description of the population, a comparison of risk factors, risk of an event, or other quantitative

result. By and large, the *estimates*, also known as the statistics, from the statistical packages will be consistent regardless of the choice of software, facilitating comparison of research from the same data. When performing the analysis, the researcher will be concerned with descriptive and inferential statistics. *Descriptive statistics* are the simplest estimates one can produce from analytic data. These include measures of frequency and distribution of characteristics of the population, for example, a mean participant age of 55 years (standard deviation of 10 years) or 45% of the population are women. The standard introductory table in a published paper – often referred to as the "Table 1" – is commonly based on descriptive statistics. If the analytic goals including inferring certain properties from the underlying data, the researcher uses *inferential statistics*, which is akin to hypothesis testing. A *hypothesis* is a concrete, testable statement about some characteristic of the population that can be tested, rejected, or upheld, via some explicit statistical model. For example, the conjecture "increased vaccination will be associated with reduced sick child visits at the pediatrician's office" is a testable hypothesis. Inferential statistics will model the relationship of vaccination to disease and produce estimates that can be used to refute or uphold the hypothesis. Studies that focus on descriptive statistics are often referred to as *hypotheses generating* studies which in turn spur *hypotheses testing* studies that use inferential statistics for the analysis.

Variables can fall into three classes of data: nominal, ordinal, and numeric. *Nominal* variables place data into categories and do not have an implied order to them, e.g., birth sex (male, female, or ambiguous) or disease status (diseased or not diseased), while *ordinal* variables have an implied order to them, e.g., annual income (<$25,000, $25,000–$50,000, >$50,000). This book treats nominal and ordinal data similarly and refers to them as *categorical* variables or data. *Numeric* variables occur on a numeric scale. When a numeric variable can be represented by a fractional number, such as weight or height, it is *continuous*. On the other hand, when the measure is represented by whole numbers, such as number of annual flu cases or people living with HIV/AIDS, it is *discrete*. Discrete measures may occasionally be analyzed as categorical variables.

The simplest way to describe categorical data are via *proportions*, and numeric data via measures of central tendency including *means* (i.e., averages) and *medians*. Variability in numeric data is typically reported as *standard deviations* or *variances* for data described by means and *interquartile range* for data described by medians. The choice to use means or medians is determined by whether the data are approximately *normal* or follow a Gaussian distribution: the so-called bell-shaped curve.

Moving from descriptive statistics to inferential statistics and hypothesis testing introduces the concept of a p-value. A *p-value* represents the likelihood the results obtained in the statistical analysis are due to chance alone, and results are typically said to be statistically significant if the likelihood is less than one in twenty, equivalent to an *alpha* of 5%. Coupled with the concept of variation is precision, often described using a confidence interval around a statistic. A *confidence interval* is used to estimate a probability of containing the population's true value in the sample, and is often accepted at 95% confidence, or 1 minus an alpha of 5%, hence the term "95% confidence interval." The choice of sample size and estimate precision are a byproduct of the *power analysis*, discussed further in Chapter 7.

When the estimates from the statistical analysis are unbiased, and therefore represent some truth about the disease or health state in the population, the results are said to be *valid*. There are a multitude of threats to the validity of an analysis, from incorrect assumptions about statistical procedures to biased data collection methods to results being confounded by extraneous variables. These are covered in detail in Chapter 9.

What EHR data look like

For those unfamiliar with EHR data, they might appear quite unlike other epidemiological sources of data, experimental, or observational. Whereas other data sources are typically well defined and orderly in their appearance, EHR data may appear quite messy. As mentioned, EHR data can be structured or unstructured. An example of an unstructured EHR entry for a John Doe appears in Box 2.1. While this style of note is highly usable to the clinician, in its present state it is near useless for a researcher, barring some sort of manual abstraction (see Chapter 4) or automated free text processing (see Chapter 12).

Box 2.1   Example of an unstructured EHR note for a single patient.

John Doe is a 50-year-old non-Hispanic white male. Patient has a history of acute bacterial sinusitis, part-time employment, limited social contact, reports of violence in the environment, social isolation, and stress. Patient is single. Patient is an active smoker and is an alcoholic. Patient identifies as heterosexual. Patient comes from a high socioeconomic background and has completed some college courses. Patient currently has coverage through Friendly Insurance Company. No Known Allergies. No Active Medications. John Doe presents to the office with a chief complaint of "sore throat for one week." Patient reports that his sore throat began last Saturday, and has been getting worse since then. He reports that his throat is very sore and it hurts to swallow. He has also developed a fever of 101 degrees Fahrenheit and a headache. He denies any other symptoms, including cough, runny nose, or congestion. He reports that he has been taking ibuprofen and drinking lots of fluids, but his symptoms have not improved.

Structured data obtained from the EHR may take many forms, depending on the exact mechanism of export, but contrast Box 2.1 with Box 2.2, where data for a Jane Doe are structured by demographics, allergies, medications, conditions, care plans, observations, procedures, and encounters. One popular EHR documentation style, known as the SOAP note, organizes a clinical note into subjective, objective, assessment, and plan sections (Podder, Lew & Ghassemzadeh, 2023). These sections may be further divided into subsections. For example, the subjective section may contain labels identifying the chief complaint, history of present illness, and review of systems. The ability to successfully parse discrete elements from a clinical note depends, in part, on how structured these data are and consistency in documentation.

Box 2.2 Example of a structured EHR export for a single patient.

Jane Doe

==================

Race: White
Ethnicity: Non-Hispanic
Gender: F
Age: 33
Birth Date: 1983-11-04
Marital Status: M

ALLERGIES: N/A

MEDICATIONS:
2013-08-22 [CURRENT]: Acetaminophen 160 MG for Acute bronchitis (disorder)
1996-05-12 [CURRENT]: Acetaminophen 160 MG for Acute bronchitis (disorder)
1995-04-13 [CURRENT]: Acetaminophen 160 MG for Acute bronchitis (disorder)
1984-01-14 [CURRENT]: Penicillin V Potassium 250 MG for Streptococcal sore throat (disorder)

CONDITIONS:
2015-10-30–2015-11-07: Fetus with chromosomal abnormality
2015-10-30–2015-11-07: Miscarriage in first trimester
2015-10-30–2015-11-07: Normal pregnancy
2013-08-22–2013-09-08: Acute bronchitis (disorder)
1985-08-07: Food Allergy: Fish

CARE PLANS:
2013-08-22 [STOPPED]: Respiratory therapy
Reason: Acute bronchitis (disorder)
Activity: Recommendation to avoid exercise
Activity: Deep breathing and coughing exercises

OBSERVATIONS:
2014-01-14: Body Weight 73.9 kg
2014-01-14: Body Height 163.7 cm
2014-01-14: Body Mass Index 27.6 kg/m^2
2014-01-14: Systolic Blood Pressure 133.0 mmHg
2014-01-14: Diastolic Blood Pressure 76.0 mmHg
2014-01-14: Blood Pressure 2.0

PROCEDURES:
2015-10-30: Standard pregnancy test for Normal pregnancy
2014-01-14: Documentation of current medications

ENCOUNTERS:
2015-11-07: Encounter for Fetus with chromosomal abnormality
2015-10-30: Encounter for Normal pregnancy
2014-01-14: Outpatient Encounter
2013-08-22: Encounter for Acute bronchitis (disorder)

Chapter 4 explores EHR data in greater detail with additional examples and screenshots from an actual EHR. Bulk data extracts from the EHR – also covered in Chapter 4 – offer the opportunity to organize the data in a more logical fashion, especially using CSV files. Figure 2.8 includes several examples of CSV files exported from a synthetic EHR by clinical module: demographics, clinical observations and measurements, diagnosed conditions, and ordered imaging studies. These sample patients were generated via Synthea, a synthetic EHR patient generator discussed further in Chapter 4 (Walonoski et al., 2018).

Patient demographics table

Id	BIRTHDATE	DEATHDATE	SSN	DRIVERS	PASSPORT	PREFIX	FIRST	LAST	SUFFIX	MAIDEN	MARITAL	RACE	ETHNICITY	GENDER
1d604da9-9a	5/25/89		999-76-6866	S99984236	X19277260X	Mr.	JosvID Eduar	GV2mez206			M	white	hispanic	M
034e9e3b-2c	11/14/83		999-73-5361	S99962402	X882754b4X	Mr.	Milo271	Feil794			M	white	nonhispanic	M
10339b10-3c	6/2/92		999-27-3385	S99972682	X73754411X	Mr.	Jayson808	Fadel536			M	white	nonhispanic	M
8d4c4326-e9	5/27/78		999-85-4926	S99974448	X40915583X	Mrs.	Mariana775	Rutherford999		Williamson7	M	white	nonhispanic	F
f5dcd418-09	10/18/96		999-60-7372	S99915787	X86772962X	Mr.	Gregorio366	Auer97				white	nonhispanic	M
72c0b9ce-7a	7/27/17		999-68-6630				Jacinto644	Kris249				white	nonhispanic	F
b1e9b0b9-da	12/13/03		999-73-2461	S99954048			Jimmie93	Harris789				white	nonhispanic	F
01207ecd-9d	5/15/19		999-81-4349											F
b58731cc-2d	5/16/70		999-90-2484	S99978036										F
cfee79fc-df0	7/4/16		999-15-5895											M
ad2e9916-45	12/19/04		999-78-4480											M
bfb6537b-53	7/3/91		999-74-9712	S99913545										F
83719bd7-7a	6/7/89		999-24-1237	S99993444										F
76982e06-f8	9/1/82		999-21-5604	S99957470										F

Conditions table

START	STOP	PATIENT		ENCOUNTER CODE	DESCRIPTION
5/1/01		1d604da9-9a	8f104aa7-4c	40055000	Chronic sinusitis (disorder)
8/9/11	8/16/11	8d4c4326-e9	9d35ec9f-35	444814009	Viral sinusitis (disorder)
11/16/11	11/26/11	8d4c4326-e9	ae7555a9-ea	195662009	Acute viral pharyngitis (disorder)
5/13/11	5/27/11	10339b10-3c	e1ab4933-07	10509002	Acute bronchitis (disorder)
2/6/11	2/14/11	f5dcd418-09	b8f76eba-77	195662009	Acute viral pharyngitis (disorder)
4/18/11	4/28/11	f5dcd418-09	640837d9-84	195662009	Acute viral pharyngitis (disorder)
11/29/11	12/13/11	f5dcd418-09	8c929690-18	444814009	Viral sinusitis (disorder)
12/31/11	1/7/12	f5dcd418-09	16300c56-a0	10509002	Acute bronchitis (disorder)
12/8/11	12/22/11	1d604da9-9a	792fae81-a0	444814009	Viral sinusitis (disorder)
12/29/16	1/5/17	034e9e3b-2c	3b639086-5f	10509002	Acute bronchitis (disorder)
8/11/11	9/1/11	10339b10-3c	470ccc46-00	444814009	Viral sinusitis (disorder)
3/20/19	4/10/19	1d604da9-9a	4e595f0c-f9	444814009	Viral sinusitis (disorder)
12/6/15	12/14/15	8d4c4326-e9	58181526-98	43878008	Streptococcal sore throat (disorder)

Observations table

DATE	PATIENT	ENCOUNTER CODE		DESCRIPTIO	VALUE	UNITS	TYPE
2012-01-23T	034e9e3b-2c	e88bc3a9-00	8302-2	Body Height	193.3	cm	numeric
2012-01-23T	034e9e3b-2c	e88bc3a9-00	72514-3	Pain severity	2 (score)		numeric
2012-01-23T	034e9e3b-2c	e88bc3a9-00	29463-7	Body Weight	87.8	kg	numeric
2012-01-23T	034e9e3b-2c	e88bc3a9-00	39156-5	Body Mass Ir	23.5	kg/m2	numeric
2012-01-23T	034e9e3b-2c	e88bc3a9-00	8462-4	Diastolic Blo	82	mm[Hg]	numeric
		c3a9-00	8480-6	Systolic Bloo	119	mm[Hg]	numeric
		c3a9-00	8867-4	Heart rate	77	/min	numeric
		c3a9-00	9279-1	Respiratory r	14	/min	numeric
		55a9-e2	8310-5	Body temper	37.1	Cel	numeric
		b7cb-13	8302-2	Body Height	165	cm	numeric
		b7cb-13	72514-3	Pain severity	1 (score)		numeric
		b7cb-13	29463-7	Body Weight	64.7	kg	numeric
		b7cb-13	39156-5	Body Mass Ir	23.8	kg/m2	numeric
		b7cb-13	59576-9	Body mass ir	71.3	%	numeric
		b7cb-13	8462-4	Diastolic Blo	70	mm[Hg]	numeric
		c3a9-00	6690-2	Leukocytes [i	9.5	10*3/uL	numeric
		339a-60	8302-2	Body Height	181	cm	numeric
		b7cb-13	8480-6	Systolic Bloo	121	mm[Hg]	numeric

Imaging studies table

Id	DATE	PATIENT	ENCOUNTER	BODYSITE_C	BODYSITE_D	MODALITY_C	MODALITY_I	SOP_CODE	SOP_DESCRIPTION
1/22/17	2/12/17	10339b10-3c							
4/23/19	5/7/19	10339b10-3c	d3e49b38-7e	2014-07-08T	b58731cc-2d	3a36836d-da	40983000	Arm	DX	Digital Radic 1.2.840.1000 Digital X-Ray Image Storage
7/3/16	7/16/16	f5dcd418-09	46baf530-49	2014-01-22T	2ffe9369-24	33b71e4b-06	40983000	Arm	DX	Digital Radic 1.2.840.1000 Digital X-Ray Image Storage
9/27/13	11/22/13	b1e9b0b9-da	f4c6c777-b5t	2005-10-10T	71e13815-5t	d067399a-b4	8205005	Wrist	DX	Digital Radic 1.2.840.1000 Digital X-Ray Image Storage
11/15/13		b1e9b0b9-da	a954c8af-9f	2017-06-07T	844d1c39-6c	bb246bbc-e3	8205005	Wrist	DX	Digital Radic 1.2.840.1000 Digital X-Ray Image Storage
5/23/18	6/20/18	72c0b9ce-7a	6156f2e6-9e	2019-11-20T	36cfc9c6-c71	b96740f2-a6	51299004	Clavicle	DX	Digital Radic 1.2.840.1000 Digital X-Ray Image Storage
10/31/17	11/14/17	b1e9b0b9-da	68010Se8-42	2008-01-13T	b2b612b0-04	9356de72-9a	51185008	Thoracic stru	CT	Computed Tc 1.2.840.1000 CT Image Storage
12/5/19	12/19/19	b1e9b0b9-da	8051710c-05	2008-02-10T	b2b612b0-04	77068c69-08	51185008	Thoracic stru	CT	Computed Tc 1.2.840.1000 CT Image Storage
11/19/18	1/3/19	72c0b9ce-7a	8c0aa29a-00	2006-06-17T	b096000e-3f	8eea95d9-at	261179002	thoracic	US	Ultrasoun 1.2.840.1000 Ultrasound Multiframe Image Storage
5/3/19	7/4/19	72c0b9ce-7a	c86b998a-66	2007-06-12T	b096000e-3f	a7d8665c-fa	261179002	thoracic	US	Ultrasoun 1.2.840.1000 Ultrasound Multiframe Image Storage
7/31/04		b58731cc-2d	75dc0d04-30	2007-12-09T	b096000e-3f	a547d3b0-4a	51185008	Thoracic stru	CR	Computed R 1.2.840.1000 Digital X-Ray Image Storage ,Ai for Pres
5/5/14	6/24/14	b58731cc-2d	1a4a4fd6-22	2007-12-09T	b096000e-3f	80b6aff5-68	261179002	Thoracic	US	Ultrasoun 1.2.840.1000 Ultrasound Multiframe Image Storage
7/8/14	9/6/14	b58731cc-2d	64f4ee98-b3	2007-12-09T	b096000e-3f	80b6aff5-68	51185008	Thoracic stru	DX	Digital Radic 1.2.840.1000 Digital X-Ray Image Storage ,Ai for Pres
3/20/16		b58731cc-2d	6ef07576-05	2011-04-25T	0f9eca6a-ce	04e78b82-84	344001	Ankle	DX	Digital Radic 1.2.840.1000 Digital X-Ray Image Storage
5/26/18	1/5/19	b58731cc-2d	68be9f41-c0	2015-06-12T	1821a44e-ba	46959f8f-13	40983000	Arm	DX	Digital Radic 1.2.840.1000 Digital X-Ray Image Storage
			daeb1573-0t	2019-12-13T	066c0f3d-90	f14e541e-18	261179002	US	Ultrasoun 1.2.840.1000 Ultrasound Multiframe Image Storage	

Figure 2.8 CSV file exports from a synthetic EHR.

Hardware and software requirements

All methods used in this book require specific software and adequate hardware for efficient operation, and any modern computer should meet these needs. It is assumed that the reader is familiar with basic computer operation as well as their preferred statistical software. This section is divided into data management and analysis requirements.

Data management

If the source data exist in a database, this may necessitate interfacing to the database to extract the data. Familiarity with structured query language (SQL) is beneficial, although not required if IT personnel are retrieving the data from the database on the researcher's behalf. Depending on the backend database and specific IT policies, Microsoft Access (Microsoft Corporation, Redmond, WA) may be required to connect to a Microsoft SQL Server database; wherever possible, direct connection from the statistical software to the database through SQL is encouraged. A spreadsheet application, such as Microsoft Excel (Microsoft Corporation, Redmond, WA), is imperative for initial data manipulation, recoding, and validation of variables and observations. Additionally, a plain text application like Windows Notepad (Microsoft Corporation, Redmond, WA), macOS TextEdit (Apple Inc., Cupertino, CA), or TextWrangler (Bare Bones Software,

North Chelmsford, MA) will be useful for data parsing and related activities. For researchers working with high-dimensional datasets, perhaps thousands of variables or millions of observations, the standard text applications may not be compatible with the sheer size of some CSV files. There are several freely available plain text applications that support large text files and can be found by an Internet search.

Data analysis and presentation

The analytic procedures described in this book require the use of *statistical software*. Statistical software include specialized procedures to analyze, and sometimes manage, quantitative data. Well-known and used statistical software include SAS (SAS Institute, Cary, NC), R (R Foundation for Statistical Computing, Vienna, Austria), SPSS (International Business Machines Corporation, Armonk, NY), and Stata (StataCorp, College Station, TX). Microsoft Excel (Microsoft Corporation, Redmond, WA) also includes the ability to analyze data through the Analysis ToolPak, though in a more limited sense than the specialized statistical software. Python (Python Software Foundation, Beaverton, OR) is increasingly being used for statistical programming, although it is primarily a general-purpose programming language and as such is not discussed in this book. Any modern statistical software will be capable of the analytic techniques used in this text.

Occasionally, the data provided for research is the result from an export from one of these software packages directly and is not in the researcher's preferred format. For example, the Centers for Disease Control and Prevention's National Health and Nutrition Examination Survey (a.k.a. NHANES) provides publicly available data in SAS transport (XPT) files (National Center for Health Statistics, 2021). In this instance, the researcher's preferred statistical software must be capable of reading this file format; otherwise, third-party software may be required to read and export the data in a more universal format, such as a CSV file. The SAS Universal Viewer (SAS Institute, Cary, NC) is capable of reading XPT files and exporting them into another format. There are third-party utilities or applications, such as Stat/Transfer (Circle Systems, Seattle, WA), that will achieve the same end goal. The choice of statistical software is largely a pragmatic one: an institutional preference, cost–benefit, knowledge of programming language, or other practical reason. While the author does not specifically endorse any software and the focus of the book is generalizable across all platforms, selected code samples are available in the appendix in R format.

Moving from analysis to publication and presentation will require a word processor, such as Microsoft Word (Microsoft Corporation, Redmond, WA) or equivalent, as well as a portable document format reader, such as Adobe Acrobat (Adobe Systems Incorporated, San Jose, CA). Presentation of research at scientific meetings may require access to a slide show presentation program, such as Microsoft PowerPoint (Microsoft Corporation, Redmond, WA) or equivalent. LibreOffice (The Document Foundation, Berlin, Germany) is an open-source alternative to the Microsoft suite of applications. Preparation of graphics can be accomplished within the statistical software or externally using graphic software applications including Adobe Photoshop (Adobe Systems Incorporated, San Jose, CA), the GNU Image Manipulation Program (The GIMP Team), or data visualization dashboards such as Tableau (Tableau Software, Seattle, WA).

References

Dolin RH, Alschuler L, Beebe C, Biron PV, Boyer SL, Essin D, Kimber E, Lincoln T, Mattison JE. The HL7 clinical document architecture. J Am Med Inform Assoc. 2001 Nov–Dec;8(6):552–69.

Ehrenstein V, Kharrazi H, Lehmann H, et al. Obtaining Data From Electronic Health Records. In: Gliklich RE, Leavy MB, Dreyer NA, editors. Tools and Technologies for Registry Interoperability, Registries for Evaluating Patient Outcomes: A User's Guide, 3rd ed., Addendum 2 [Internet]. Rockville, MD: Agency for Healthcare Research and Quality (US); 2019 Oct. Chapter 4. Available from: https://www.ncbi.nlm.nih.gov/books/NBK551878/

National Center for Health Statistics. National Health and Nutrition Examination Survey Frequently Asked Questions (FAQs). https://wwwn.cdc.gov/nchs/nhanes/continuous-nhanes/faq.aspx?BeginYear=2015#Q5 (accessed December 8, 2021), 2021.

Pendergrass SA, Crawford DC. Using electronic health records to generate phenotypes for research. Curr Protoc Hum Genet. 2019 Jan;100(1):e80.

Podder V, Lew V, Ghassemzadeh S. SOAP Notes. In: StatPearls [Internet]. Treasure Island, FL: StatPearls Publishing; 2023. Available from: https://www.ncbi.nlm.nih.gov/books/NBK482263/

Pollard T, Dernoncourt F, Finlayson S, Velasquez A. Data Preparation. In: Secondary Analysis of Electronic Health Records. Cambridge, MA: Springer, 2016.

Rae-Dupree J. How Fast Can A New Internet Standard For Sharing Patient Data Catch Fire? Kaiser Health News. https://khn.org/news/how-fast-can-a-new-internet-standard-for-sharing-patient-data-catch-fire/ (accessed December 8, 2021), 2020.

Richesson RL, Hammond WE, Nahm M, Wixted D, Simon GE, Robinson JG, Bauck AE, Cifelli D, Smerek MM, Dickerson J, Laws RL, Madigan RA, Rusincovitch SA, Kluchar C, Califf RM. Electronic health records based phenotyping in next-generation clinical trials: A perspective from the NIH health care systems collaboratory. J Am Med Inform Assoc. 2013 Dec;20(e2):e226-e231.

Sohn S, Wang Y, Wi CI, Krusemark EA, Ryu E, Ali MH, Juhn YJ, Liu H. Clinical documentation variations and NLP system portability: A case study in asthma birth cohorts across Institutions. J Am Med Inform Assoc. 2018 Mar 1;25(3):353–359.

Tahir D. Embedded Bias: How Medical Records Sow Discrimination? Kaiser Health News. https://kffhealthnews.org/news/article/electronic-medical-records-doctor-bias-open-notes-treatment-discrimination/ (accessed September 30, 2022), 2022.

Thacker SB. Centers for disease control and prevention. Epidemiology and Public Health at CDC. MMWR Suppl. 2006 Dec 22;55(2):3–4.

Walonoski J, Kramer M, Nichols J, Quina A, Moesel C, Hall D, Duffett C, Dube K, Gallagher T, McLachlan S. Synthea: An approach, method, and software mechanism for generating synthetic patients and the synthetic electronic health care record. J Am Med Inform Assoc. 2018 Mar 1;25(3):230–238.

Wei WQ, Denny JC. Extracting research-quality phenotypes from electronic health records to support precision medicine. Genome Med. 2015 Apr 30;7(1):41.

Section I

EHR Data for Research

3   Planning for Electronic Health Record Research

The first section of this book describes the development of a research database that can be used for epidemiological analyses, which is the focus of the second section of the book. Whether this database exists already or is developed *de novo*, the research database is dependent upon several factors: namely familiarity with the research process; data availability and accessibility; data privacy, security, and human subjects protection; and study funding and sponsorship; all discussed in the present chapter. The chapter also includes an example *research planner*, which may prove useful when undertaking secondary data analyses from the EHR.

Many of the examples in this book are derived from an example dataset of risk factors associated with low birthweight of infants, *birthwt*, available in the *MASS* package (Venables & Ripley, 2002) in the R statistical software (R Core Team, 2020). This example dataset is conceived as an extract of EHR data, and more details concerning this dataset and its use are found in section II of this book. While users of other statistical software can import this dataset into other applications, readers may also learn by applying the methods in this book to their data, as the methods are intentionally presented generically and applicable to all analytic software. For users of R, Appendix 2 includes specific code examples used throughout the book, and will be referenced in line with the text as appropriate. Example code to load the *birthwt* dataset from the *MASS* package and save it as a universally readable CSV file can be found in Appendix 2 (Code #3.1).

The research process

The research process is iterative: the researcher moves sequentially between steps, and the end product results in a feedback loop (Figure 3.1). To begin with, a *research question* is identified, and in fact likely already exists in the investigator's mind. First and foremost, this question must be answerable using EHR data. It needs to be clear and concise to motivate the rest of the process. A well-defined research question defines the target population by person, place, and time; identifies the health state being measured; and implies the measure of occurrence for

DOI: 10.4324/9781003258872-5

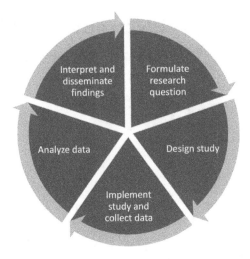

Figure 3.1 The research process.

analysis (Lesko, Fox & Edwards, 2022). For example, consider the following two research questions for an inpatient hospital:

1 *Research Question #1*: How do we protect our patients against hospital-acquired infections?
2 *Research Question #2*: What is the frequency of hospital-acquired infections, and how effective is our infection control program?

While the first question is concise, it is not clear from a research perspective. The second question, although less concise, is more answerable and indicates unambiguous directions for research: first, to quantify how often hospital-acquired infections are occurring, and second, to determine the effectiveness of the hospital's infection prevention activities. Research question #2 can be further refined for clarity, as follows. First, we can specify which types of hospital-acquired infections we are interested in studying, and second, we can identify what types of infection prevention activities are relevant. Third, the timeframe for the study also needs to be indicated. Last, in the spirit of brevity, this research question is probably better stated as two independent research questions:

1 *Research Question #2a*: What is the frequency of *Clostridoides difficile* infection for the past year?
2 *Research Question #2b*: How effective is the use of ultraviolet-C light in inpatient rooms at destroying *Clostridoides difficile* spores?

The answer to these two questions can then be used to describe the clinical epidemiology of *Clostridoides difficile* infection at the hospital, improve the infection prevention program of the hospital, and help advance the scientific field of hospital-acquired infections in general. Contrast these improved research questions with the original research question #1 – "How do we protect our patients against hospital-acquired infections?" This question is ambiguous and open-ended, requiring substantial refinement, and potential conjecture, before it becomes answerable through a research study. Further, research questions #2a and b set the stage for hypothesis formation, the next step in the process.

A *hypothesis* is a concrete, testable statement that can either be supported or refuted as a result of the analysis. Consider research questions #2a and b from earlier. There are two main hypotheses contained within. First, for question #2a, to quantify the frequency of *Clostridoides difficile* infection for the past year, and second, for question #2b, to measure the effectiveness of ultraviolet-C light in inpatient rooms to destroy *Clostridoides difficile* spores. To move from the research question to the testable hypothesis, we need to specify a belief about the direction – or magnitude – of its effect. Continuing with our example, consider the following two competing hypotheses for research question #2b:

1 *Hypothesis #1*: Ultraviolet-C light will be effective at destroying *Clostridoides difficile* spores.
2 *Hypothesis #2*: Use of ultraviolet-C light will result in a 40% reduction in *Clostridoides difficile* spores in inpatient rooms.

The second hypothesis is preferred as it sets the stage for statistical analysis by defining an *a priori* threshold level. Through statistical analysis, this hypothesis can be tested, resulting in two dichotomous outcomes: no demonstrable germicidal effect at the 40% level (the *null hypothesis*) or support of the 40% reduction in spores (termed the *alternative hypothesis*). The null and alternative hypotheses are necessarily competing: either one may be rejected – or more specifically, failed to be accepted – through analytic testing. *It is customary to establish the null hypothesis as no effect and the alternative hypothesis as effect.* Hypothesis #2, stated as a null and alternative hypothesis, looks like:

1 *Null hypothesis (H_0)*: Use of ultraviolet-C light will not reduce *Clostridoides difficile* spores by 40% or more in inpatient rooms.
2 *Alternative hypothesis (H_a)*: Use of ultraviolet-C light will reduce *Clostridoides difficile* spores by 40% or more in inpatient rooms.

The challenge in crisp, testable hypothesis formation is bringing prior knowledge on the direction or magnitude of effect. While in some cases this prior knowledge may be based on one's own experience – or in the very rare case, an epiphany – most of the prior knowledge is cemented in the *literature review* process. Although presented here as part of the hypothesis formation step in the research process, the literature review likely started concurrent with formulating the research question. The goal of the literature review is twofold: first, to survey the field for the state of the science, and second, to examine gaps in the literature and opportunities for additional work. In other words, the literature review determines what is and is not known on a subject, or at least what has been published.

Once a testable hypothesis is formed and agreed upon by the research team, the study is designed, the data are collected, and subsequently analyzed. The goal of analysis depends upon the research question and hypothesis. In strictly exploratory work, there may be no hypothesis posited, and the research question may be used to describe a population, process, or phenomenon. In more sophisticated work, such as identification of risk factors or disease etiology, measures of association often involve hypothesis testing and statistical inference. In all cases, the analytic procedures are conducted within the statistical software and the results generated inform the research question. The results are interpreted and the researcher decides to accept or reject a hypothesis if the goal was inferential statistics or decides if patterns in studied characteristics are meaningful if the work was exploratory.

The final step in the process is the dissemination of findings. Whether the results feed back into the investigator's own research as part of the continuum or inform others who are conducting similar research elsewhere, proper presentation of results is essential to move the science forward while avoiding miscommunication or misrepresentation of the findings. Even if the results are contrary to the association hypothesized, these should still be disseminated to the field. Dissemination of results may occur in the traditional scientific forms of published articles or meeting presentation, or to nonscientific audiences through other mediums. Each of these forms of dissemination present their own challenges and are discussed in more detail in Chapter 13.

Data availability and accessibility

Data availability

A crucial factor in research planning is the availability of data that can answer the research question(s) and test the hypothesis(es). Using EHR data as a secondary data source implies the data already exist. This is both an advantage and a disadvantage for the researcher. As an advantage, no primary data collection can translate into a more efficient study, both in terms of time and financial cost, yet a major disadvantage is that the research is confined to the data at hand. Occasionally existing data in the EHR can be supplemented with primary data collected via a substudy. However, before undertaking additional data collection, the following requirements should be considered: (1) funding and resources are available, (2) participants are available, and (3) the substudy is worthwhile, practical, and ethical. After the substudy is conducted, the data are merged with the original EHR data. The process of data merging is covered in detail in Chapter 5.

Regardless of the source of the data, the research question(s) and hypothesis(es) must be answerable from these data. This should make intuitive sense; for example, one would not recruit a cohort of adults from a pediatric practice. Yet sometimes the distinction is subtle and requires rumination to determine the plausibility of the research. Additionally, even with availability of the seemingly "correct" variables, the actual data contained in these variables can differ from expectations. After all, EHR data are optimized to answer clinical questions not epidemiological needs. In short, while there may be an abundance of the data in the EHR, usable data for research may be much less (Weiskopf et al., 2013). Several examples can drive home this point.

Consider the nebulous concept of socioeconomic status (SES) (Braveman et al., 2005), which is often used in health disparities research. A host of factors contribute to SES (American Psychological Association, 2017), and perhaps the researcher is forced to use patients' insurance as a proxy for SES. This is straightforward to do as payer information is recorded in the EHR but, by doing so, carries important limitations when used as a proxy for SES. For example, assuming that individuals who are uninsured are lower SES may lead to erroneous conclusions if individuals chose to forgo insurance but otherwise had access to the healthcare, such as being in a direct primary care model. Similarly, assuming those with private insurance are higher SES does not elicit other factors that may in fact place these individuals in poverty, such as having a low-paying job that includes a health insurance benefit. In the U.S., researchers have observed low correlation between Medicaid (as a proxy for SES) and traditional measures of SES, such as education and income (Casey et al., 2018). Nevertheless, the use of Medicaid may reveal disparities in health outcomes when better measures of SES are not available in the EHR.

Another example is inferring the sociologic concept of gender from an EHR variable corresponding to biologic sex. Sex and gender may mismatch if transgender or gender nonconforming individuals are included in the EHR (Blosnich & Boyer, 2022). In a related concept of sexuality, assuming lack of disclosure of sexual minority status in the EHR equates to heterosexual orientation will be misleading. Perhaps only individuals who have specific risk factors, such as a history of sexually transmitted infections, were asked their sexual orientation which was then documented in the EHR. More appropriate measures of sexual orientation and gender identity are beginning to be incorporated in the EHR (IOM, 2013), but retrospective studies may be subject to the data limitations described thus far.

One final example is the common use of "social determinants" of health in epidemiological studies, including the previously discussed measures of SES. As with sexual and gender identity, recommendations exist for the capture of social determinants in the EHR (IOM, 2015) and there have been calls to standardize this across EHRs (Cantor & Thorpe, 2018). Among the 12 social and behavioral measures enumerated in the 2015 IOM report (race and ethnicity, tobacco use, alcohol use, residential address, educational attainment, financial resource strain, stress, depression, physical activity, social isolation, intimate partner violence, and neighborhood median-household income), only a small subset may be typically collected as discrete data in the EHR, most likely race and ethnicity, tobacco use, alcohol use, and residential address. However, even seemingly straightforward variables to record in the EHR may not align with reality. Consider race and ethnicity: in one study of an EHR in New York City, 66% of patients reported race and ethnicity collected via a paper survey differently from what was captured in the EHR (Polubriaginof et al., 2019). Also consider homelessness: researchers have identified six areas in the EHR where this might be captured, including the (1) encounter note, (2) problem list, (3) patient's address, (4) social history, (5) care plan, and (6) housing status (Kaiser et al., 2022). The incorporation of additional social determinants in the EHR will benefit researchers in the long run (Chen, Tan & Padman, 2020), yet until this occurs, and especially when considering retrospective EHR-based studies, use of these variables is subject to measurement error, misclassification, and residual confounding (see Chapter 9). Understanding the conditions surrounding original data acquisition by speaking with those who enter the data in the EHR is an important step to help mitigate biases during analysis.

Ideally, a data dictionary would be available that defines the data elements in the EHR, but the unfortunate reality is this rarely exists. As such, we as researchers need to consult with our informatics and clinical colleagues to fully appreciate the data in the EHR. Similar issues of variable ambiguity can occur under circumstances where the patient's records are entered secondhand by staff other than the patient's provider, or, for example, the units of a measurement are unclear (weight entered as pounds when one expects kilograms). Interviewing data entry personnel can alleviate these issues. Often variables that may not appear as part of the normal clinical workflow exist in the background and can be obtained by consulting with the informatics group. Sometimes, documentation obtained from the EHR vendor may substitute for a data dictionary, while keeping in mind that EHRs are highly customized to each institution and clinical practice.

One final consideration in terms of data availability is the number of observations accessible to the researcher. This depends on the catchment of the institution, the longevity of the EHR, and whether paper records have been imported in the EHR. The number of observations can diminish rapidly once the study inclusions and exclusion criteria are applied, which then reduces the study sample size and statistical power of the study. Abstracting data from the EHR is discussed in Chapter 4 and sample size and power issues are discussed in Chapter 7. Related to this consideration is the temporal nature of data in the EHR, and more specifically, recent data. Real-time research from the EHR may be hampered by the time lag from observation to data entry and availability, especially billing or procedure codes. One study of mechanical ventilation procedure codes at the Veterans Health Administration found that "54% of the [ventilation] events existed in the EHR by 1-week post ventilation, 74% by 2 weeks, 87% by 3 weeks, 94% by 4 weeks" (Gastby, 2018).

Data accessibility

Intertwined with data availability is data accessibility. Whereas availability implies the data exist, accessibility means the researcher can access and subsequently use the EHR data. Accessing data from an EHR presents unique challenges. External collaborators may receive extremely limited datasets, as institutions are required to protect their data for privacy and security concerns, and possibly intellectual property reasons. Before any EHR data are requested, the process for obtaining data must be satisfied, which may include institutional review board (IRB) approval and/or legal data use or sharing agreements. The path of least resistance to obtaining data from a specific EHR is to identify an internal collaborator who can champion the work. This internal collaborator can then serve as the point person for all data requests and assist with identifying additional institutional contacts that can move the data request forward through clinical, legal, and information technology hurdles. The ideal internal collaborator is someone who has both requested and obtained EHR data for prior research. A full treatment of EHR data sources can be found in Chapter 4 and more detail regarding IRBs and legal agreements can be found later in this chapter.

The IT or informatics group should also be engaged in the process as early as possible, as there are often special, and perhaps lengthy, considerations for retrieving data from the EHR. Depending on whether the EHR is hosted internally to the organization or externally may require liaising with different groups, and possibly, the EHR vendor. Once a data request is initiated, the researcher should provide a comprehensive list of the patients and variables needed for the project, for example, all patient records for a certain timeframe or all patients meeting one or more clinical criteria. The EHR research planner presented at the conclusion of this chapter can help with the data request.

Data privacy, security, and human subjects protection

Privacy and security are sometimes conflated. Privacy ensures that patients in the EHR are not identifiable, while security ensures that the EHR data are inaccessible to nonauthorized personnel. Confidentiality is an assurance that private information will not be disclosed.

Depending on the location of the researcher, there are various privacy and security laws and regulations of relevance: the General Data Protection Regulation in the European Union, the Personal Information Protection and Electronic Documents Act in Canada, and Health Insurance Portability and Accountability Act (HIPAA) in the United States. In the U.S., HIPAA governs basic protections for using health information for research purposes, including protected health information (U.S. Department of Health & Human Services, 2015). There are 18 "identifiers" of protected health information (PHI) enumerated in HIPAA and shown in Table 3.1. Most identifiers are not relevant for typical EHR-based research projects, although a small number are frequently used. For example, dates, such as admission, discharge, diagnosis, or procedure dates, are useful for defining inclusion and exclusion criteria or studying temporal processes. Geographic location data obtained from the patient's address may be used if performing a geospatial analysis or linking individual-level data to community-level data. The medical record number is also frequently used as an identifier, possibly for data

Table 3.1 Protected health information identifiers enumerated in the Health Insurance Portability and Accountability Act

Identifier	Relevance to EHR research	Allowed in limited dataset
Person names	Low, unless used for linkage	No
Geographic subdivisions of a state[a]	High, for geospatial analyses	Yes
Dates	High	Yes, plus age
Telephone numbers	Low	No
Vehicle identification	Low	No
Fax numbers	Low	No
Device identifiers	Low	No
Email addresses	Low	No
Web addresses	Low	No
Social security numbers	Low, unless used for linkage	No
Internet addresses	Low	No
Medical record numbers	High	No
Biometric identifiers	Low	No
Health plan beneficiary numbers	Low	No
Full-face photographs	Low	No
Account numbers	Low, unless used for linkage or to identify individual encounters	No
Certificate or license numbers	Low, unless used for linkage	No

Note:
[a] Researchers working with geographies from the EHR should consult reference (U.S. Department of Health & Human Services, 2015) for further details.

linkage; however, this number should be removed from any analytic datasets, especially before sharing.

HIPAA requires an ethics board or IRB to make determinations about the use of PHI for research purposes, although certain exemptions to informed consent are possible. In general, working with secondary data from the EHR is usually a more streamlined pathway to IRB review. Before engaging the IRB, the researcher should be able to answer these two questions: is the work necessary and is the study ethical? The IRB will require a justification for both. Reviewing the literature, identifying gaps, and consulting funding sources for current trends in research are critical steps in addressing the question of necessity. Familiarity with the research aims, data collection process, protection of the participants identity, and minimizing risk to the participants are all part of the informed consent process that the IRB will review. The guidance provided herein should not be substituted for advice received from your own IRB, nor is intended to supersede any IRB, as each may have its own requirements.

Most institutions have an internal IRB or have contracted with an external IRB. As a researcher, if you need to ask whether or not to consult an IRB, the answer is probably "yes." IRBs exist not only to protect patients, but also to protect researchers; therefore, they are available to serve you. If your institution does not have an IRB, this does not exempt the research from the review process; instead, the researcher must identify an external IRB that will be responsible for the review process. For multi-site studies, or studies under the purview of multiple IRBs (for example, the EHR data are obtained from a different institution than the investigators'), the onus is on the researcher to coordinate across all IRBs. A primary IRB, typically the owner of the data, should be identified and approval sought from that IRB first. Any secondary IRBs will likely expedite review contingent upon approval from the primary IRB. Requesting *letters of reliance* is way to simplifying multiple IRBs, provided they are amenable to this. A letter of reliance indicates that one IRB is deferring to another IRB, and as such, separate IRB approvals are unnecessary.

In general, secondary data from the EHR will fall under one of two IRB review distinctions: exempt or expedited. If the research requires primary data collection to supplement existing data, then full IRB review will be necessary. Retrospective single-institution EHR-based studies may receive an exempt status as (1) data were captured for clinical care, not research, (2) data will be de-identified during research to remove PHI, (3) data will not leave the institution, and (4) patients will not be contacted, nor can be contacted once de-identified. Such minimal risk studies of secondary EHR data can apply for a waiver of informed consent and a HIPAA authorization waiver. Review of your institution's notice of privacy practices should yield the specific stipulations. The notice of privacy practices, required by law under the HIPAA, may contain specific information regarding use of health data for research.

As mentioned, if the research occurs in house (a *covered entity*), uses existing data in the health record, and does not require identifiable information (that is, de-identified), the data may be used for research without consent from the patients (U.S. Department of Health & Human Services, 2018). If the research requires protected health information or patient contact, signed permission from each study participant is required per the HIPAA authorization for research privacy rule (National Institutes of Health, 2004), and will likely necessitate full IRB review. The HIPAA privacy rule "Safe Harbor" provision provides a list of identifiers that must be removed from data prior to use, while the security rule stipulates administrative, physical, and technical safeguards required of electronic health information (U.S. Department of Health & Human Services, 2015).

As part of preparing the research database, identifiable health information may be required. Fortunately, the HIPAA privacy rule contains specific provisions for this circumstance, including documented IRB approval, with minimal risk to participants without alternatives. Any identifiable health information in the research database must reside on a password protected, and ideally encrypted, share accessibly only by the research team. The researcher's institution may have their own requirements and safeguards against data breach, defined by the IT group. As proposed in this book, the analytic dataset will fall under the *limited dataset* provision in the privacy rule. Under this provision, a data use agreement is entered between the researcher and the sponsoring institution, and states that the dataset excludes most PHI (Table 3.1), carries sufficient safeguards against data breach, and will not be disseminated to individuals outside of the research group.

Data use or data license agreements are often required when a researcher external to the covered entity is collaborating. As defined by HIPAA, the *data use agreement* (DUA) enumerates the permitted uses and sharing of the data, limits who can use or receive the data, requires appropriate safeguards of the data, provides a mechanism for notice of violation of the agreement, and reaffirms no contact with individuals in the dataset (U.S. Department of Health & Human Services, 2018). There are a variety of DUA templates publicly available on the Internet should the researcher need to draft such an agreement or review the requirements, and consulting with general counsel or a lawyer is prudent. The DUA should not be confused with a similar sounding agreement: the confidentiality or nondisclosure agreement (CDA or NDA). The intention of the CDA/NDA is to protect the intellectual property of an individual or organization and is typically agreed upon prior to any work commencing. This way should the research arrangement dissolve, the parties may not disclose the research details to others for some period of time, as stipulated in the CDA/NDA.

Common sense can go a long way toward ensuring data privacy and security, for example, by not sending medical data through email or storing it on an external USB drive that can easily be misplaced or stolen. Separating identifiers from the analytic data protects the privacy of individuals should a disclosure of the data invertedly occur. A *crosswalk* spreadsheet, stored on an encrypted drive or in a locked cabinet, maps between an arbitrary (random) identifier in the dataset from a known identifier in the EHR, such as the medical record number (see Chapter 5 for more details and an example). Any identifier that is considered PHI (Table 3.1) should be separated from the analytic datasets. There are also approaches for separating the data from the analysis to ensure privacy and security (Goldstein & Sarwate, 2016) including the idea of "tokenization" that is used to construct aggregated real-world databases (Dagenais et al., 2022). Should you have the need to share data externally, many organizations have encryption or secure email solutions available to specifically protect health information; consult with your IT group.

Lastly, the IRB will stipulate the amount of time that researchers are permitted to retain the EHR data. This typically extends for three to five years beyond the end of the research project to allow ample time for research dissemination. It is incumbent upon the researcher to destroy the data once this time has elapsed, or otherwise request an extension from the IRB.

Study funding and sponsorship

Having motivated and vested sponsors and collaborators increases the chances of successful research. In the context of secondary data, sponsorship may mean assistance with funding applications (discussed next), IRB documentation, data use requests, analysis, and dissemination of findings. For data derived from an EHR, sponsors may require a staff clinician who works directly with the EHR data or clinical leadership within the EHR group. Research building upon previous work or utilizing complex methodology may necessitate additional collaboration including biostatisticians and epidemiologists. Potential collaborators can be identified from past publications and faculty or clinical profiles on institutional websites. Sponsorship is not always necessary if the work is small in scope or the researcher's institution owns the EHR data. In these cases, many of the hurdles to data availability and accessibility have been cleared, and while analysis and publication are still major tasks to be completed, these tasks can be handled by the primary researcher or delegated to the research team. If the sponsor is also the study funder, it is essential for the researcher to understanding the funding process.

Funding and research go hand in hand, especially in academia, and, depending on the researcher's institution and arrangement, may be commensurate with salary or require internal or external awards. Internal or intramural awards are more frequently found in academic institutions or larger healthcare systems and are an attractive funding source for the researcher. Intramural awards are particularly relevant when the EHR data were collected in the same covered entity as the researcher. External or extramural awards are obtained through organizations or entities outside of the researcher's institution and typically, though not always, are more time consuming and difficult to obtain. If your institution has an Office of Sponsored Programs, you may need to work with them anytime funding is being sought.

There are different types of funding categories, including grants, cooperative agreements, and contracts. Grants and cooperative agreements both provide funding for a research project, the difference being cooperative agreements have substantial involvement from the funder, while grants afford greater flexibility and autonomy. Contracts are typically smaller in scope, more well-defined, and less flexible. For the remainder of this section, we will focus on grants, but the points are germane to all funding types.

Depending on the career level of the researcher, the approaches to obtaining funding differ. For students, many organizations offer training grants, which financially support the student as they complete their degree program. Recent graduates holding terminal degrees may also take advantage of grant opportunities specifically targeted toward postgraduate trainees, which are intended to support the awardee during their path toward research independence. Grants such as these require not only a well-developed research plan, but also a strong training plan for professional and career development that includes institutional and academic support. Outside of training grants, recent graduates may also take advantage of "early career" research awards designed to support the funding of researchers who have not had time to develop a history of funded projects as the principal investigator.

Grant funding may include support for the researcher's time, dubbed *effort*, the effort of collaborators and consultants, payment to participants if incentivized, and any materials or supplies needed for the research program including data collection, analysis, and results dissemination. Each grant has specific rules governing monetary expenditure, and it is the responsibility of the researcher to thoroughly explore the funding stream that best fits their project. Some grants are only designed to support the collection of data and may explicitly prohibit payment of stipends or salaries, although the collection of data could include a variety of activities and their associated costs such as mailed surveys, collecting specimens, laboratory testing on specimens, or paying for existing data, especially if EHR data need to be purchased (discussed in Chapter 4). When the EHR data were collected in the same covered entity as the researcher, costs for data collection should be low or nonexistent and researchers should target grants which will support their salary and other costs associated with the analysis, publication, and presentation.

When preparing a budget, it is important to work with your Office of Sponsored Programs, grants analyst, or business manager. Budgets can range from a few thousand dollars on small intramural awards to several millions of dollars on large extramural awards. When working with collaborators outside of your institution, subaward or subcontract budgets will be needed, so ample lead time is suggested. Depending in the funding source, budgets may include both direct and indirect costs. Direct costs are those required to pay for the investigator's effort, data collection, and personnel needed to conduct the research. Indirect costs, the amount of which varies by institution and are also known as facilities and administrative or overhead, cover expenses related to the research support not covered by direct costs. The details of the budgets are enumerated in a *budget justification* document.

Identifying appropriate grants and applying for those grants is no small task. EHR researchers can consider a variety of sponsors, including government agencies, foundations, nonprofit healthcare or academic systems, or industry. In terms of government funding, the National Institutes of Health (NIH) is perhaps the most widely recognized funding source for health-related research in the U.S. There are 26 federal grant-making agencies in the U.S., and researchers should explore the central database of federal grants – Grants.gov (https://www.grants. gov) – to learn about the variety of opportunities to federally fund their research. Importantly, researchers should also explore active grants to appreciate the type of work that has (and has not) been funded. The NIH RePORTER (https:// reporter.nih.gov/) allows prospective investigators to search the portfolio of NIH-funded projects. Figure 3.2 is a screen capture of a RePORTER search using the keywords "electronic health record." The search results can be used to ascertain agencies who fund relevant work, institutions and investigators who have received funds, synopses of the research, publications resulting from the work, as well as related grants.

Another major government funder of EHR-based research is the National Science Foundation (NSF). As with NIH RePORTER, NSF maintains its own database of funded projects (https://www.nsf.gov/awardsearch/). There are other government funders of EHR research in the U.S., including the Centers for

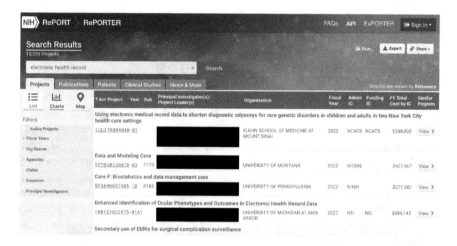

Figure 3.2 NIH RePORTER search for the keywords "electronic health record." Investigator names have been redacted.

Disease Control and Prevention (https://www.cdc.gov/funding/resources/index.html) and the Agency for Healthcare Research and Quality (https://www.ahrq.gov/funding/index.html); however, a full enumeration is outside the scope of this chapter.

Identifying nongovernment funders such as foundations, nonprofit healthcare or academic systems, and industry is more laborious. EHR-relevant societies can help identify funders, for example, the American Medical Informatics Association (https://amia.org) or the Healthcare Information and Management Systems Society (https://www.himss.org). There are also nongovernmental, nonprofit funders of EHR research, such as the Patient-Centered Outcomes Research Institute (https://www.pcori.org/funding-opportunities). To aid the researcher, there are several databases and clearinghouses for foundation awards, including Pivot (ProQuest, LLC, Ann Arbor, MI), the Foundation Center (Candid, New York, NY), and Funding Institutional (Elsevier, Amsterdam, Netherlands). These are subscription-based services, and access to them may depend on your institutional affiliations.

Regardless of the funder, grant applications tend to follow a standard structure, including

1 *Specific aims.* A concise statement of the research objectives. All other parts of the grant support the accomplishment of these aims. In writing the specific aims, the objectives need to remain relevant to the scope of the project, and avoid a phenomenon known as "scope creep" where the aims change or grow during the research. The mnemonic acronym SMART can assist the researcher when developing the objectives, in that the aims need to be Specific, Measurable, Achievable, Relevant, and Timely (Bogue, 2005).

2 *Research and analysis plan.* This section serves as the roadmap for activities conducted under the grant and includes an explicit and exhaustive discussion of the methods for conducting literature reviews, collecting data, designing the study, analyzing data, and reporting the results.

3 *Detailed timeline.* As an addendum to the research and analysis plan, the timeline includes estimated completion dates for major work products or milestones. Timelines can and likely will need to be revised, especially if the project is long-term. Depending on the length of the grant period, the timeline may be presented monthly, quarterly, or semi-annually.

4 *List of study personnel.* This includes identifying of the principal investigator(s), co-investigators, and other collaborators or consultants. Typically, qualifications of study personnel follow the NIH biographic sketch (a.k.a biosketch) format (National Institutes of Health, 2021). The publicly available SciENcv tool (http://www.ncbi.nlm.nih.gov/sciencv/) automates the creation of NIH-compliant biosketches.

5 *Resources and environment.* This section of the application details the resources available to the research team at the participant institutions. Boilerplate language for this section may be available from the investigators' institutions but should always be tailored specific to the application.

6 *Letters of support.* Although not always required, having letters of support from collaborators outside of the principal investigator's institution demonstrates a strong commitment to the success of the research. As with the resources and environment, these letters should always be tailored specific to each collaborator.

7 *Budget.* The funding agency will want to know exactly how the researcher will use the grant money. Sometimes budget items are straightforward, one-time costs. However, if the project includes data collection, the costs may be dependent on the total number of samples or surveys, and the total cost will only be an estimate. Estimate the cost as realistically as possible based on the plan and timeline outlined; typically, one wants to estimate within 80% of the actual costs. As detailer earlier, money may include direct and indirect costs; working with your institutions sponsored programs office will ensure the budget is correctly completed.

   If the funding will be coming from a training grant,[1] there are additional areas that need to be described in the application.

8 *Academic and institutional support.* If training is one of the purposes of funding, the researcher must show that the availability of appropriate resources and mentors to ensure successful training. This includes defining a mentoring team of faculty and other researchers who are available to help the trainee accomplish the research goals and resolve any unforeseen challenges. A team with a proven history of funding and mentoring experience will be an asset, and some grants may specifically require appointment of a seasoned mentor as the principal investigator.

9 *Career goals.* The funders may want a description of short- and long-term career goals and how this project – and specifically this funding – will further career advancement. The researcher should make a clear case for the necessity

of funding for the success of the work, inferring what would be difficult or impossible to achieve without it.

Funding depends not only on the quality of the application, but also on the funding available to that organization and the number of other applicants. This necessitates creativity in the approach, called grantsmanship, and many investigators use figures, tables, and text formatting tricks to make key points evident to the readers.

Once an application is submitted, it typically undergoes peer review. In some instances, prior to a full application being submitted, a concise "letter of interest" is requested. In these instances, if the funder identifies the proposed research as high priority based on this brief letter, a full proposal is invited. After the application's review, if feedback is provided and a resubmission allowed, it will behoove the researcher to systematically address all points raised during the review and provide a cover letter explicating the changes.

Ultimately it matters less where the money comes, more so the researcher's ability to conduct and disseminate research. Once funding is received, the money needs to be managed. Sometimes the funds are appropriated to you as an individual, as in the case of a contract, but more often they will go through the researcher's institution. The researcher should be in constant contact with their institution before and throughout the application process so that they are prepared to help manage the award.

EHR research planner

Given the complexity of EHR research, an EHR research planner is provided in Appendix 1 that can help capture the pertinent details to ensure a successful project. This planner can be filled out on a per-analysis basis or generically for multiple studies and analyses. Table 3.2 is an example planner that has been completed for research on low-birthweight neonatal outcomes and will be referenced in Section II of the book.

Table 3.2 EHR research planner for a study on neonatal outcomes associated with low birthweight

Study aims	*Chapter 3*
Lead researcher (PI):	*Lead researcher's name*
Co-investigator(s):	*Co-investigator names, if any*
Other key personnel:	*Other key personnel*
Research question(s) or specific aim(s):	*Are very low-birthweight infants more likely to have or staph infections compared to nonvery low-birthweight infants?*
Hypothesis(es):	*Infants less than 1,500g will be at an increased risk of staph infections.*
IRB needed:	__X__ Yes _____ No
IRB review type:	__X__ Exempt _____ Expedited _____ Full
IRB (primary):	*Local institution*
IRB (secondary):	*None*

(Continued)

Table 3.2 (Continued)

Funding				*Chapter 3*
Needed:	__X__ Yes _____ No			
Anticipated budget:	*$10,000*			
Funding type:	__X__ Grant/Agreement _____ Contract _____ Other			
Potential funders:	*Hospital provided internal grant for local research*			
Competing interests:	*None*			

EHR data source(s)			*Chapter 4*
Data source:	__X__ Single institution	_____ Multi-institution	
	_____ Claims database	_____ Other	
Export method:	_____ Chart review	_____ Reporting tool	
	__X__ Direct connection	_____ Existing extract	
Data location:	__X__ Internal	_____ External	_____ Other
Data Interface:	__X__ SQL	_____ Data file	_____ Other
Source description:	*Neonatal intensive care unit electronic health record; data reside on a SQL Server database run by the IT group*		
Institution/location(s):	*Academic medical center NICU, City, State/Country*		
EHR data point person:	*IT group database manager's name and contact*		
Supplementary sources:	*Hospital inpatient medical record for maternal perinatal history and birth record*		

Data description			*Chapters 4 and 5*
Type of data:	__X__ Cross-sectional	_____ Longitudinal	
Data organization:	__X__ Wide	_____ Long	
Merge/link required:	_____ Merging	__X__ Linking	_____ Both
Merge/link description:	*Linkage from the neonatal record to the inpatient record will be done by hospital MRN; data needed from both systems and will be manually joined*		
Population description:	*Infants that are admitted to the hospital's neonatal intensive care unit (NICU)*		
Years of data:	*2001–present*		
Num. subjects:	*~10,000*		
Num. observations:	*~12,000*		
Additional denominator Considerations:	*Multiple admissions to the NICU for some infants*		

Variables		*Chapters 4 and 5*
Unique identifier:	*Infants MRN*	
Primary exposure(s):	*Very low birthweight (<1500g)*	
Primary outcome(s):	*New cases of staph infection in the NICU*	
Potential confounder(s):	*Maternal and pregnancy risk factors*	
	Delivery method	
	Maternal infections	
	Infant comorbidities	
	Invasive produces performed in the NICU	
Potential mediator(s):	*None*	
Potential modifier(s):	*None*	
Other core variables:	*Infant sex*	
	Race/ethnicity	
	Mother's marital status	
	Maternal age	
Variables not available:	*Maternal infections*	
	Family socioeconomic status	

(Continued)

Table 3.2 (Continued)

Epidemiology		*Chapters 7 and 8*
Study design:	_____ Cross-sectional	__X__ Cohort
	_____ Case–control	_____ Longitudinal
	_____ Multi-level	_____ Other
Inclusion criteria:	*Infants admitted to the NICU during 2001–2020*	
Exclusion criteria:	*Infants not born in the local hospital, but transferred from another facility*	
Power analysis:	*For 80% power, 200 very low-birthweight infants and 200 nonvery low-birthweight infants to demonstrate a twofold increase in risk*	
Matching:	_____ Yes	__X__ No
Matching factor(s):	*None*	
Disease measures:	__X__ Incidence	_____ Prevalence
	__X__ Risk comparison	_____ Survival

Analysis			*Chapters 10 and 11*
Missing data:	_____ Yes	__X__ No	
Missing data type:	_____ MCAR	_____ MAR	_____ MNAR
Imputation:	_____ Yes	__X__ No	
Estimate type:	_____ Crude	__X__ Adjusted	
Analytic technique:	_____ Descriptive	_____ Other	
	__X__ Regression	Specify type: _Logistic_	
	_____ ML	Specify type: _____	
Regression assumptions:	__X__ Normality	__X__ Independence	
	__X__ Linearity	__X__ Equal variance	
Sensitivity analysis:	*What if we considered other infections, and not just staph?*		
Unexpected deviations:	*In consultation with a neonatologist, learned that NICU admission criteria changed mid-way through study; perhaps stratify analysis by this time*		

Publication and Presentation		*Chapter 13*
Dissemination:	__X__ Publication	__X__ Presentation
Target journal:	*Pediatrics*	
Open access:	_____ Yes	__X__ No
Target conference:	*Pediatric Academic Societies Annual Meeting*	
Abstract deadline:	*October 15th*	
Abstract type:	_____ Talk	_____ Poster	__X__ Either
Other mechanisms:	*Share results with hospital PR group to promote on blog and through email to research staff*	

Note

1 For readers who may be pursuing an NIH career development award, they are referred to this series of blog posts by the author that describe his experience with the process: https://www.goldsteinepi.com/blog/ajuniorepidemiologistsexperiencewithsubmit tingacareerdevelopmentawardpart1/index.html.

References

American Psychological Association.Education and Socioeconomic Status. https://www.apa.org/pi/ses/resources/publications/education (accessed December 2, 2021), 2017.

Blosnich JR, Boyer TL. Concordance of data about sex from electronic health records and the national death index: Implications for transgender populations. *Epidemiology.* 2022 May 1;33(3):383–385.

Bogue RL. Use S.M.A.R.T. goals to launch management by objectives plan. TechRepublic. http://www.techrepublic.com/article/use-smart-goals-to-launch-management-by-objectives-plan (accessed December 2, 2021), 2005.

Braveman PA, Cubbin C, Egerter S, Chideya S, Marchi KS, Metzler M, Posner S. Socioeconomic status in health research: One size does not fit all. JAMA. 2005 Dec 14;294(22):2879–2888.

Cantor MN, Thorpe L. Integrating data on social determinants of health into electronic health records. Health Aff (Millwood). 2018 Apr;37(4):585–590.

Casey JA, Pollak J, Glymour MM, Mayeda ER, Hirsch AG, Schwartz BS. Measures of SES for electronic health record-based research. Am J Prev Med. 2018 Mar;54(3):430–439.

Chen M, Tan X, Padman R. Social determinants of health in electronic health records and their impact on analysis and risk prediction: A systematic review. J Am Med Inform Assoc. 2020 Nov 1;27(11):1764–1773.

Dagenais S, Russo L, Madsen A, Webster J, Becnel L. Use of real-world evidence to drive drug development strategy and inform clinical trial design. Clin Pharmacol Ther. 2022 Jan;111(1):77–89.

Gastby E. Today is not tomorrow's yesterday: combining data sources can mitigate delays in EHR data availability. Abstract. Society of Epidemiologic Research Annual Meeting. 2018. Baltimore, MD.

Goldstein ND, Sarwate AD. Privacy, security, and the public health researcher in the era of electronic health record research. Online J Public Health Inform. 2016 Dec 28;8(3):e207.

Institute of Medicine (IOM) Board on the Health of Select Populations. Collecting Sexual Orientation and Gender Identity Data in Electronic Health Records: Workshop Summary. Washington, DC: National Academies Press (US); 2013.

Institute of Medicine (IOM) Committee on the Recommended Social and Behavioral Domains and Measures for Electronic Health Records; Board on Population Health and Public Health Practice. Capturing Social and Behavioral Domains and Measures in Electronic Health Records: Phase 2. Washington, DC: National Academies Press (US); 2015 Jan 8.

Kaiser P, Pipitone O, Earl A, Miller M. Identifying homelessness from EMRs: standard and custom approaches. Society for Epidemiologic Research Annual Meeting. 2022. Chicago, IL.

Lesko CR, Fox MP, Edwards JK. A framework for descriptive epidemiology. Am J Epidemiol. 2022 Nov 19;191(12):2063–2070.

National Institutes of Health. Biosketch Format Pages, Instructions and Samples. https://grants.nih.gov/grants/forms/biosketch.htm (accessed January 13, 2022), 2021.

National Institutes of Health. HIPAA Authorization for Research. https://privacyruleandresearch.nih.gov/authorization.asp (accessed December 2, 2021), 2004.

Polubriaginof FCG, Ryan P, Salmasian H, Shapiro AW, Perotte A, Safford MM, Hripcsak G, Smith S, Tatonetti NP, Vawdrey DK. Challenges with quality of race and ethnicity data in observational databases. J Am Med Inform Assoc. 2019 Aug 1;26(8–9):730–736.

R Core Team. R: A Language and Environment for Statistical Computing. Vienna: R Foundation for Statistical Computing, 2020. https://www.R-project.org/.

U.S. Department of Health & Human Services. Guidance Regarding Methods for De-identification of Protected Health Information in Accordance with the Health Insurance Portability and Accountability Act (HIPAA) Privacy Rule. https://www.hhs.gov/hipaa/for-professionals/privacy/special-topics/de-identification/index.html. (accessed January 12, 2022), 2015.

U.S. Department of Health & Human Services. Research. https://www.hhs.gov/hipaa/for-professionals/special-topics/research/index.html (accessed December 2, 2021), 2018.

Venables WN, Ripley BD. Modern Applied Statistics with S. Fourth Edition. Springer, New York, NY, 2002.

Weiskopf NG, Hripcsak G, Swaminathan S, Weng C. Defining and measuring completeness of electronic health records for secondary use. J Biomed Inform. 2013 Oct;46(5):830–836.

4 Accessing Electronic Health Record Data

The motivation of this chapter is to build a research database. Such a database may already be available to you as a researcher, nevertheless reviewing the concepts in this chapter will help appreciate the structure of EHR data. To construct this research database first requires an in-depth understanding of using EHRs as a data source, as well as the use of non-EHR data as a supplement. For those researchers who will be "hands-on" with the data, we will also discuss the process of accessing and extracting EHR data, focusing on several methods, including chart review, reporting tools, direct database interfacing, and previously abstracted data sources. It is the goal that by the end of this chapter, the EHR data will be clearly identifiable and accessible to the researcher for planning the epidemiological analyses.

As a reminder of several important concepts from previous chapters, patient encounters with a health system may be inpatient or outpatient, and each of these may generate different types of data. Inpatient data represent a small snapshot of a patient's overall life but capture rich clinical data during the hospitalization (depth, not breadth of data). In contrast, outpatient data may represent a better longitudinal view of the patient's health, but without the same level of detail as an inpatient admission (breadth, not depth of data). Of course, these are only generalizations that may not always hold true. Patient data are also organized in a hierarchy in the EHR, where each visit with the health system generates new encounter-level data.

Dagenais et al. (2022) provide a categorization of "real-world" observational data sources, many of which are derivatives of data collected in the healthcare setting. They classify these sources broadly as administrative, EHR-based, patient-driven, diagnostic, and other, such as vital statistics or surveillance-based. Many of these data sources are covered in this chapter, but readers are referred to Table 1 in Dagenais et al. (2022) for a list of EHR and non-EHR data sources with relevant examples. Readers should keep in mind that this is an active and evolving area and the appearance (or disappearance) of any specific vendor or product is not uncommon. The extent of the uniqueness of these data sources also needs to be evaluated.

DOI: 10.4324/9781003258872-6

Data sources

Institutional EHRs

By institutional EHRs, we mean EHRs that are found within the patient care setting that are directly accessible to the researcher. In the simplest case of EHR-based research, the researcher is embedded within the institution and has access to the EHR data, most likely through a health information management or informatics group. This represents the most streamlined path toward obtaining data. For researchers who are external to the institution but still wish to access EHR data, Chapter 3 provided an overview of the process including identifying a collaborator within the institution and establishing data use agreements. There may also be previously abstracted, pre-existing EHR datasets available to the researcher, obviating the need for the institution, discussed later.

Recognizing that patients *sometimes* have a choice or need to seek care at different practices, single institutional EHRs may be missing important data for the research project. For example, assessing hospital re-admission rates or visits to outpatient clinics may miss encounters that were outside of the health system, and as such, data may be captured in different EHRs. This missing data problem is widely recognized in EHR research and will be discussed further in Chapter 6.

To account for the missing visit challenge in EHR research, one may consider cross-institutional EHR linkage or leveraging data stored in health information exchanges (HIEs). HIEs – also referred to as health information networks – link patient data across disparate health systems. Yet because these exchanges vary by region, researchers will need to consult their specific network's enabling legislation or health department for data accessibility and permissibility.[1] Further, some HIEs only allow clinical care data uses and may forbid research data uses unless all parties agree to release data explicitly for this purpose. Linkage across EHRs requires participating and collaborating with health systems, as well as the ability to identify patients uniquely and reliably. The process of data linkage is found in Chapter 5. Some of the larger healthcare systems and networks, as well as insurers, create their own aggregated views of multiple EHRs for analytic purposes, discussed later, although doing so among disparate entities is a further challenge. Indeed, this was exemplified during the COVID-19 pandemic when researchers sought to create a clearinghouse of research data from multiple EHRs (Schulte, 2020).

In a related notion of population health management, some commercial software vendors, healthcare systems, and health departments have begun to assemble longitudinal views of patients' healthcare encounters through innovative data linkage across multiple EHRs. For example, MDPHnet, of the Massachusetts Department of Public Health, brings together health indicators for the entire state via data linkage from hospitals' and clinics' EHRs (Massachusetts Technology Collaborative, 2018). To protect patient privacy and promote security, the data all reside within the original EHRs, and only the linkage is provided.

MDPHnet is discussed further in Chapter 14. There are a variety of commercial vendors offering EHR-agnostic population health management platforms, including Cerner[2] (Cerner Corporation, Kansas City, MO), Health Catalyst[3] (Health Catalyst, Salt Lake City, UT), Philips[4] (Philips Healthcare, Andover, MA), and i2i[5] (i2i Population Health, Franklin, TN).

Multi-institution EHR studies have certain implications for research. There are many EHR differences between institutions including care delivery and documentation practices. The choice of EHR vendor is site-specific, and even among institutions that use the same vendor, EHRs are highly customized to reflect local practices and cultures. Reassuringly, the meaningful use incentive of the HITECH act (see Chapter 1) has led to the collection of standardized data points in EHRs – the *common clinical data set* – but there are variations even within the prescribed data points. One implication of these site-to-site differences is the notion of database heterogeneity, where the same study research question analyzed in different databases may yield different results (Madigan et al., 2013). This heterogeneity motivates the need for a common data model.

The Observational Medical Outcomes Partnership (OMOP) Common Data Model (CDM) is a database schema for aggregating data from disparate observational databases, including EHRs (Figure 4.1) (Observational Health Data Sciences and Informatics, 2021a). Once data are organized using the OMOP CDM, open-source tools are available to analyze population-level characteristics (Observational Health Data Sciences and Informatics, 2021b). Other CDMs have been proposed, including PCORnet (National Patient-Centered Clinical Research Network, 2022), openEHR (openEHR Foundation, 2022), Sentinel (U.S. Food and Drug Administration, 2022), and FHIR (Health Level Seven International, 2022).

Before using any standardized model, the researcher needs to consider the return-on-investment: will the added work of standardizing the data improve the efficiency and quality of research? The research database proposed in this book does not use a CDM, instead relying on a simpler approach focusing on a single institution EHR. Those affiliated with multiple institutions, large academic medical centers, or disparate data sources and who need to design a research database, data mart, or data warehouse may wish to consider a CDM. For an application of an EHR-derived clinical data repository using the PCORnet CDM, see Hurst et al. (2020), and for an application using the OMOP CDM, see Lamer et al. (2021). For a comparison of various CDMs for representing longitudinal EHR-derived data, see Garza et al. (2016). An applied example can be found in Arterburn et al. (2018), where the authors longitudinally examined weight loss following bariatric surgery among nearly 50,000 patients seen at 41 healthcare systems part of PCORnet. A bariatric case phenotype was developed in collaboration with PCORnet using data elements from their CDM.

One final comment on institutional EHRs as a data source, while EHRs are accessible to providers within the walls of the institutions, that does not necessarily imply the data themselves reside within the institutions. For example, EHR data may reside in offsite servers, sometimes referred to as cloud computing if the

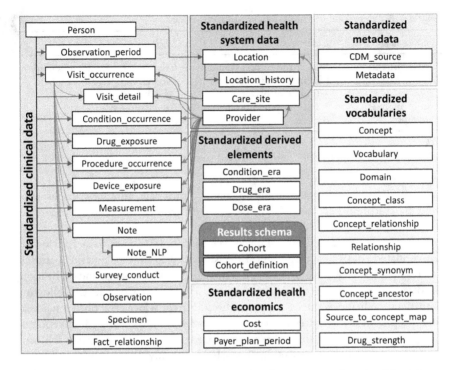

Figure 4.1 Observational Medical Outcomes Partnership Common Data Model v.6.0.

data are hosted on the Internet. One such example of this is Epic (Epic Systems Corporation, Verona, WI) being hosted on Amazon Web Services (Amazon.com, Inc., Seattle, WA) (Amazon Web Services, 2022). Data are extracted from an onsite EHR and sent to AWS in real-time or near real-time. The implication of offsite data storage is that a data use agreement between the institution and Amazon may be required. An advantage of working in a virtual environment is that the analysis can run directly on the cloud for resource-intensive operations as well as to ensure data privacy and security. Alternatively, the data may be able to be saved locally in the more conventional analytic paradigm. Your health information management or informatics groups can assist in this process.

Non-institutional EHRs

By non-institutional EHRs, we mean EHRs that are not directly accessible to the researcher within an institution. This is a rather broad categorization and may include the previously mentioned population health management and health information exchange data sources, health systems and insurer aggregated databases, clinical data registries, commercialized and syndicated databases, open

Table 4.1 A comparison of claims data versus EHR data

Consideration	Claims data	EHR data
Primary intention	Billing and reimbursement	Clinical care and documentation
Representativeness	Patients with insurance (public or private)[a]	Patients who have accessed healthcare
Unit of analysis	A reimbursement claim	An encounter
Geography	Broader	Narrower

Note:
[a] Largely dependent on the source database.

access EHR data, and even insurance benefits claims data, although this last type must be distinguished from EHR data. Many of the same caveats regarding multi-institutional EHR data apply here as well.

Let us begin by distinguishing *claims data* from EHR data as these two are often conflated. EHRs capture clinical decisions and healthcare practice patterns, whereas claims data capture coverage (reimbursement) decisions and utilization; the data capture processes differ (summarized in Table 4.1). Consider the following outpatient medicine example. Suppose a healthcare provider prescribed a medication to a patient that required three refills every 30 days. Assuming patient compliance, claims data would show three dates approximately 30 days apart each time the patient fulfilled the prescription. The EHR may only show a single medication prescribed to the patient without any indication of the order being fulfilled, unless the EHR was linked to the pharmacy. As such, the types of research possible in each of these data sources differ. As delineated in Madigan et al. (2013), "each [of these data sources] reflects a different source population with varied patient demographics, underlying disease severity, and length of longitudinal data capture. Patients may receive care from different health-care systems and over different periods of time, so differences in geographic and temporal quality of care could alter data captured for those individuals" and thus impact the research findings.

Claims data have been linked to EHR data to supplement the strengths and address the limitations of each data source. Previous research has demonstrated how using claims data alone may be subject to misclassification, and when supplemented with EHR data, reveal a more accurate picture (Angier et al., 2014). As an example, the OneFlorida Data Trust is a centralized research database covering approximately 20 million individuals who have received healthcare in Florida, and incorporates data from EHRs, claims data, vital statistics, and disease registries (Hogan et al., 2021). The database is built using the PCORnet CDM and access to the data for research purposes requires the submission of an application.[6] Researchers contemplating linking claims data to EHR data for the purpose of studying drug effectiveness and safety should consult Lin and Schneeweiss (2016).

The distinction between claims data and EHR data is not always apparent. The commercial Premier Healthcare Database (Premier Inc., Charlotte, NC) is one frequently used option for purchasing healthcare data. This database captures

US-based inpatient and outpatient encounter-level data for over 200 million unique patients based on standard hospital discharge billing summaries (Premier Applied Sciences, 2020). Other popular options for acquiring healthcare data include IBM MarketScan[7] (International Business Machines, Armonk, NY), Optum Claims Data[8] (Optum, Inc., Eden Prairie, MN), Kaiser Permanente Research Bank[9] (Kaiser Permanente, Oakland, CA), PCORnet[10] (Patient-Centered Outcomes Research Institute, Washington, DC), IQVIA[11] (IQVIA, Danbury, CT), Cerner Real-World Data[12] and Learning Health Network[13] (Cerner Corporation, Kansas City, MO), and MedRIC[14] (Acumen, LLC, Burlingame, CA), to name a few. These databases, in a general sense, combine information from disparate sources, and may include claims data and EHR data. They capture different populations, from healthcare-specific systems and private insurers, such as Kaiser Permanente, to Medicare and Medicaid patients, such as MedRIC. Tokenization, or the linkage of multiple data sources via a nonidentifiable "token," has further blurred the distinction in the types of data available in these aggregated sources. Products such as HealthVerity MarketPlace[15] (HealthVerity, Inc., Philadelphia, PA), Datavant[16] (Datavant, San Francisco, CA), and Gravitas[17] (LexisNexis Risk Solutions Inc., Alpharetta, GA) have the capacity to construct large de-identified real-world datasets built from observational data that include EHRs.

There are non-commercial options to obtain EHR and claims data as well. Some of the previously mentioned databases, such as MedRIC, may be freely available depending on the scope of research. Others may have tiered data access depending on the level of data needed. The Medical Information Mart for Intensive Care (MIMIC) database[18] is a publicly available database comprising de-identified health-related data for over 40,000 intensive care unit patients at the Beth Israel Deaconess Medical Center (Boston, MA). MIMIC is further described in Johnson et al. (2016). The eICU Collaborative Research Database[19] is another publicly available resource comprising de-identified health-related data for over 200,000 intensive care unit admissions. As compared to the single-center MIMIC database, the eICU database includes multiple facilities across the continental United States participating in the Philips Healthcare eICU telehealth program (Philips Healthcare, Andover, MA). eICU is further described in Pollard et al. (2018). The National Health Service in the United Kingdom maintains an open data portal for their data,[20] and the U.S. National Institutes of Health's *All of Us* research program includes publicly available aggregated data from surveys, wearables, biospecimens and physical measurements, and EHRs from a sample of the population.[21] Data scientists have also publicly released limited, de-identified exports of institutional EHR data for other researchers.[22]

There are even freely available synthetic EHR data generators (Buczak, Babin & Moniz, 2010; Choi et al., 2017; Walonoski et al., 2018). To describe one of these in more detail, Synthea[23] can model over 90 different diseases and conditions, capturing longitudinal inpatient and outpatient encounters spanning from birth through death (Walonoski et al., 2018). EHR modules in the synthetic data include patient-specific data, such as demographics, conditions, allergies, medications, vaccinations, clinical observations and vital sign assessment, labs, procedures, and care plans, as well as payers and providers data. Structured data can be generated in a variety of formats including plain text and CSV. By default, simulated patients are representative of either the US overall or the Commonwealth of Massachusetts, but other geographic or geopolitical locations are possible.

Select societies, organizations, and consortiums may collect EHR data through member-based clinical data registries. For example, the Vermont Oxford Network maintains several databases[24] of neonatal care and outcomes that cover over a thousand submitting entities. The American College of Cardiology runs ten registries[25] that collate records from more than 2,400 hospitals and 8,500 outpatient providers. The Rheumatology Informatics System for Effectiveness[26] run by the American College of Rheumatology includes data on over 1,000 rheumatology clinicians and 2.4 million patients. The Pediatric Health Information System database[27] run by the Children's Hospital Association includes inpatient, ambulatory surgery, emergency department, and observation unit data from over 50 pediatric hospitals in the United States. Many other examples exist: PsychPRO[28] of the American Psychiatric Association, Clinical Emergency Data Registry[29] of the American College of Emergency Physicians, PRIME Registry[30] of the American Board of Family Medicine, to name but a few. There are also commercialized registry options for obtaining data such as CorEvitas[31] (CorEvitas, LLC, Waltham, MA) and Target RWE[32] (Target RWE, Durham, NC). The ability to retrieve individual-level deidentified patient data as opposed to aggregated reports must be ascertained on a per-registry basis.

Finally, there are initiatives that are attempting to create decentralized marketplaces of EHR data that depend on the patient to release their records (dHealth Network, 2021). Patient-driven data are increasingly available via personal health records, consumer genetic testing, and biometric devices (Dagenais et al., 2022). This is an active area of development as of writing and in some cases may already be incorporated into the tokenized real-world datasets introduced earlier.

In short, the landscape of commercial and noncommercial options for EHR data is vast, complex, and constantly evolving. Regardless of the data source, having a sense of the catchment of and contributors to these databases is critical for identifying issues with data validity, representativeness, and generalizability, all discussed further in Chapters 6 and 9.

Non-EHR

It may seem paradoxical to include a section on non-EHR data sources in an EHR research book, but the ability to link EHR data to non-EHR data can allow the researcher to address a wider range of questions. There are numerous examples in the literature of EHR data being supplemented with data derived from pharmacies, disease registries, immunization information systems, vital statistics, government censuses, genomics registries, environmental and built-environment sources, as well as existing research cohorts embedded within a healthcare system. Shortreed et al. (2019) includes citations for many of these examples. There is even a book cataloging secondary data sources for health researchers (Boslaugh, 2007). Below, we briefly discuss a few examples linking non-clinical data sources.

As mentioned, linking EHR data to census data is a popular option. This linkage occurs based on the patients' addresses that are recorded in the EHR and allows the researcher to link area-level data to individual-level data. The process of linking EHR data to census data is covered in Chapter 5 with additional caveats detailed in Chapter 6. Linking census data can allow the researcher to build area-level profiles of patients' socioeconomic classes, such as measures of unemployment, education, poverty, income, government assistance, and so on. In fact, the *area deprivation index* is one standardized measure built from census data that may be useful to describe the neighborhood milieu of patients in the EHR (Messer et al. 2006). An example of linking EHR data to the area deprivation index may be found in Goldstein et al. (2021).

Another example of bridging EHR and non-EHR data is the linkage to population-based biobanks. Biobanks store biological specimens, such as from residual blood after laboratory diagnostics, and have been used for genome-wide and phenome-wide association studies (see Chapter 12). Linking these data to patient-level EHR data allows for a richer exploration of disease risk factors and prognosis, as well as treatment targets and sensitivity. A review of EHR-linked biobank data is available in Wolford, Willer and Surakka (2018). One hospital system's EHR-linked biobank in New York City seeks to recruit one million people by 2027, with a lofty goal of offering genetic sequencing to every consenting patient, and subsequently the de-identified data available to researchers (Mount Sinai Health System, 2022).

Which data belong in the research database?

The first question one may ask is, "Why subset, why not take all of the data?" There are practical and theoretical reasons. From a practical standpoint, data may be inaccessible, may include superfluous information, or may be missing. Furthermore, obtaining all data from an EHR will likely result in a database that is excessively large and unwieldly for the researchers. EHRs and other complex healthcare applications encompass numerous supporting functions invisible to the end user, but are apparent when accessing the backend data. Such backend data are of little utility to the researcher[33] and will only complicate the research database. A final practical reason comes from the institutional review board, as only the minimal data necessary to answer a research question will typically be approved.

From a theoretical standpoint, there is simply no need for all the data. For example, one does not need to study the entire US population to quantify the population's health via the use of random sampling techniques. The goal of the research database is a core set of the necessary observations and variables that can answer the research questions: in other words, a parsimonious database. Including extraneous information induces complexity in the extraction process,

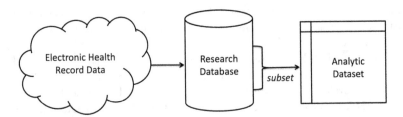

Figure 4.2 Relationship of the EHR to the research database and analytic dataset.

increases the size of the database, and may introduce scope creep or the tendency to examine associations extraneous to the research aims. The question then becomes, "What data do I need?" The research planner introduced in Chapter 3 is one starting point, but to better answer this question, let us revisit the goal of the research database.

As conceived herein, the research database represents a rolling snapshot of the EHR and is used to create the individual analytic datasets for a given analysis or research aim (Figure 4.2). As such, the research database should contain the variables and observations needed for all the research aims. As each individual analytic dataset is created, the inclusion and exclusion criteria of that study are applied to limit the observations and variables required for analysis.

Which observations?

By observations, we mean records in the EHR, whether at the practice level, patient level, or encounter level. The short answer to this question is, "All that are needed for answering your research questions." For example, consider an EHR implemented in a metropolitan hospital that covers patient care since 1990 and contains 10,000,000 patient-level records. Suppose the data prior to 2000 are stored offsite and are only accessible for legal or disaster recovery purposes, or perhaps the records from 1990 through 2000 are scanned paper charts where the only digital information is the demographic attributes of the name, date of birth, medical record number, and address. In such instances, there is a major barrier in accessing these historic records. If the research question is dependent on these data, the study aims may need to be reassessed. Furthermore, suppose the goal of the research database was to quantify the prevalence of various exposures or outcomes in the EHR. Is there a public health or clinical need to describe prevalence rates that are several decades old? Therefore, it may be easiest to initially restrict the research database to a more contemporary timeframe and only obtain recent records.

Defining the denominator – that is, the total population of interest in the EHR – is complicated by the nature of patient encounters with the healthcare system, as introduced in Chapter 2. For example, in an outpatient study, we may wish to only retrieve "active" patients and what constitutes an active patient can differ between healthcare systems, or even practice-to-practice within a single healthcare system. An active patient may be defined as a patient with one or more encounters in the past two years; however, using a fixed threshold may result in an unintended bias in the data, and thus need to be varied in a sensitivity analysis to assess the impact on the analysis (see Chapter 9). Furthermore, even active patients may have recently moved, left the practice, or died, or are concurrently receiving care elsewhere, exacerbating selection or measurement issues. On the other hand, overly active patients may also bias the results given that their health and healthcare-seeking behavior can systematically differ from the general population. Cocoros et al. (2019) examined how changing the definition of an active patient in the EHR impacted prevalence estimates of several chronic conditions and noted that "[these estimates] varied by more than 20 percent for some conditions depending on the choice of denominator." However, there was no single optimal definition revealed during the study.

Revisiting the research planner and discussing the research agenda with the various stakeholders can help identify a start year for the database as well as the denominator. When forming the analytic datasets from the research database, a sample size and power calculation may help to determine the minimum number of data points needed for a given level of statistical certainty, however these calculations have limited utility for secondary data. Sample size and power calculations are discussed in Chapter 7.

Which variables?

The choice of which variables to include in the research database will be more difficult to answer than which observations, as often there is a practical restriction on the number of observations one has access to while there are seemingly unlimited number of variables. As stated earlier, EHRs contain modules specific to departmental needs that may have little bearing on clinical research. The research planner can be used to identify variables for a given study, that is, the analytic dataset, and the sum-total of these variables belong in the research database. As before, there are theoretical and practical reasons to include or exclude certain data points. Starting with a theoretical justification for variables will ensure that the research database is not overly rich with variables that will either be unusable or have little bearing on the research question.

To start, it makes sense to revisit the literature review conducted in the formation of the research question(s) to identify relevant papers and enumerate the variables modeled in those studies. This can serve as a baseline for the wish list of variables. Next consider the core categories of variables in the EHR as defined in Chapter 2 (Pollard et al., 2016): demographics, laboratory, medical imaging, physiologic measurements, medications, diagnosis and procedural codes, and caregiver and procedure notes. Ensure that the research database has coverage in these core areas as aligned with the following categories (Miettinen, 1985): administrative information for patient identification, substantive information for assessing study eligibility criteria, exposures, outcomes, effect modifiers or mediators, confounders, and any other characteristics that may impact external validity. When forming the wish list of variables, engaging the informatics

1. DOES YOUR RESEARCH USE [THE REGISTRY] FOR POPULATION OR INDIVIDUAL (PATIENT SPECIFIC) LEVEL STUDIES?

____ POPULATION   ____ INDIVIDUAL   ____ BOTH

2. WHAT ARE THE PATIENT AGE(S) IN THE STUDY COHORTS THAT YOU MOST COMMONLY USE?

3. DO YOU NEED TO FOLLOW PATIENT COHORTS OVER TIME? THAT IS, WILL YOU TRACK THE SAME GROUP OF PATIENTS FROM YEAR TO YEAR?

____ YES   ____ NO

IF YES, PLEASE PROVIDE AN IDEA OF THE TIME INTERVAL TYPICALLY LOOKED AT:

4. WHAT INTERNAL/EXTERNAL DATA SETS ARE NECESSARY FOR YOUR RESEARCH IN [THE REGISTRY]?

____ VITAL RECORDS   ____ IRIS ____ CASES   ____ MEDICAID

____ RECALL

PLEASE INDICATE ANY OTHER DATA SETS THAT ARE NOT LISTED ABOVE:

5. FROM THE DATA SET(S) YOU IDENTIFIED ABOVE, SPECIFICALLY WHAT INFORMATION IS BEING USED (E.G., BIRTH CERTIFICATE NUMBER, BIRTH ATTENDANT, RECALL POSTCARD DATA, ETC.)?

Figure 4.3 Research database survey example.

groups as well as those who enter data in the EHR will help to identify whether the wish list aligns with the actual data available in the EHR. Finally, consult experts in the field, including the research stakeholders, and administer a survey to ascertain the variables necessary for research. Figure 4.3 is an excerpt from a survey used to build a research database from an immunization registry.

The research database is inherently identifiable, meaning it contains protected health information, such as patient name, data of birth, address, or medical record identifiers. This is necessary for linkage to other databases or datasets, therefore, when assembling the list of variables to include, be sure to include all potential variables used for linkage. Typically, these would include some combination of medical record number, name, date of birth, gender, and address history. Chapter 5 presents specific requirements and approaches to data linkage in the EHR.

When requesting data from the EHR, one needs to guard against conflating data and analysis. For example, suppose a researcher is tasked with assessing the proportion of patients screened for HIV in an outpatient clinic for the past two years. There is no variable in the EHR corresponding to "proportion screened for HIV." Rather, this is an analysis of the data in this patient population. As such, the researcher would need to identify data to form the numerator, for example, number of HIV tests that resulted during the last two years, and the denominator, for example, number of unique patients for this same period. Relatedly, data recorded in the EHR may differ from data needed for modeling. Miettinen (1985) discusses four principles for ensuring the correct data are retrieved:

1 *Primary* data are obtained as opposed to inferential information. For example, individual values of blood pressure are obtained rather than the diagnosis of hypertension.
2 *Detailed* information allows arbitrary categorizations to occur. For example, obtaining weight and height allows the calculation of body mass index and categorization into obese versus not obese, or underweight, normal, overweight, and obese, and so on.
3 *Objectivity* and *judgment* may be equally important. In some cases, it may be better to use the measure of clinical judgment, whereas, in others, the objective measure may be preferred.
4 *Justification* must drive the inclusion of variables into the research database. In other words, data that are retrieved must be needed to answer the research question(s) as described earlier in this section.

Some researchers may be surprised to learn that a variable that should be seemingly obvious to retrieve may not be present in the underlying EHR data. For example, in a traditional epidemiologic analysis, one may examine the presence or absence of a health state to identify correlates of protection or risk. Yet there may be no dichotomous health state variable – that is, the presence or absence of this condition – that can be directly obtained from the EHR. Rather the researcher may need to construct this latent condition from the manifest variables available including signs, symptoms, laboratory results, medications administered, billing codes, and so forth; in other words, operationalizing the clinical phenotype (Richesson et al., 2021). This not only applies to health states but also to risk factors. For example, Kaiser et al. (2022) relied on six areas in the EHR to construct a latent homeless variable: the (1) encounter note, (2) problem list, (3) patient's address, (4) social history, (5) care plan, and (6) housing status. When operationalizing summary indicators of complex health conditions, the notion of "differential item functions" becomes a possibility, whereby a summary indicator of the health phenomenon may differ from group to group (Jones, 2019). Before developing a phenotype definition *de novo*, researchers are advised to search for existing and validated clinical phenotypes; the NIH Pragmatic Trial Collaboratory has cataloged several entities[34] who have previously defined phenotypes.

In forming the list of potential variables, some variables may be available as discrete, coded data points, while others occur as unstructured data, namely "free text." The delineation between these two is important. Consider again Table 2.1 from Chapter 2. Suppose a researcher needed a variable corresponding to family history of cerebral palsy. A free text note to this effect could take countless forms, for example, "family history of cerebral palsy," "hx of CP," "brother is GFMCS-IV." and so on. On the other hand, an ICD or SNOMED code capturing the same information should only take one of a few possible values. As another example, a free text diagnosis of "STI" is open to several possible interpretations including "soft tissue injury" or "sexually transmitted infection," whereas a corresponding code is unambiguous. In general, one should work with codes as opposed to their meaning or interpretation. Nevertheless, narrative-free text as typed or dictated by the clinical provider contributes substantially to the value of data in the EHR but is more difficult for the researcher to operationalize. According to one estimate, 70% of data in the EHR is unstructured free text (Linguamatics, 2022). Researchers are most likely to encounter free text in areas of the EHR corresponding to discharge summaries; laboratory and imaging reports; lifestyle, behavioral, and social factors; call center notes; patient histories and physical findings; progress notes related to care, especially behavioral or mental health notes; and external referral notes. Box 2.1 in Chapter 2 displayed a hypothetical encounter note for reference. Previous research has suggested that even in the presence of structured data entry options, free text entry still occurs (Zheng et al., 2011; Zhou et al., 2012). Chapter 12 provides an overview of several options for dealing with free text in the EHR including performing qualitative research on the free text, machine learning, and natural language processing to create discrete data.

The bulk of data requested from the EHR are likely to be time-varying variables, in that the value depends on when the measurement was performed. This could be true for measures taken from a physical examination, laboratory diagnostics, medications administered, and so forth. Figure 4.4 depicts four measurements of a vital sign for a hypothetical patient. Regardless of whether this was an inpatient with repeated measures during their hospitalization or an outpatient with repeated measures across encounters, the right measurement must be obtained at the right time for valid epidemiological inference. In a repeated measures analysis, all values may be necessary to obtain (and stored in long or wide format, discussed in Chapter 5), whereas in a cross-sectional analysis only a single measure may be needed. The choice as to which measure(s) to obtain is informed by the parameters of the study and the theoretical window of time that

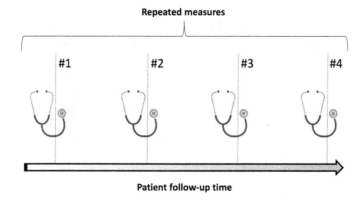

Figure 4.4 Four measurements of a vital sign for a hypothetical patient.

CPT Code List

Code	Category	Description
86704	Pathology	Hepatitis B core antibody (HBcAb); IgG and IgM test.
86705	Pathology	IgM antibody - Hepatitis B core antibody test.
86706	Pathology	Hepatitis B surface antibody (HBsAb) test.
86707	Pathology	Hepatitis Be antibody (HBeAb) test.
86708	Pathology	Hepatitis A antibody (HAAb); IgG and IgM test.
86709	Pathology	Hepatitis A Antibody Test, IgM.
86803	Pathology	Hepatitis C Antibody Test.
86804	Pathology	Hepatitis C Antibody; confirmatory test (eg, immunoblot).
87340	Pathology	Infectious agent antigen detectiion by enzyme immunoassay technique, qualitative or semiquantitat
87350	Pathology	Infectious agent antigen detectiion by enzyme immunoassay technique, qualitative or semiquantitat
87380	Pathology	Infectious agent antigen detectiion by enzyme immunoassay technique, qualitative or semiquantitat
87515	Pathology	Infectious agent detection by nucleic acid (DNA or RNA); hepatitis B virus, direct probe technique.
87516	Pathology	Infectious agent detection by nucleic acid (DNA or RNA); hepatitis B virus, amplified probe techniqu
87517	Pathology	Infectious agent detection by nucleic acid (DNA or RNA); hepatitis B virus, quantification.
87520	Pathology	Infectious agent detection by nucleic acid (DNA or RNA); hepatitis C virus, direct probe technique.
87521	Pathology	Infectious agent detection by nucleic acid (DNA or RNA); hepatitis C virus, amplified probe techniqu
87522	Pathology	Infectious agent detection by nucleic acid (DNA or RNA); hepatitis C virus, quantification.
87525	Pathology	Infectious agent detection by nucleic acid (DNA or RNA); hepatitis G virus, direct probe technique.

Figure 4.5 Current procedural terminology codes for viral hepatitis.

is of greatest relevance. This may be complicated by EHRs where the problem list is separate from the encounter, and thus not updated at each visit.

Variables derived from external provider orders, including medical imaging studies and laboratory requisitions, require further consideration. An EHR with computerized provider order entry makes it straightforward to capture such orders; on the other hand, the results of these studies can be reported in numerous ways, evolving over time. Consider an order for a hepatitis C test, antibody, and viral load, with orders using Current Procedural Terminology (CPT) codes and results using Logical Observation Identifiers Names and Codes (LOINC). There are only a handful of CPT codes for hepatitis C tests (Figure 4.5). On the other hand, there are many possible LOINC codes for the laboratory to use in order to report the results to the provider (Figure 4.6). Further complicating this may be the lab-to-lab differences in assay equipment and reporting convention as well as results being provided as subjective interpretations as opposed to objective measures. See the earlier discussion regarding data versus analysis for suggestions on how to approach this complexity.

Aside from the traditional data mined from the EHR (see earlier discussion of Pollard et al., 2016), researchers may also consider non-traditional EHR data. Ehrenstein, Kharrazi and Lehmann (2019) described several emerging data types found in the EHR, including healthcare utilization metrics, biosamples, genetic information, social data, patient-generated data such as health communications, community, and geospatial data such as through census linkage (Chapter 5), survey and screening instrument results, and clinical workflow data. Variables can be operationalized based on any or all of these categories. Hirsch et al. (2017) demonstrated the use of EHR audit data to capture patient patterns and clinical workflow in the hospital to ascertain differences in patient time spent waiting, with a nurse, and with a physician. They noted important differences in time by demographic and clinical features of the patients. Goldstein et al. (2017) mined the EHR for documentation events to reconstruct the patient care network of

LOINC	LongName	Component
88453-6	HIV 1 RNA+Hepatitis C virus RNA+Hepatitis B virus DNA [Presence] in Se	HIV 1 RNA+Hepatitis C virus RNA+Hepatitis B virus DNA
51656-7	Hepatitis C virus Ab Signal/Cutoff in Body fluid	Hepatitis C virus Ab Signal/Cutoff
48159-8	Hepatitis C virus Ab Signal/Cutoff in Serum or Plasma by Immunoassay	Hepatitis C virus Ab Signal/Cutoff
82380-7	Hepatitis C virus genotype 1 NS5a gene mutations detected [Identifier]	Hepatitis C virus genotype 1 NS5a gene mutations detected
82381-5	Hepatitis C virus genotype 1 NS5b gene mutations detected [Identifier]	Hepatitis C virus genotype 1 NS5b gene mutations detected
82514-1	Hepatitis C virus genotype 3 NS5a gene mutations detected [Identifier]	Hepatitis C virus genotype 3 NS5a gene mutations detected
81116-6	Hepatitis C virus core Ab+Ag [Presence] in Serum	Hepatitis C virus core Ab+Ag
54914-7	Hepatitis C virus core Ag [Units/volume] in Serum by Immunoassay	Hepatitis C virus core Ag
49846-9	Hepatitis C virus core Ag [Presence] in Blood or Marrow from Donor	Hepatitis C virus core Ag
79189-7	Hepatitis C virus core Ag [Presence] in Serum or Plasma by Immunoassay	Hepatitis C virus core Ag
22328-9	Hepatitis C virus superoxide dismutase Ab [Presence] in Serum	Hepatitis C virus superoxide dismutase Ab
11077-5	Hepatitis C virus superoxide dismutase Ab [Presence] in Serum by Immun	Hepatitis C virus superoxide dismutase Ab
59052-1	HIV 1+Hepatitis C virus RNA+Hepatitis B virus DNA [Presence] in Serum c	HIV 1+Hepatitis C virus RNA+Hepatitis B virus DNA
48574-8	Hepatitis C virus genotype [Identifier] in Blood by NAA with probe detectio	Hepatitis C virus genotype
32286-7	Hepatitis C virus genotype [Identifier] in Serum or Plasma by NAA with pro	Hepatitis C virus genotype
49607-5	Hepatitis C virus genotype [Identifier] in Tissue by NAA with probe detectic	Hepatitis C virus genotype
48575-5	Hepatitis C virus genotype [Identifier] in Unspecified specimen by NAA wit	Hepatitis C virus genotype
73654-6	Hepatitis C virus NS3 gene mutations detected [Identifier] by Genotype me	Hepatitis C virus NS3 gene mutations detected
73655-3	Hepatitis C virus NS5 gene mutations detected [Identifier] by Genotype me	Hepatitis C virus NS5 gene mutations detected
60279-7	IL28B gene associated variant rs12979860 [Presence] in Blood or Tissue	IL28B gene associated variant rs12979860
23870-9	Hepatitis C virus 100+5-1-1 Ab [Presence] in Serum by Immunoblot	Hepatitis C virus 100+5-1-1 Ab
22324-8	Hepatitis C virus 100-3 Ab [Presence] in Serum	Hepatitis C virus 100-3 Ab
9608-1	Hepatitis C virus 100-3 Ab [Presence] in Serum by Immunoblot	Hepatitis C virus 100-3 Ab
22327-1	Hepatitis C virus Ab [Units/volume] in Serum	Hepatitis C virus Ab
5198-7	Hepatitis C virus Ab [Units/volume] in Serum by Immunoassay	Hepatitis C virus Ab

Figure 4.6 Logical observation identifiers names and codes for viral hepatitis.

infants in the neonatal intensive care unit for the purposes of identifying intervention points for hand hygiene. Projects such as these demonstrate the application of traditional and non-traditional EHR data to improve patient care practices in the healthcare setting.

Toward construction of the research database

Up to this point, the research database has been treated as an abstract concept. This section marks the division between abstract and concrete. In building the research database, one has several options to consider. Will this database reside locally on the researcher's computer or virtually on a shared drive? Will the database be accessible to more than one researcher? How will the database be secured, encrypted, and password protected? Will a CDM be used or will this be a one-off homegrown solution? Who will retrieve the data from the EHR? Who will update the research database with new EHR data? Does a research database or clinical data warehouse for research purposes already exist? These questions must be answerable to proceed.

Should a research database already exist, such as a clinical data warehouse or previously extracted EHR dataset, much of what remains in this chapter may be moot. Nevertheless, the reader may still find this material helpful in understanding the process of constructing an EHR-based research database as well as the potential limitations of the data therein.

There are a variety of technological solutions for building a research database. On the one hand, this database could reside natively within the statistical software, on a Microsoft Access (Microsoft Corporation, Redmond, WA) database, or in a Microsoft Excel (Microsoft Corporation, Redmond, WA) spreadsheet. These options are straightforward with minimal technical requirements and may be ideal for small-scale projects. On the other hand, a complex or extremely large research database may require an enterprise-wide solution such as Microsoft SQL Server (Microsoft Corporation, Redmond, WA) or REDCap (Vanderbilt University, Nashville, TN).[35]

REDCap (Research Electronic Data Capture) is a popular option for storing research data. As of this writing, there are nearly 6,000 institutions using RED-Cap for over 1,400,000 projects. REDCap is a self-managed, secure, web-based solution designed to support data collection strategies for research studies (Harris et al., 2009; Harris et al., 2019). There are numerous benefits to using a previously vetted solution such as REDCap, such as integrated analysis, data standardization and quality assurance, user access control, automated data dictionary, ease of data entry, data import and export, and HIPAA and IRB compliance. Furthermore, via the REDCap application programming interface, one can automate data import and export operations, even directly from statistical software, such as R (Nutter & Lane, 2020). Regardless of the specific technology used for the research database, what follows will still be germane to its construction.

The rolling snapshot model

The research database is conceived as a rolling snapshot that can be updated on a recurring basis, useful for when new observations or variables are added over time. Therefore, it is not necessary to initially include every observation or variable that may be potentially useful. Rather, it may be easiest to start with a core set of variables and observations that more closely align the research database to the analytic dataset, and then expand it overtime. The initial "turn" of the database, defined herein as process of connecting to EHR data and updating the research database, will consist of its initial construction. It may be useful to think of this initial turn as the proof of concept: will this research database model work for the type of research being conducting? If so, then it can be updated, including more observations, and expanded, including more variables, the next time the database is turned. If possible, nominate a data manager who will be responsible for all aspects of the research database construction and dissemination.

Turning the research database can be done cumulatively or iteratively. In the cumulative approach, the entire database is regenerated each time an update is initiated. The advantage of this approach is consistency in data coding and the inclusion of new variables for all observations. The disadvantage is the time required to regenerate the data, particularly for large or intensive operations, or slow network connections. Unique identifiers must be preserved to allow for data linkage, reconciliation, and reproducibility. An iterative update to the research database, where only the new observations are added or appended, significantly reduces the burden of updating the database. However, any new variables that are added will only be available from a given time point, unless special consideration is given to historic observations. Furthermore, if data have changed in the underlying EHR, this may result in data inconsistencies across time without the researcher's awareness.

Methods for data extraction

The methods for data extraction will vary by the source of EHR data. In this section, we will consider the following four data export methods: (1) manual chart review, (2) EHR reporting tools, (3) EHR direct connection, and (4) existing data extraction. If the EHR is institutional, as defined at the start of this chapter, methods #1–3 are most applicable; if the EHR is non-institutional, method #4 may be the only possibility. Although these methods are presented separately, they may be used in a complementary fashion. For example, following an automated extraction of EHR data via a reporting tool, one may consider auditing the data through a manual chart review to ensure data integrity.

As an aside and up to this point in the book, the words "export" and "subset" have been used interchangeably. It is now worthwhile to make a distinction between the two: exporting is the act of extracting data from a source and saving it in a new location, whereas subsetting limits the data extracted. Furthermore, exporting has a specific connotation. If the source is a database, the term export makes intuitive sense, as the data are the result of a literal export operation performed by the user. On the other hand, if the source is a spreadsheet, technically the export operation has already occurred upstream when the spreadsheet was created. Yet the word (re-)export is used here to mean data that are subsequently copied or saved from the spreadsheet to another location: the research database. Understanding this use of the word export will help in the rest of the discussion.

In this section, we perform both export and subset operations concurrently. Later, we will exclusively be subsetting the data when forming the analytic dataset. At this point, no distinction is made based on the type of data (i.e., cross-sectional or longitudinal) and whether the observations are unique per person or multiple per person. Data organization is the focus of Chapter 5. At the end of this section, the exported and subsetted data may be stored in the research database directly, a CSV file, or natively within the preferred statistical software. All formats are treated equally in subsequent chapters and consequently the output format should be governed by the methods used to arrive at the extracted data. The general flow of data from the EHR to analysis is shown in Figure 4.7, which is an expansion of Figure 4.2.

Manual chart review

Manual chart review can take several forms, but essentially involves abstracting EHR data directly via the user interface and entering the data into the research database. This type of data abstraction is common practice (Alzu'bi, Watzlaf & Sheridan, 2021) and may occur by manually typing data from the EHR into the research database, or perhaps copying and pasting from the EHR into the research database. The advantages of this approach include confidence in obtaining the correction information – provided the abstracter has familiarity with the EHR – and ease to which the information is available. If data are stored in free

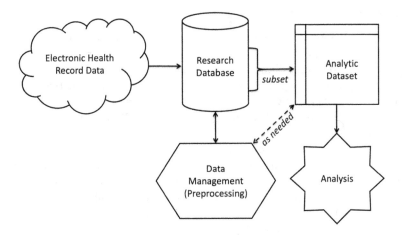

Figure 4.7 Flow of data from the EHR to analysis.

text as opposed to discrete elements, real-time interpretation of the information is possible, especially if working with the clinicians who entered the patient data. (Free text was covered earlier in the chapter). For studies with few patients and few variables, this can also be an efficient approach. However, the need to obtain anything other than a small number of observations and variables places a huge burden on the data abstractor introducing the possibility of transcribing errors in the process. An existing literature has found notable differences in manual versus electronic data abstraction (Brundin-Mather et al., 2018; Knake et al., 2016; Yin et al., 2022). Furthermore, the availability of the end-user view of the EHR may not be an option for many researchers; more likely, these researchers may be accessing a deidentified clinical data warehouse. If a manual chart review is occurring from the data warehouse, the same caveats apply.

For researchers who are limited to chart review as the method for data abstraction, there are several approaches to limiting data entry errors. First, the data abstractor should be trained by someone with familiarity with data entry in the EHR. Second, the use of multiple abstractors with redundant coding can reveal if there are data points that are more complex or nuanced to be captured. This dual-coding approach does not have to occur on all observations and variables, but rather a (random) subset. One can then compute an inter-abstractor reliability measure, such as percent agreement or kappa (to take into account random variation), to identify discordance in data entry. Third, researchers may want to consider auditing the data that were manually abstracted. As before, this does not need to be done for the entire data set, but a random sample can be taken and used to approximate the overall error rate. An *a priori* threshold can be set, such as 10%, where an error rate more than this threshold requires re-abstraction. If re-abstraction is necessary, further investigation may reveal if there are patterns by certain patients or variables, and thus re-abstraction can be more targeted.

EHR reporting tools

The use of an automated approach to abstract data from the EHR standardizes the process and improves coding accuracy and efficiency. There are many reporting tools available depending on the EHR and the ability to connect to it via an application programming interface. Most EHRs will include a native reporting tool for abstracting patient-level data, for example, Cerner's PowerInsight (Cerner Corporation, Kansas City, MO) or Epic's Reporting Workbench (Epic Systems Corporation, Verona, WI). Institutional EHR users should consult with their informatics or health information technology groups to obtain access to a reporting tool for data extraction. Crystal Reports (SAP, Waldorf, Germany) is a popular third-party software application that connects to many EHR databases and can be used for data abstraction. There are also numerous consulting companies that specialize in EHR data extraction: a simple Internet search will yield ones with EHR vendor-specific experience.

If the EHR data are accessible via an application programming interface or reside in a clinical data warehouse, this introduces additional data extraction options including open-source tools such as i2b2 (Murphy et al., 2010), Leaf (Dobbins et al., 2020), EMERSE (Hanauer et al., 2015), and ReviewR (Mayer et al., 2022). For clinical data warehouses, there may also be built-in reporting tools the research can leverage similar to the integrated EHR reporting tools. As these will be vendor and site-specific, researchers are advised to consult with their respective informatics or health information technology groups.

Regardless of the tools and technologies used, the research can either directly import the data into the research database through the use of an application programming interface, or save the exports as a CSV file as an intermediate step.

EHR direct connection

A direction EHR connection is the most flexible method while being the most challenging to implement. Under this method, the EHR database or clinical data warehouse must be accessible via a network connection with the appropriate user access rights. The connection with the database will occur via an application programming interface, such as using one of the reporting tools described above, an SQL interface, or a native programming interface, for example, the Cerner Command Language (Cerner Corporation, Kansas City, MO). As the use of reporting tools and a native programming interface are vendor-specific, the balance of this section will focus on SQL interfaces. Nevertheless, the comments are still applicable to all direct connections.

An SQL interface allows user queries to the database using a special-purpose programming language – the structured query language – and can be thought of as an automated copy and paste of only desired observations and variables from the underlying database tables. There are several requirements before an SQL connection can be obtained. First, as mentioned, the database must be accessible via a network. Second, the investigator must have a user account that can access the database server. For example, under Microsoft Windows (Microsoft Corporation, Redmond, WA), the Windows' user account can be enabled with database access permissions; otherwise, a special user account can be created on the database to allow investigator access. Third, the proper software must be installed on the investigator's computer. Connecting to the database via statistical software allows for both data retrieval and data processing to occur (data processing is discussed in Chapter 5). SAS (SAS Institute, Cary, NC), R (R Foundation for Statistical Computing, Vienna, Austria), SPSS (IBM Corporation, Armonk, NY), and Stata (StataCorp, College Station, TX) all can issue SQL queries. Example code demonstrating an SQL query to a database using R can be found in Appendix 2 (Code #4.1). Another option is to use a third-party application. For example, Microsoft Access and Excel (Microsoft Corporation, Redmond, WA) can both query a database using SQL.

There are two general options for creating an SQL interface to a database. The most straightforward option is to setup an open database connectivity (ODBC) data name source, which serves as a shortcut to the database. A second option is to reference the database directly in the SQL connection, bypassing the need for an ODBC. Bypassing the need for an ODBC entry allows real-time configuration changes and may obviate the need for an operating system-specific change on the investigator's computer. Depending on the connection type, the SQL code will either reference the data source name or the ODBC protocol directly. At this point, an SQL query can be issued to the database to both export and subset the data in a single step, but this requires familiarity with the SQL programing language. There are different implementations of SQL and while there are many commands in common, including most of the core operations, a full introduction to the programming language is outside the scope of this book. The reader is referred to any number of website references (e.g., W3Schools, 2021), or books on the subject (Kline, 2008), although one specific to the statistical software's SQL implementation will be of most value. What follows is a high-level overview of using SQL to extract data from a database.

A basic SQL command for data retrieval will take the shape of "SELECT <variables> FROM <table>". Suppose all the observations and variables are contained in a single table or pre-programmed query called **patient demographics**. The corresponding SQL can be as simple as "SELECT * FROM [patient demographics]." To subset either the variables or observations will require modifying the SQL query. For example, suppose we wish to retrieve only the "patient ID," "name," "gender," and "address" variables from the **patient demographics** table from Figure 4.8. The asterisk, which requested the database to return all variables from the **patient demographics** table, is now replaced with the requested variable names. These variable names need to match the names in the database and thus require knowledge of the database schema, as shown in Figure 4.8. The modified SQL query will be "SELECT [patient id], [patient name], [gender], [address] FROM [patient demographics]." The correct use of capitalization and spaces will be specific to the database.

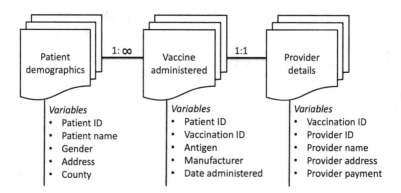

Figure 4.8 An immunization database.

To subset the observations, the SQL query is further modified to specify one or more constraints on the returned data. For example, suppose we wish to retrieve patient data for a given county – Philadelphia County – for the same set of variables "patient ID," "name," "gender," and "address." The SQL query will include the WHERE keyword as follows, "SELECT [patient id], [patient name], [gender], [address] FROM [patient demographics] WHERE [county]='Philadelphia County'." This export command is a basic example of subsetting based on both variables and observations.

Considering one of the core principals of efficient database design is the use of a relational structure, that is, segregating similar data into separate tables, multiple tables may need to be referenced in the SQL query. For example, to retrieve vaccination event data for each person will require "joining" the **vaccine administered** table to the **patient demographics** table. Building upon the previous query restricting the variables and observations, but adding the "antigen" and "date administered" variables yields the following query, "SELECT [patient id], [patient name], [gender], [address], [antigen], [date administered] FROM [patient demographics] LEFT JOIN [vaccine administered] ON [patient demographics].[patient id]= [vaccine administered].[patient id] WHERE [county]='Philadelphia County'." These queries quickly become quite complex! As such, the researcher should inquire if a pre-programmed query can be created to minimize the load on the database and complexity of the SQL command. It may also be possible to build the SQL statement using a graphical user interface, such as Microsoft Access's Query Design tool and then view the underlying SQL syntax. One may also decide to perform separate queries specific to each database table and then manually join them as explained in Chapter 5. Once output from SQL SELECT commands is obtained, these data can either be directly imported the data into the research database, thereby preserving any data types that have been automatically assigned as a result of the SQL query, or saved as a CSV file as an intermediate step before importing to the research database.

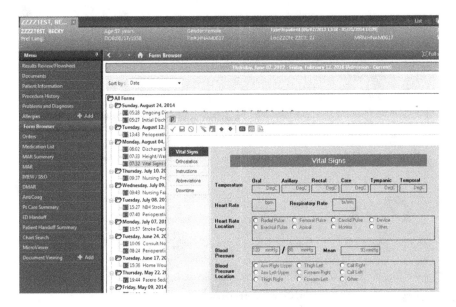

Figure 4.9 An example screenshot from Cerner PowerChart.

[Image used with permission from Cerner Corporation.]

As has been alluded to several times, when undertaking a direct connection to the EHR, one will encounter the complexity of the data stored in these systems. From the end user's perspective, such as the clinician, it may be readily apparent which data are needed for a study. For example, consider the researcher interested in obtaining vital sign information for a cohort of patients. Figure 4.9 is a screenshot from Cerner PowerChart (Cerner Corporation, Kansas City, MO), which clearly show the needed vital sign data on a medical charting form. Manual abstraction of these data is trivial.

On the other hand, mapping the front-end display to the back-end variable is difficult. Not only may this differ vendor to vendor, but this may also differ from patient to patient, depending on the exact source of the information. In our example, we will need to know how the availability of vital sign data in the front end of the EHR corresponds to the actual vital sign variables in the backend database. Furthermore, in the backend database, there may not be clearly defined variables corresponding to systolic and diastolic blood pressure, temperature, heart rate, respiratory rate, oxygen saturation, and so forth. So how do we know which variables to query? One option is to make a list of the front-end data that are needed and inquiring with the institutional informatics group or contacting the EHR vendor directly. Another option is to use a reporting tool, if available, because when creating an EHR report the variable names may be indicated. Figure 4.10 is a screenshot of the Cerner PowerInsight (Cerner Corporation, Kansas City, MO) reporting tool that interfaces with the PowerChart database. When using this tool to construct a report abstracting vital sign data it becomes apparent which

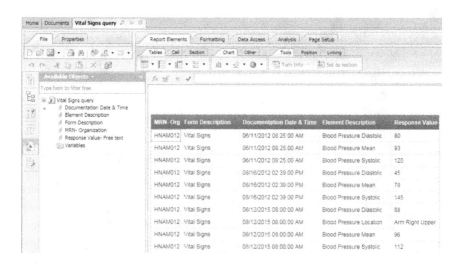

Figure 4.10 An example screenshot from Cerner PowerInsight.

[Image used with permission from Cerner Corporation.]

variables correspond to systolic and diastolic blood pressure. The variable names can now be copied into the SQL statement that live queries the database.

Existing data extract

If the EHR data are not accessible to the researcher but instead are obtained through other channels, the data may require manipulation before importing into the research database. Given the breadth of possible data sources – databases, spreadsheets, statistical software export, and proprietary and other data formats – each of these data source formats will be treated separately below, as they all have their own requirements. If possible, the most compatible format for obtaining non-institutional EHR data is through a shared CSV file.

Data that exist in a database not accessible to the researcher will require a third party to handle the data export and subset operations. In this scenario, the EHR architecture and variable names are likely unknown to the researcher and will require the third party to translate the data request. To facilitate this request, the researcher can become familiar with the front end of the database and make the request for data using the front-end variable labels. In Figure 4.9, a vital sign form from Cerner PowerChart shows the blood pressure of a patient. By requesting "blood pressure," the researcher relies upon the third party to select the relevant variables. The onus is on the researcher to request the appropriate data and perform integrity and quality assurance checks to ensure the data appear "correct." Should one request systolic blood pressure but receive diastolic blood pressure, performing exploratory data analysis will hopefully reveal this discrepancy. To organize this data request to the third party, a simple table can be assembled and organized by the forms or reports from the front-end of the

EHR, and columns or field names indicating the variables to retrieve. This can then be provided in combination with criteria for patient selection, such as all discharges since the year 2005, for an export and subset as a single request. The data file should be requested in the universal CSV format.

Data that exist in a spreadsheet format are typically encountered as the result of a prior export of EHR data. This is a common type of EHR-derived data and conveniently depicts all observations (rows) and variables (columns) in a single view. Before importing into the research database, exploratory analysis can occur within the spreadsheet itself to perform the previously mentioned quality assurance checks. Any extraneous variables or observations can be removed by simply deleting the appropriate column or row. Microsoft Excel (Microsoft Corporation, Redmond, WA) is particularly useful for such data clean-up and processing operations, and is discussed in more detail in Chapter 5, although extremely large datasets may exceed Excel's capabilities. In the case of a spreadsheet with multiple sheets, each sheet will need to be saved as a separate CSV file and then joined in the data linkage step explained in the next chapter. In some instances, CSV files may be provided along with accompanying import scripts to assist in building the research database: this is the case with the previously mentioned MIMIC database[36] and eICU database.[37]

Data that exist in a statistical software format have similar considerations as to the spreadsheet format. The export operation has already occurred, the available variables and observations are visible, and any extraneous data can be removed by deleting variable(s) or observation(s). Unlike data provided in a CSV file, data provided in a statistical software export may already have the data types and missing data properly encoded, saving time and potentially avoiding coding errors. If the analysis will not use the same statistical software as has been provided, the researcher may need to convert the data to the preferred software format. If the source statistical software is available, converting the data can often be accomplished using the integrated "Save as..." or "Export" commands and selecting the preferred statistical software format or a CSV file. Alternatively, the researcher's statistical software may have an integrated "Import" command that can read other statistical data formats. In the event that neither the desired format is available within the software, nor the import command accepts the provided format, a third-party utility such as Stat/Transfer (Circle Systems, Seattle, WA) may be needed to convert between statistical software's native file formats.

Lastly, when data exist in a proprietary or another unknown format, the end goal is to convert the data file to a CSV file that is universally compatible. If proprietary data are suspected, contact the data provider to inquire if any other formats, preferably spreadsheet or statistical software, are available.

Notes

1 As of this writing, there was no centralized list of HIEs across the U.S. All states have such exchanges, many states have more than one exchange, and some are also interconnected to form regional exchanges. Frequently, HIEs are accessible via a website.; for example, information about the Delaware Health Information Network is available

at: https://dhin.org. Civitas Networks for Health (https://www.civitasforhealth.org) is a member driven organization promoting health information exchanges and covers approximately 95% of the U.S. population.

2 https://www.cerner.com/solutions/population-health-management
3 https://www.healthcatalyst.com/offerings/population-health/
4 https://www.usa.philips.com/healthcare/medical-specialties/population-health/what-is-population-health-management/
5 https://www.i2ipophealth.com
6 https://onefloridaconsortium.org/front-door/research-infrastructure-utilization-application/
7 https://www.ibm.com/products/marketscan-research-databases
8 https://www.optum.com/business/solutions/life-sciences/real-world-data/claims-data.html
9 https://researchbank.kaiserpermanente.org/our-research/for-researchers/
10 https://pcornet.org/data/
11 https://www.iqvia.com/insights/the-iqvia-institute/available-iqvia-data
12 https://www.cerner.com/solutions/real-world-data
13 https://www.cerner.com/solutions/learning-health-network
14 https://www.medric.info
15 https://healthverity.com/solutions/healthverity-marketplace/
16 https://datavant.com/product/
17 https://risk.lexisnexis.com/products/gravitas
18 https://mimic.mit.edu
19 https://eicu-crd.mit.edu
20 https://opendata.nhsbsa.net/pages/about
21 https://databrowser.researchallofus.org
22 https://www.kaggle.com/datasets?search=ehr
23 https://synthea.mitre.org
24 https://public.vtoxford.org/data-and-reports/
25 https://cvquality.acc.org/NCDR-Home/registries
26 https://rheumatology.org/about-rise-registry
27 https://www.childrenshospitals.org/content/analytics/product-program/pediatric-health-information-system
28 https://www.psychiatry.org/psychiatrists/research/registry
29 https://www.acep.org/cedr/
30 https://primeregistry.org
31 https://www.corevitas.com/data-sources#registries
32 https://www.targetrwe.com/services/data-solutions/registries/
33 Occasionally, backend data may prove useful, such as the use of EHR logging data to track patient care and workflow. See, for example, Hirsch et al. (2017), discussed later in this chapter.
34 https://rethinkingclinicaltrials.org/chapters/conduct/electronic-health-records-based-phenotyping/finding-existing-phenotype-definitions/
35 https://www.project-redcap.org
36 https://mimic.mit.edu/docs/gettingstarted/local/
37 https://eicu-crd.mit.edu/gettingstarted/dbsetup/

References

Alzu'bi AA, Watzlaf VJM, Sheridan P. Electronic health record (EHR) abstraction. Perspect Health Inf Manag. 2021 Mar 15;18(Spring):1g.

Amazon Web Services. Epic on AWS. https://aws.amazon.com/health/solutions/epic/ (accessed January 20, 2022), 2022.

Angier H, Gold R, Gallia C, Casciato A, Tillotson CJ, Marino M, Mangione-Smith R, DeVoe JE. Variation in outcomes of quality measurement by data source. Pediatrics. 2014 Jun;133(6):e1676–e1682.

Arterburn D, Wellman R, Emiliano A, Smith SR, Odegaard AO, Murali S, Williams N, Coleman KJ, Courcoulas A, Coley RY, Anau J, Pardee R, Toh S, Janning C, Cook A, Sturtevant J, Horgan C, McTigue KM; PCORnet Bariatric Study Collaborative. Comparative effectiveness and safety of bariatric procedures for weight loss: A PCORnet cohort study. Ann Intern Med. 2018 Dec 4;169(11):741–750.

Boslaugh S. Secondary Data Sources for Public Health. New York, NY: Cambridge University Press, 2007.

Brundin-Mather R, Soo A, Zuege DJ, Niven DJ, Fiest K, Doig CJ, Zygun D, Boyd JM, Parsons Leigh J, Bagshaw SM, Stelfox HT. Secondary EMR data for quality improvement and research: A comparison of manual and electronic data collection from an integrated critical care electronic medical record system. J Crit Care. 2018 Oct;47:295–301.

Buczak AL, Babin S, Moniz L. Data-driven approach for creating synthetic electronic medical records. BMC Med Inform Decis Mak. 2010 Oct 14;10:59.

Choi E, Biswal S, Malin B, Duke J, Stewart WF, Sun J. Generating Multi-label Discrete Patient Records Using Generative Adversarial Networks. In Machine Learning for Healthcare Conference, 2017 Nov 6 (pp. 286–305).

Cocoros NM, Ochoa A, Eberhardt K, Zambarano B, Klompas M. Denominators matter: Understanding medical encounter frequency and its impact on surveillance estimates using EHR data. EGEMS. 2019 Jul 23;7(1):31.

Dagenais S, Russo L, Madsen A, Webster J, Becnel L. Use of real-world evidence to drive drug development strategy and inform clinical trial design. Clin Pharmacol Ther. 2022 Jan;111(1):77–89.

dHealth Network. Public Blockchain Framework for Healthcare. https://uploads-ssl.webflow.com/62434be6096bbb00e80dbf0d/6253e75695e36ce5aa800dd8_Whitepaper-dHealth-Network.pdf (accessed May 10, 2022), 2021.

Dobbins NJ, Spital CH, Black RA, Morrison JM, de Veer B, Zampino E, Harrington RD, Britt BD, Stephens KA, Wilcox AB, Tarczy-Hornoch P, Mooney SD. Leaf: An open-source, model-agnostic, data-driven web application for cohort discovery and translational biomedical research. J Am Med Inform Assoc. 2020 Jan 1;27(1):109–118.

Ehrenstein V, Kharrazi H, Lehmann H, et al. Obtaining Data From Electronic Health Records. In: Gliklich RE, Leavy MB, Dreyer NA, editors. Tools and Technologies for Registry Interoperability, Registries for Evaluating Patient Outcomes: A User's Guide, 3rd Edition, Addendum 2 [Internet]. Rockville, MD: Agency for Healthcare Research and Quality (US), 2019 Oct., Chapter 4. Available from: https://www.ncbi.nlm.nih.gov/books/NBK551878/.

Garza M, Del Fiol G, Tenenbaum J, Walden A, Zozus MN. Evaluating common data models for use with a longitudinal community registry. J Biomed Inform. 2016 Dec;64:333–341.

Goldstein ND, Eppes SC, Mackley A, Tuttle D, Paul DA. A network model of hand hygiene: How good is good enough to stop the spread of MRSA? Infect Control Hosp Epidemiol. 2017 Aug;38(8):945–952.

Goldstein ND, Kahal D, Testa K, Burstyn I. Inverse probability weighting for selection bias in a Delaware community health center electronic medical record study of community deprivation and hepatitis c prevalence. Ann Epidemiol. 2021 Aug;60:1–7.

Hanauer DA, Mei Q, Law J, Khanna R, Zheng K. Supporting information retrieval from electronic health records: A report of university of Michigan's nine-year experience in developing and using the electronic medical record search engine (EMERSE). J Biomed Inform. 2015 Jun;55:290–300.

Harris PA, Taylor R, Minor BL, Elliott V, Fernandez M, O'Neal L, McLeod L, Delacqua G, Delacqua F, Kirby J, Duda SN; REDCap Consortium. The REDCap consortium: Building an international community of software platform partners. J Biomed Inform. 2019 Jul;95:103208.

Harris PA, Taylor R, Thielke R, Payne J, Gonzalez N, Conde JG. Research electronic data capture (REDCap)–a metadata-driven methodology and workflow process for providing translational research informatics support. J Biomed Inform. 2009 Apr;42(2):377–381.

Health Level Seven International. Welcome to FHIR. http://hl7.org/fhir/ (accessed August 15, 2022), 2022.

Hirsch AG, Jones JB, Lerch VR, Tang X, Berger A, Clark DN, Stewart WF. The electronic health record audit file: The patient is waiting. J Am Med Inform Assoc. 2017 Apr 1;24(e1):e28–e34.

Hogan WR, Shenkman EA, Robinson T, Carasquillo O, Robinson PS, Essner RZ, Bian J, Lipori G, Harle C, Magoc T, Manini L, Mendoza T, White S, Loiacono A, Hall J, Nelson D. The OneFlorida data trust: A centralized, translational research data infrastructure of statewide scope. J Am Med Inform Assoc. 2021 Oct;19:ocab221.

Hurst JH, Liu Y, Maxson PJ, Permar SR, Boulware LE, Goldstein BA. Development of an electronic health records datamart to support clinical and population health research. J Clin Transl Sci. 2020 Jun 23;5(1):e13.

Johnson AE, Pollard TJ, Shen L, Lehman LW, Feng M, Ghassemi M, Moody B, Szolovits P, Celi LA, Mark RG. MIMIC-III, a freely accessible critical care database. Sci Data. 2016 May 24;3:160035.

Jones RN. Differential item functioning and its relevance to epidemiology. Curr Epidemiol Rep. 2019 Jun 15;6:174–183.

Kaiser P, Pipitone O, Earl A, Miller M. Identifying homelessness from EMRs: standard and custom approaches. Society for Epidemiologic Research Annual Meeting. 2022.

Kline K. SQL in a Nutshell, 3rd Edition. Sebastopol, CA: O'Reilly Media, Inc, 2008.

Knake LA, Ahuja M, McDonald EL, Ryckman KK, Weathers N, Burstain T, Dagle JM, Murray JC, Nadkarni P. Quality of EHR data extractions for studies of preterm birth in a tertiary care center: Guidelines for obtaining reliable data. BMC Pediatr. 2016 Apr 29;16:59.

Lamer A, Abou-Arab O, Bourgeois A, Parrot A, Popoff B, Beuscart JB, Tavernier B, Moussa MD. Transforming anesthesia data into the observational medical outcomes partnership common data model: Development and usability study. J Med Internet Res. 2021 Oct 29;23(10):e29259.

Lin KJ, Schneeweiss S. Considerations for the analysis of longitudinal electronic health records linked to claims data to study the effectiveness and safety of drugs. Clin Pharmacol Ther. 2016 Aug;100(2):147–159.

Linguamatics. Social Determinants of Health (SDoH). https://www.linguamatics.com/solutions/social-determinants-health-sdoh (accessed July 29, 2022), 2022.

Madigan D, Ryan PB, Schuemie M, Stang PE, Overhage JM, Hartzema AG, Suchard MA, DuMouchel W, Berlin JA. Evaluating the impact of database heterogeneity on observational study results. Am J Epidemiol. 2013 Aug 15;178(4):645–651.

Massachusetts Technology Collaborative. MDPHnet. https://mehi.masstech.org/mdphnet (accessed January 20, 2022), 2018.

Mayer DA, Rasmussen LV, Roark CD, Kahn MG, Schilling LM, Wiley LK. ReviewR: a light-weight and extensible tool for manual review of clinical records. JAMIA Open. 2022 Aug 3;5(3):ooac071.

Messer LC, Laraia BA, Kaufman JS, Eyster J, Holzman C, Culhane J, Elo I, Burke JG, O'Campo P. The development of a standardized neighborhood deprivation index. J Urban Health. 2006 Nov;83(6):1041–1062.

Miettinen O. Theoretical Epidemiology. New York, NY: John Wiley & Sons, Inc., 1985.

Mount Sinai Health System. Mount Sinai Launches Large-Scale Genetic Sequencing Project with the Regeneron Genetics Center. https://www.mountsinai.org/about/newsroom/2022/mount-sinai-launches-large-scale-genetic-sequencing-project-with-the-regeneron-genetics-center (accessed November 4, 2022), 2022.

Murphy SN, Weber G, Mendis M, Gainer V, Chueh HC, Churchill S, Kohane I. Serving the enterprise and beyond with informatics for integrating biology and the bedside (i2b2). J Am Med Inform Assoc. 2010 Mar-Apr;17(2):124–130.

National Patient-Centered Clinical Research Network. Data. https://pcornet.org/data/ (accessed January 21, 2022), 2022.

Nutter B, Lane S. redcapAPI: Accessing Data from REDCap Projects Using the API. R Package Version 2.3. 2020. https://github.com/nutterb/redcapAPI/wiki.

Observational Health Data Sciences and Informatics. OMOP Common Data Model. http://www.ohdsi.org/data-standardization/the-common-data-model/ (accessed December 2, 2021), 2021a.

Observational Health Data Sciences and Informatics. Analytic Tools. https://www.ohdsi.org/software-tools/ (accessed December 2, 2021), 2021b.

openEHR Foundation. openEHR Specifications. https://specifications.openehr.org (accessed August 16, 2022), 2022.

Pollard T, Dernoncourt F, Finlayson S, Velasquez A. Data Preparation. In Secondary Analysis of Electronic Health Records. Berlin: Springer, 2016.

Pollard TJ, Johnson AEW, Raffa JD, Celi LA, Mark RG, Badawi O. The eICU collaborative research database, a freely available multi-center database for critical care research. Sci Data. 2018 Sep 11;5:180178.

Premier Applied Sciences. Premier Healthcare Database: Data That Informs and Performs. https://products.premierinc.com/downloads/PremierHealthcareDatabaseWhitepaper.pdf (accessed January 21, 2022), 2020.

Richesson R, Wiley LK, Gold S, Rasmussen L; for the NIH Health Care Systems Research Collaboratory Electronic Health Records Core Working Group. Electronic Health Records–Based Phenotyping: Introduction. In: Rethinking Clinical Trials: A Living Textbook of Pragmatic Clinical Trials. Bethesda, MD: NIH Health Care Systems Research Collaboratory. Available at: https://rethinkingclinicaltrials.org/chapters/conduct/electronic-health-records-based-phenotyping/electronic-health-records-based-phenotyping-introduction/. Updated July 27, 2021 (accessed December 8, 2021).

Schulte F. As coronavirus strikes, crucial data in electronic health records hard to harvest. Kaiser Health News. April 30, 2020. https://khn.org/news/as-coronavirus-strikes-crucial-data-in-electronic-health-records-hard-to-harvest/.

Shortreed SM, Cook AJ, Coley RY, Bobb JF, Nelson JC. Challenges and opportunities for using big health care data to advance medical science and public health. Am J Epidemiol. 2019 May 1;188(5):851–861.

U.S. Department of Veterans Affairs. Computerized Patient Record System (CPRS) User Guide: GUI Version. https://www.va.gov/vdl/documents/Clinical/Comp_Patient_Recrd_Sys_(CPRS)/cprsguium.pdf (accessed December 2, 2021), 2021.

U.S. Food and Drug Administration. Sentinel Common Data Model. https://www.sentinelinitiative.org/methods-data-tools/sentinel-common-data-model (accessed August 15, 2022), 2022.

W3Schools. SQL Tutorial. http://www.w3schools.com/SQl/default.asp (accessed December 2, 2021), 2021.

Walonoski J, Kramer M, Nichols J, Quina A, Moesel C, Hall D, Duffett C, Dube K, Gallagher T, McLachlan S. Synthea: An approach, method, and software mechanism for generating synthetic patients and the synthetic electronic health care record. J Am Med Inform Assoc. 2018 Mar 1;25(3):230–238.

Wolford BN, Willer CJ, Surakka I. Electronic health records: The next wave of complex disease genetics. Hum Mol Genet. 2018 May 1;27(R1):R14–R21.

Yin AL, Guo WL, Sholle ET, Rajan M, Alshak MN, Choi JJ, Goyal P, Jabri A, Li HA, Pinheiro LC, Wehmeyer GT, Weiner M; Weill Cornell COVID-19 Data Abstraction Consortium, Safford MM, Campion TR, Cole CL. Comparing automated vs. manual data collection for COVID-specific medications from electronic health records. Int J Med Inform. 2022 Jan;157:104622.

Zheng K, Hanauer DA, Padman R, Johnson MP, Hussain AA, Ye W, Zhou X, Diamond HS. Handling anticipated exceptions in clinical care: Investigating clinician use of 'exit strategies' in an electronic health records system. J Am Med Inform Assoc. 2011 Nov-Dec;18(6):883–889.

Zhou L, Mahoney LM, Shakurova A, Goss F, Chang FY, Bates DW, Rocha RA. How many medication orders are entered through free-text in EHRs?–A study on hypoglycemic agents. AMIA Annu Symp Proc. 2012;2012:1079–1088.

5   Data Management

This chapter presents some of the most crucial aspects of assembling a research database: data organization, linkage, cleaning, and operationalization. Broadly speaking, this is known as data management or data preprocessing. The data will be organized in a logical fashion and, if necessary, joined with other datasets to create the master repository of variables and observations for EHR research. We then discuss the manipulation of variables, observations, and the final database.

Based on the previous chapter, the beginnings of a research database have taken shape. The source of EHR data was identified, the records abstracted, and then subset into a workable database or dataset. At this stage, research data may exist in a CSV file, in the statistical software, or in a database, although the methods discussed in this chapter will require the use of statistical software or Microsoft Excel (Microsoft Corp., Redmond, WA). At the conclusion of this chapter, the research database will be complete with respect to the available variables and observations, and only require basic data manipulations before beginning the epidemiological analyses.

Data organization

In the research planner, we identified the type of data as being cross-sectional or longitudinal. Cross-sectional data represent a single point or period in time and may contain immutable characteristics of the individual (e.g., date of birth) or a single measure of a characteristic that changes over time (e.g., weight or blood pressure). When we only have a single measure, particularly a single outcome measure, the data are said to be cross-sectional as they represent a cross-section of the patient's health. Many surveys used in public health are cross-sectional in nature. Cross-sectional data are appealing because they are easy to collect and analyze, but they have certain limitations for demonstrating trends over time, particularly as the result of some intervention.

If an EHR contains only single encounters with providers, such as for an acute problem, the patient-level data are cross-sectional. When the study follows patients over time with repeated measurements, the data are said to be longitudinal. By design, longitudinal data will contain multiple measures and therefore can make data organization a challenge, particularly if the type of analysis is unknown

DOI: 10.4324/9781003258872-7

at this stage. Routine preventive health or chronic disease outpatient visits stored in an EHR are one example of longitudinal data. In these examples, a patient has multiple encounters with a provider alongside multiple measurements input to the EHR. An inpatient visit can also generate multiple measurements over time and be considered longitudinal for the duration of the hospitalization. Multiple encounters may be treated cross-sectionally if we ignore the multiple measurements, or on the other hand, longitudinally if the repeated measurements are important to the research question. Note that the data we collect on that patient does not need to be obtained at the same absolute time, such as at a single clinical encounter, but cross-sectional data are analyzed as such.

A fundamental decision needs to be made about the organization of the data: will the data be stored in long or wide format? This question is apropos more so to longitudinal data as cross-sectional data are inherently wide. This distinction will become more apparent after reading the following sections. For all types of data, we assume that a patient represents a single unit of analysis. That is, each patient contributes EHR data to the database and the unit of analysis for statistical inference is the person.

Wide format

When data are stored in *wide* format, each person represents a distinct observation: one row per patient. All the data that this patient has contributed toward the study is stored in distinct variables, and consequently, the more data that was gathered on the patient, the more variables that exist. In other words, the data are wide. Figure 5.1 depicts a simplified database where each observation is a unique person.

In this trivial example, the data are cross-sectional in nature. We do not have multiple measurements for the variables: only a single name, gender, and address are recorded. Let us extend this example to a more real-world application of an

ID	Name	Gender	Address
1	Person #1	F	Address for person #1
2	Person #2	M	Address for person #2
3	Person #3	F	Address for person #3
4	Person #4	M	Address for person #4
5	Person #5	F	Address for person #5
6	Person #6	M	Address for person #6
7	Person #7	M	Address for person #7
8	Person #8	F	Address for person #8
9	Person #9	F	Address for person #9
...			
...			

Figure 5.1 Demographic database with one observation per person.

immunization database that was presented in Chapter 2, where we wish to include individual vaccination events. If we are tracking the number of vaccines received over time, the data become longitudinal, as there are multiple vaccination measurements for each person and there is the potential to capture a newly administered vaccine at each clinical encounter. One possible way of storing these data is to create a new variable for each possible vaccine a person may receive (for simplicity, assume a maximum of two vaccines in this example), along with the corresponding variables that capture the delivery of that vaccine, namely, the date administered. The hypothetical database would be as follows:

Note that we still only have one observation per patient and the data are captured in a wide format, despite this being a longitudinal study. The advantage of organizing the data in wide format is it is intuitive to grasp and relatively simple to analyze. The drawback is we need to anticipate the maximum number of vaccine variables that a patient may need, and the structure may become quite unwieldy for many vaccines. Furthermore, if we wish to analyze the data longitudinally, the data will need to be transformed into a long format first.

As an aside, capturing repeated measurements can be done on a per-encounter basis or all at once. One can conceivably capture all immunizations to date at a single point in time, such as during a patient interview. If this is the case, there are still multiple vaccination events to record but we likely have a better appreciation for the hypothetical maximum number of vaccines an individual could have received if we are storing data in a wide format. Once all of the immunization data have been gathered, we are able to assess the maximum number of immunizations and create the appropriate number of variables to replicate the longitudinal design stored in a wide format (Figure 5.2). Indeed, this is the case when transforming data from long format to wide format.

ID	Name	Gender	Address	Antigen1	Date1	Antigen2	Date2
1	Person #1	F	Address for person #1	MMR	1/1/2016	HepB	1/1/2016
2	Person #2	M	Address for person #2	HepB	3/1/2016	HepB	5/1/2016
3	Person #3	F	Address for person #3	DTaP	6/1/2016	IPV	6/1/2016
4	Person #4	M	Address for person #4	IPV	1/1/2016	MMR	2/1/2016
5	Person #5	F	Address for person #5	MMR	9/1/2016	DTaP	9/1/2016
6	Person #6	M	Address for person #6	HepB	7/1/2016		
7	Person #7	M	Address for person #7	DTaP	3/1/2016	HepB	1/1/2016
8	Person #8	F	Address for person #8	HepB	4/1/2016		
9	Person #9	F	Address for person #9	IPV	12/1/2016	DTaP	12/1/2016
...							
...							

Figure 5.2 Demographic and vaccine-wide database with one observation per person.

If researchers are undertaking retrospective analysis of existing EHR data, the issue of an unknown maximum number of variables is moot. If the researchers are designing a research database that will capture prospective EHR data, the issue of the maximum number of variables must be considered if designing a wide database. For simplicity, unless specifically mentioned in the text, data are assumed to be in wide format.

Long format

Now consider an alternative strategy for organizing the data assuming we do not know the maximum number of vaccines a patient can receive. As such, we will need to create a new record in the database each time a patient receives a vaccine. The data are stored in *long* format. Under this strategy, we will only need a single vaccine antigen variable and a vaccine date administered variable; however, we now need multiple observations per patient (Figure 5.3). As can be seen, some of the data are redundant per observation – gender and address – and some are unique per observation – antigen and date administered. The exact structure can take many possible forms. In this example, the repeating values for the variable "ID" link the data together, in that we know person #1 has had two vaccines: an MMR administered on 1/1/2016 and a HepB administered on the same date. If person #1 had only a single vaccine, such as person #6, she would have only a single row (i.e., observation) in this database.

Transforming from long-to-wide format

Consider the example database in long format presented in Figure 5.3, and the target wide format presented in Figure 5.2. Moving from one vaccination event per observation to multiple vaccination events per observation will require two

ID	Name	Gender	Address	Antigen	Date
1	Person #1	F	Address for person #1	MMR	1/1/2016
1	Person #1	F	Address for person #1	HepB	1/1/2016
2	Person #2	M	Address for person #2	HepB	3/1/2016
2	Person #2	M	Address for person #2	HepB	5/1/2016
3	Person #3	F	Address for person #3	DTaP	6/1/2016
3	Person #3	F	Address for person #3	IPV	6/1/2016
4	Person #4	M	Address for person #4	IPV	1/1/2016
4	Person #4	M	Address for person #4	MMR	2/1/2016
5	Person #5	F	Address for person #5	MMR	9/1/2016
5	Person #5	F	Address for person #5	DTaP	9/1/2016
6	Person #6	M	Address for person #6	HepB	7/1/2016
...					

Figure 5.3 Demographic and vaccine long database with multiple observations per person.

vaccine variables – antigen and date administered – for each vaccine an individual receives, up to the maximum number of vaccines an individual received in the database. We can determine this maximum number from the number of duplicate entries by some person-level identifier, in this case, ID. Suppose, we have determined that individuals can only have received a maximum of two vaccinations. The number of total vaccine variables needed in the wide format will be $2 \times 2 = 4$.

This type of data transformation is a common task included in the core functionality of statistical software. Users of R have access to the "reshape" command included in the base distribution, as well as many packages that provide extended capabilities. Example code and output can be found in Appendix 2 (Code #5.1). Users of SAS should refer to the "transpose" procedure (UCLA: Statistical Consulting Group, 2021a), SPSS refer to the "casestovars" command (UCLA: Statistical Consulting Group, 2021b), and Stata to the "reshape" command (UCLA: Statistical Consulting Group, 2021c). An overview of the long-to-wide transformation algorithm is:

1 Initialize a new wide database with variables for "ID", "Name", "Gender", and "Address".
2 Initialize four vaccine variables: "Antigen1", "Date1", "Antigen2", "Date2".
3 Set an index for number of vaccines to 1, and person to 1.
4 Loop through each observation (1–10).

   a If the person ID has not changed take the vaccine from the current observation and copy it to the appropriate antigen and date variables in the wide database, determined by the vaccine index.
   b Increment the vaccine index.
   c If the person ID has changed, reset the vaccine index, copy the "ID", "Name", "Gender", and "Address" variables to the wide database, and update the person index.

5 Repeat step 4 until all observations have been processed.

Transforming from wide-to-long format is a matter of reversing this operation to collapse multiple variables into a single variable while creating a unique identifier to denote the duplicate observations. Note that this operation creates some additional complexities to ensure that all variables being collapsed share the same data type. Typically, one would want to transform wide-to-long format when undertaking a longitudinal analysis. As before, this common type of data transformation is built into the core functionality of the statistical software.

Data merging

This text makes a didactic difference between merging and linkage. As used herein, *merging* represents the addition of observations to a database (also known as an *append* operation), whereas *linkage* represents the addition of variables to a database. Merging is only needed if there are observations in multiple datasets to be joined to create the research database. If the research database is organized in wide format, it is assumed that all the data to be merged are also in wide format. Similarly, if the research database is organized in long format, it is assumed that all the data to be merged are also in long format.

Merging without linkage occurs when the observations are found in multiple files. This may be the case for a variety of reasons including the EHR export was too long for a single file or patient data are coming from disparate systems that share the same set of variables. If the list of variables is identical, they can be readily joined together, either by a manual copy and paste of the records in the raw datasets or performing a merge or append command within the statistical software. If the list of variables is not identical, placeholder variables can be created in both datasets to align the list. Placeholder variables are variables without data that are created to ensure the list of variables in both datasets to be merged are the same. For example, consider Figure 5.4, where one dataset contains a variable "Address" whereas another contains a variable "Phone." For simplicity, these data are stored in a wide format. To align these two datasets, we will need to create a placeholder variable "Phone" in the top dataset and "Address" in the bottom dataset.

When performing a merge operation, care needs to be taken to ensure a unique identifier is correctly assigned. Otherwise, a byproduct of merging

ID	Name	Gender	Address	Antigen	Date
1	Person #1	F	Address for person #1	MMR	1/1/2016
2	Person #2	M	Address for person #2	HepB	3/1/2016
3	Person #3	F	Address for person #3	DTaP	6/1/2016
4	Person #4	M	Address for person #4	IPV	1/1/2016
5	Person #5	F	Address for person #5	MMR	9/1/2016
...					
...					

+

ID	Name	Gender	Phone	Antigen	Date
11	Person #11	F	(555) 555-5555	HepB	1/1/2016
12	Person #12	M	(555) 555-5555	HepB	5/1/2016
13	Person #13	F	(555) 555-5555	IPV	6/1/2016
14	Person #14	M	(555) 555-5555	MMR	2/1/2016
15	Person #15	F	(555) 555-5555	DTaP	9/1/2016
...					
...					

Figure 5.4 Merging two datasets where the variable lists do not align.

datasets may be the creation of duplicate records or records that convey the same information or have the same unique identifier. If duplicate records exist during analysis, they may cause errors in model estimation or bias the results. In the case of Figure 5.4, prior to the merge operation, we should check to ensure the "ID" variable is unique across the two datasets. If the data in Figure 5.4 were stored in a long format, the duplicate IDs may in fact be necessary to identify multiple vaccinations per patient. Data reconciliation including the handling of duplicate observations is covered in more detail later in the chapter.

Data linkage

Data linkage is paramount in EHR research. The linkage may be needed between outpatient encounters, between inpatient encounters, between inpatient and outpatient encounters or vice versa, between disparate inpatient or outpatient systems, from research cohort to EHR data, from EHR data to non-EHR data such as census data covered later in this chapter, and so on. Data linkage is a complex process and texts have been written exclusively on the subject. Presented here are a few core methods for common scenarios when working with secondary data derived from the EHR. Linkage is only needed if there are multiple datasets to be joined to create the research database, where each dataset contains similar (or identical) observations but with different variables. For simplicity, we also assume the data are in wide format with one row per unique observation. The researcher's comfort level with programming and the availability of identifiers will likely influence the choice of the following methods:

- The same unique identifier is available in all datasets to be joined or can be created in the datasets to be joined. This is known as *exact matching*.
- The same unique identifier is not available in one or more datasets to be joined nor cannot be created. This is known as *fuzzy matching*.

In exact matching, a unique identifier is available that matches a given observation in one dataset to a given observation in another dataset, where both datasets have the same identifier available. To be more precise, the unique identifier will identify the person in the first dataset to be matched to the person in the second dataset and then the variables from the second dataset can be imported to the first dataset. If the data were stored in long format, a unique identifier may have multiple matches between datasets given the redundancy of identifiers to denote more than one observation per patient.

A *unique identifier*, as its name implies, uniquely identifies an observation in the data. Frequently, unique identifiers are sequential or random numbers that have no inherent meaning to them and are coded as a single variable, for example, the "ID" variable in Figure 5.1. In EHRs, commonly used unique identifiers include medical record numbers (MRNs) or social security numbers at the patient-level and financial or visit numbers at the encounter level. Note how a unique identifier at one level – encounter – may be duplicated at

ID	Name	Gender	Address	Name+Gender
n/a	Person #1	F	Address for person #1	Person1-F
n/a	Person #2	M	Address for person #2	Person2-M
n/a	Person #3	F	Address for person #3	Person3-F
n/a	Person #4	M	Address for person #4	Person4-M
n/a	Person #5	F	Address for person #5	Person5-F
n/a	Person #6	M	Address for person #6	Person6-M
n/a	Person #7	M	Address for person #7	Person7-M
n/a	Person #8	F	Address for person #8	Person8-F
n/a	Person #9	F	Address for person #9	Person9-F
...				
...				

Figure 5.5 Creation of a unique identifier for the demographic database.

another level – patient. As discussed in Chapter 3, the unique identifier may include protected health information (Table 3.1), and as such, should be treated carefully.

In the absence of a unique identifier and where data linkage is required, one may be able to create a unique identifier by concatenating other variables. For example, suppose in Figure 5.1 the "ID" variable was absent. Conceivably in this toy database, we can concatenate person name and gender to create a unique identifier (Figure 5.5). This unique identifier of "Name+Gender" does not have an inherent meaning, other than it serves to uniquely identify each person in the database. Given the small number of observations this works well, however, in real applications more thought must be put into this approach.

In a fuzzy matching approach, the same identifier is not available in both datasets nor cannot be readily created. Therefore, we must resort to a best-guess, probabilistic approach to matching records. For example, we may try to match observations by variables corresponding to last name, gender, and date of birth. However, suppose in one of the datasets to be joined the last name contained a misspelling. Perhaps we consider the match to be "close enough," and, therefore, join the data if the spelling was only off by a letter or two. The corollary is that we discard the potential match if it was off by more than a couple of letters. Unfortunately, name changes will fail to match using this approach, so we would need to incorporate additional potential identifiers in the fuzzy matching algorithm. This will be discussed further in the fuzzy match section.

For simplicity, we will assume linking occurs between two and only two data sets at a time in wide format. If there are more than two datasets to be joined, they must be done hierarchically, as shown in Figure 5.6. Depending on the software used to perform the linkage, an arbitrary number of datasets may be able to be joined concurrently. Regardless, the same principles discussed apply. In addition,

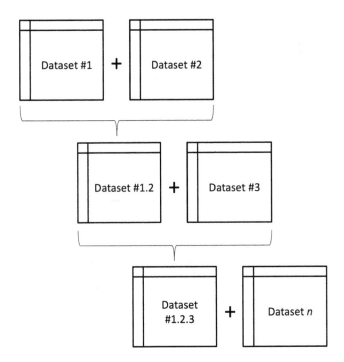

Figure 5.6 A hierarchical approach to linking more than two datasets.

as the data are in wide format, each observation (or person) from one dataset can match at most one observation (or person) from a second dataset. When this assumption does not hold, such as if the data are in long format, the same methods can be expanded upon to iterate over all matches. In all cases and regardless of the linkage type, the data should be spot checked in a manual review to ensure the link operation worked as expected.

Exact matching

Exact matching is a deterministic approach to linking data. There is no ambiguity in the matching identifier and this identifier is unique per observation in the data; at the person-level, this could be their MRN. Suppose we wish to link datasets of vaccination records where the same person appears in both datasets but the vaccine events were recorded separately. Building on top of the example in Figures 5.2 and 5.3, where there were at most two vaccines per individual, one can imagine two separate datasets each with one vaccine (Figure 5.7).

We can then join these datasets together based on the unique "ID" variable, copying the additional variables from the second dataset over to the first dataset. The choice in this case to make the first dataset the primary or *master* database was arbitrary as both datasets contained the same variables. This may not always be

ID	Name	Gender	Address	Antigen	Date
1	*Person #1*	F	*Address for person #1*	MMR	1/1/2016
2	*Person #2*	M	*Address for person #2*	HepB	3/1/2016
3	*Person #3*	F	*Address for person #3*	DTaP	6/1/2016
4	*Person #4*	M	*Address for person #4*	IPV	1/1/2016
5	*Person #5*	F	*Address for person #5*	MMR	9/1/2016
...					
...					

+

ID	Name	Gender	Address	Antigen	Date
1	*Person #1*	F	*Address for person #1*	HepB	1/1/2016
2	*Person #2*	M	*Address for person #2*	HepB	5/1/2016
3	*Person #3*	F	*Address for person #3*	IPV	6/1/2016
4	*Person #4*	M	*Address for person #4*	MMR	2/1/2016
5	*Person #5*	F	*Address for person #5*	DTaP	9/1/2016
...					
...					

Figure 5.7 Two datasets to be linked.

the case, and in general, it is easiest to make the master database the one with the most data, to minimize the burden of copying variables. An outline for the exact match linkage algorithm may look like:

1   In the first dataset, initialize two new variables to store the vaccine and date administered from the second dataset, e.g., "Antigen.2" and "Date.2".
2   For each observation in the first dataset, check if the "ID" occurs in the second dataset.
3   If a match is found, copy the two vaccine variables from the second dataset back to the first.
4   Repeat steps 2–3 until all observations have been checked.

This approach has a key limitation. It considers only potential matches from the first dataset matched to the second. Suppose the first dataset was incomplete and was missing some individuals included in the second dataset. We have two potential options. The easiest approach is to ignore the other additional observations. This makes sense when the first dataset is deemed the master database and we know in advance that any additional observations in the second dataset are irrelevant. The second approach is to append the unmatched observations to the first dataset. This requires a slight modification to the proposed linkage algorithm to incorporate a merge operation, as follows:

1 In the first dataset, initialize two new variables to store the vaccine and date administered from the second dataset, e.g., "Antigen.2" and "Date.2".
2 In the second dataset, initialize a new variable that records whether this record was matched into the first dataset, e.g., "Match" and set all values to false.
3 For each observation in the first dataset, check if the "ID" occurs in the second dataset.
4 If a match is found, copy the two vaccine variables from the second dataset back to the first and set the "Match" variable in the second dataset to true.
5 Repeat steps 2-3 until all observations have been checked.
6 Copy any observations from the second dataset where the "Match" variable equals false to the first dataset.
7 Check for and remove duplicate observations.

For users of R, see Appendix 2 for example code and output using an integrated merge function to perform the linkage (Code #5.2), and for example code demonstrating a manual implementation of the modified linkage algorithm (Code #5.3).

To complicate this approach a bit further, suppose "ID" did not exist, as in Figure 5.5, and therefore we need to create a unique identifier. There are many potential options, even for a small number of variables. For example, a dataset with four variables (e.g., first name, last name, gender, and date of birth) will have 15 possible combinations of variables. This can be calculated as the number of combinations choosing one variable + the number of combinations choosing two variables + the number of combinations choosing three variables + the number of combinations choosing four variables = 4 + 6 + 4 + 1 = 15, as shown in Table 5.1.

Some of these combinations can be immediately discarded (first name alone, first name + gender) but others are not as clear (last name + gender + date of birth versus first name + last name + gender + date of birth) therefore the process of unique identifier creation is both an art and a science. In general, one would want to avoid using variables that may change over time, such as names or addresses. Date of birth is an excellent candidate combined with another feature that rarely would change, such as gender. It is important to note that the unique identifiers described herein are for data linkage; in operationalizing a unique identifier in the research database one would not want to include personally identifiable details in such an identifier, such as a patient's date of birth or social security number. This ensures that the data can be anonymized while preserving the unique identifier. This was discussed further in Chapter 3.

When concatenating variables, text standardization should be employed including adjusting the case (all UPPERCASE or lowercase) and removing non-alphanumeric characters (e.g., hyphens or apostrophes in names). After the new identifier is created, checking for duplicates can assess its uniqueness. In addition,

Table 5.1 Possible combinations of four variables (first name, last name, gender, and date of birth) to create a unique identifier

Option number	Number of variables concatenated	Resulting combination
1	1	First name
2	1	Last name
3	1	Gender
4	1	Date of birth
5	2	First name + Last name
6	2	First name + Gender
7	2	First name + Date of birth
8	2	Last name + Gender
9	2	Last name + Date of birth
10	2	Gender + Date of birth
11	3	First name + Last name + Gender
12	3	First name + Last name + Date of birth
13	3	First name + Gender + Date of birth
14	3	Last name + Gender + Date of birth
15	4	First name + Last name + Gender + Date of birth

Note that some of these combinations are unreasonable for a unique identifier.

the use of the entire variable may not be necessary; only the first few letters from the first and last names may be sufficient to avoid duplicates.

Fuzzy matching

When the uniqueness of an identifier cannot be assured and exact matching is not plausible, fuzzy matching is needed to link the datasets. Fuzzy matching is a probabilistic operation meaning that candidate matches are given a probability of being "correct" controlled by a threshold value to adjust the level of certainty required. Suppose a threshold of 80% certainty is needed for a match to be deemed correct. If the candidate match resulted in a score of 79% or lower, the observations would not be linked together, whereas a score of 80% or higher would result in the observations being linked.

Suppose we are building a proposed unique identifier using last name + gender + date of birth and we wish to perform a fuzzy match against a second dataset with the same variable concatenation. If the variables match exactly, then a link operation is obvious and exact matching can occur. However, if there were a misspelling of the last name or a typo in the date of birth, the match would fail in the exact match paradigm, therefore we need to allow some ambiguity to the matching. In lieu of a percentage of certainty approach, we may wish to say that if the misspelling is two characters or less, or the date of birth varies by a single digit, the match is correct, and therefore a link operation can be performed.

One implementation of this strategy uses the *Levenshtein* distance measure, which defines the number of character changes between two strings (Wang et al. 2005). Continuing with the previous example, a Levenshtein distance less than three would indicate a match on last name and a distance less than two would indicate a match on date of birth. Last name and date of birth are treated separately in this example, as a distance less than four for the entire concatenated identifier would not be equivalent, because the three-character change could occur in last name or date of birth alone. Example code for creation of a unique identifier and a fuzzy matching approach using the Levenshtein distance can be found in Appendix 2 (Code #5.4).

Fuzzy matching algorithms can be challenging to understand, complex to implement, and time-consuming (expensive) to run on large EHR-derived datasets. If the researcher lacks the expertise or time to program his or her own matching solution, there are many options available in the public domain. Table 5.2 is a summary and comparison of select fuzzy matching software.

Table 5.2 A comparison of select fuzzy matching software

Software	API	GUI	Linkage	Deduplication	Supervised learning	Unsupervised learning	Active learning
Atyimo[a]	PySpark	N	Y	Y	N	N	N
Dedupe[b]	Python	N	Y	Y	Y	N	Y
fastLink[c]	R	N	T	?	N	Y	N
FEBRL[d]	Python	Y	Y	Y	N	N	N
FRIL[e]	Java	Y	Y	N	?	Y	N
FuzzyMatcher[f]	Python	N	Y	N	N	Y	N
JedAI[g]	Java	Y	Y	?	Y	?	?
PRIL[h]	SQL	N	Y	?	?	?	?
Python Record Linkage Toolkit[i]	Python	N	Y	Y	Y	Y	N
RecordLinkage (R)[j]	R	N	Y	Y	Y	Y	N
RELAIS[k]	N	Y	Y	?	?	Y	N
ReMaDDer[l]	N	Y	Y	Y	N	Y	N
Splink[m]	PySpark	N	Y	Y	N	Y	N
The Link King[n]	N	Y	Y	Y	?	Y	N

API application programming interface, *GUI* graphical user interface

This table is reprinted from https://github.com/J535D165/data-matching-software (by Jonathan de Bruin) under the CC-BY-SA 3.0 license. No claim is made about the accuracy of the contents.

Notes:
a   https://github.com/pierrepita/atyimo
b   https://github.com/dedupeio/dedupe
c   https://cran.r-project.org/web/packages/fastLink/index.html
d   https://sourceforge.net/projects/febrl/
e   http://fril.sourceforge.net/
f   https://pypi.python.org/pypi/fuzzymatcher
g   http://jedai.scify.org/
h   https://github.com/LSHTM-ALPHAnetwork/PIRL_RecordLinkageSoftware
i   https://github.com/J535D165/recordlinkage
j   https://cran.r-project.org/web/packages/RecordLinkage/index.html
k   https://www.istat.it/en/methods-and-tools/methods-and-it-tools/process/processing-tools/relais
l   http://remadder.findmysoft.com/
m   https://github.com/moj-analytical-services/splink
n   http://www.the-link-king.com/

Linking census data

The notion of linking census data to EHR data using patients' addresses was introduced in Chapter 4. Herein, we will discuss the process specific to the United States and in Chapter 6, we will discuss the limitations and potential complications of this linkage.

The first thing one needs to understand about census data is how the geography is defined. Census estimates are produced for various geographical units that are interrelated in a hierarchy (Figure 5.8). The smallest census unit is known as a block. This forms the basis for all estimates and other geographic units that arise from census surveys. All areas of the United States can ultimately be broken down into these blocks, and likewise, all larger geographic types are aggregates of individual blocks. As such, census geographies can be readily transformed between units using predefined relationship files.[1] Yet one does not always need to start at the block level; census data can be retrieved for a variety of the levels seen in Figure 5.8.

The question of which geographic unit to consider is an important one for both statistical and causal inference. From a statistical standpoint, selecting a unit that is too small will translate to less power to detect statistical differences in areas, especially for nested multilevel data. From a causal inference standpoint,

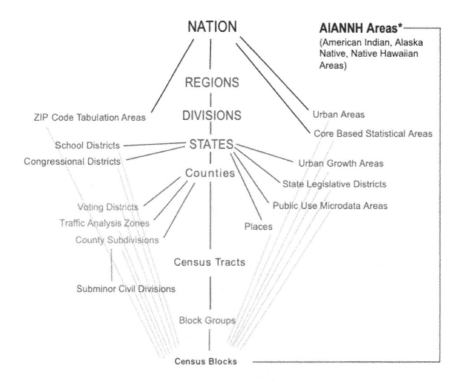

Figure 5.8 Standard hierarchy of US Census Bureau geographic entities.

one needs to be aware of what census geographies represent. For example, census blocks are defined based on "visible features, such as streets, roads, streams, and railroad tracks, and by nonvisible boundaries, such as selected property lines and city, township, school district, and county limits and short line-of-sight extensions of streets and roads" (Rossiter, 2011). This definition will not necessarily apply to how people live, work, eat, socialize, play, and so on, important factors in public health. Therefore, it may be necessary to transform contextual units into ones that are more appropriate for inference.

To obtain census data, researchers can use automated tools, if available, within the statistical software, such as *tidycensus* in R (Walker, 2020), or manually download data from https://data.census.gov. There are myriad censuses and surveys conducted by or on behalf of the US Census Bureau; a comprehensive list of surveys can be found here.[2] Below are four surveys that are of particular importance to public health:

- **American Community Survey (ACS)**. This is an annually updated cross-sectional survey at the community level, intended to focus on the changing dynamics within a given area. Community statistics can be obtained for a single-year or multi-year (3- or 5-year) periods. Single-year estimates are available from 2005 on, and 5-year estimates started in 2010.
- **American Housing Survey**. Although the ACS includes some information about housing, the American Housing Survey is a more comprehensive look at a wide range of housing subjects. Its longitudinal design allows the researcher to track trends and changes within the same group of respondents.
- **Decennial Census**. This once every ten-year census primarily serves for measuring population size and growth for the purposes of redistricting – altering, adding, or removing geopolitical boundaries – based upon population change. The decennial census includes abundant data on sociodemographic and economic characteristics of an area.
- **Population Estimates**. This survey is particularly useful for obtaining the "denominator" data for various epidemiological measures of health, including measures of births, deaths, and migration by age, sex, race, and Hispanic origin. While population denominator data can be found in the ACS, it is the Population Estimates program that yields the official estimates.

Once census data are identified the linkage can commence. There are several approaches for data linkage: the approach presented here is based on the census geographic identifiers (GEOIDs).[3] Census data will always include a GEOID regardless of the geography. These GEOIDs follow a similar hierarchy to Figure 5.8; each smaller unit of geography is concatenated with the larger unit of geography to form the ID. GEOIDs also include a human-readable representation of the geography. For example, suppose we wish to identify a specific census tract (#2231) in Harris County, Texas. Texas is represented by the two-digit code "48" and Harris County by the three-digit code "201." Thus GEOID "482012231" is census tract #2231 in Harris County, Texas. A full listing of GEOIDs is available here.[4]

Further suppose that we wish to link EHR data on patients' addresses to census data. From a typical address in the United States we can perform an exact match on state or ZIP code[5]; one would just need to download the census data at the correct geography to allow this data linkage. On the other hand, a typical address in the EHR will not include geographies such as census tract or county. To link at these other geographic levels, the address data must first be geocoded.

Geocoding is the process of obtaining the latitude and longitude of a given address. There are a variety of geocoding solutions available, from commercial software such as ArcGIS (Esri, Redlands, CA) to publicly available geocoders, including the US Census Bureau.[6] Geocoding address data from the EHR must be done in such a manner as to protect the patient's privacy, since address data are protected health information. After geocoding, the latitude and longitude can be mapped into the appropriate census geography, and then linked using an exact match to the census data. A full treatment of geocoding is outside the scope of this text; users of R are referred to these two articles which provide an overview of geocoding and linking addresses to census data at various geographies (Goldstein, 2015; Goldstein, Auchincloss & Lee, 2014). As mentioned at the start of this section, there are many assumptions and challenges in working with geographic data. The most relevant ones for EHR research are discussed in Chapter 6. A review of challenges in working with geospatial data may be found in Delmelle et al. (2022).

Manipulating variables

Assigning data types

Up until this point, variables have been regarded as generic, nonspecific types. *Data types* allow specific operations on variables that otherwise would be cumbersome or impossible. For example, it is not possible to add two "strings" together; that is an operation reserved for numbers. Likewise, software cannot calculate how many calendar days have elapsed between two numbers; that is an operation reserved for dates. When operationalizing variables, having the correct data type helps to ensure valid analysis.

For our purposes, there are only a few core data types that are pertinent to EHR research: (1) text strings, (2) numbers, (3) dates, and (4) coded categories. Text strings are the least restrictive data type and can be used to capture free text (introduced in Chapter 4) or other clinical documentation that is not intended for data analysis but exists rather for descriptive purposes. If the data stored in a text string are needed for analysis, they must be parsed, such as through natural language processing (discussed in Chapter 12). Numbers, on the other hand, are computer-interpretable and may represent decimal values, such as reported in many laboratory test results, or whole numbers, such as integers representing weight in kilograms. Dates, as the name implies, are computer-interpretable calendar dates, useful for when examining trends over time or conducting before and after analyses. Finally, coded categories represent discrete text or numeric data

ID	Name	Gender	Address	Antigen	Date	Dose #
1	Person #1	F	Address for person #1	MMR	1/1/2016	1
2	Person #2	M	Address for person #2	HepB	3/1/2016	2
3	Person #3	F	Address for person #3	DTaP	6/1/2016	4
4	Person #4	M	Address for person #4	IPV	1/1/2016	1
5	Person #5	F	Address for person #5	MMR	9/1/2016	2
...						
...						

Figure 5.9 A hypothetical research database.

that have only a limited number of possible values, and therefore tend to repeat many times in a database. For example, a race/ethnicity variable with possible values of non-Hispanic Caucasian, non-Hispanic African American, non-Hispanic Asian, Hispanic Caucasian, Hispanic African American, Hispanic Asian would be considered a coded category/categorical variable with six options.

If the data imported to the research database originated from a CSV file, then the variables are most likely encoded as text strings or possibly numeric types. If the data were imported from another type of interface, the data type may have been preserved in the original export operation. Loading the data into your preferred statistical software will facilitate checking the variable data types to ensure data integrity. For example, Figure 5.9 depicts a small database that has some of the most common types of variables: "Name," "Gender," "Address," and "Antigen" are all character or text strings; "Date" is a calendar date; and "Dose #" and "ID" are numeric integers as they represent whole numbers.

Before assigning data types, we must ensure that all data stored in each variable conform to the data type requirements, otherwise, during the *casting* process of assigning the data types, the method may fail or corrupt the data. For data that are categorical and have only a limited number of values, the use of frequency tables allows for a manual inspection of all values encountered in the dataset. Frequency tables on variables such as "Gender," "Antigen," or "Dose" will quickly identify observations that do not conform to a specific data type.

Continuing with this example, suppose the researcher identified an observation that had the dose number variable recorded as the letter "A". This clearly represents an error in transcription or translation and will cause a numeric casting operation to fail. Each observation that has an erroneous value must be corrected, perhaps by deleting that data point or, if possible, updating it with the correct value. For variables that have many potential values, including person name, address, or date, frequency tables may prove less useful. In such instances, one can assign a data type and observe if any error occurs.

Once all data in the variables conform to the proposed data types, the casting operation can proceed: calendar dates as *date* variables, numbers as *numeric* variables, text as *string* variables, and so on. When in doubt, leave the variable in a string data type, as casting to a specific data type that is inappropriate may result in data corruption. Furthermore, always cast existing variables into new variables rather than overwriting the existing variable, thereby preserving the original data. Example R code for casting variable data types can be found in Appendix 2 (Code #5.5).

Regardless of the data type, some variables will contain categorical data, or data that represent distinct concepts. Assigning these variables as "categorical" has several benefits. First, it ensures data integrity as only the predetermined categories are allowed, and second, it ensures valid statistical inference, as certain variables need to be recognized as categories for proper analysis. Depending on the software, the assignment of data types and categories can be done within the graphical user interface or command line.

Renaming and recoding variables

When working with secondary data abstracted from the EHR, the variables are rarely in the desired format or adhere to preferred naming conventions. As such, recoding of variables is one of the most common variable-level operations performed. The primary purpose of recoding variables is to standardize their interpretation for proper analysis, and a side benefit to clearly coded and named variables is that new users will be easily assimilated to your research database.

Each researcher has his or her preferred method for naming variables: some appreciate short concise variable names while others advocate for longer descriptive names. At one point this decision was largely dictated by the architecture of the statistical software, as eight characters may have been the maximum number for a variable name. This has largely disappeared as a software limitation, now allowing much more descriptive variable names. In general, the more descriptive the variable name, the easier it will be to avoid ambiguity and assimilate new users. On the other hand, longer variable names mean less efficient coding.

Consider the variable names in Figure 5.9: "ID," "Name," "Gender," "Address," "Antigen," "Date," and "Dose #." While these are relatively clear for this contrived example, if there were hundreds or thousands of variables, these names would become less obvious and useful. Further, the use of the "#" sign in "Dose #" may not be allowed in certain statistical software, and therefore should be renamed. One way of ensuring unique variable names that are readily identified is by prefixing the variable name with the source of that variable. Assume "Name," "Gender," and "Address" came from the **Demographic** table and "Antigen," "Date" and "Dose #" from the **Immunization** table. More descriptive names would be "Demographic_name," "Demographic_gender," "Demographic_address," "Immunization_antigen," "Immunization_date," and "Immunization_dose_num." To further clarify the type of the variables, a suffix can also be applied to indicate special data types or re-codes, for example "Immunization_antigen_category," if we choose to enforce that only certain preselected antigens are allowed. Changing variable names is a nondestructive process and therefore does not necessitate creating a new variable with the improved name. The original name can be safely modified without fear of losing data, although some prefer to always keep the original variable as-is.

Recoding variables can take many forms, from correcting misspellings in existing data to combining many variables into one[7] (or vice versa), but regardless of the reason, recoding is generally done for improved clarity and interpretation, or for a specific analytic goal. As the focus of the present chapter is on the research database, we will revisit recoding for analysis later in the book. Therefore, the goal of recoding variables for the research database is primarily for clarity and interpretation. Table 5.3 depicts several common scenarios and examples that warrant variable recoding.

Many recoding operations use logic statements, such as if-then-else, with Boolean comparisons (and, or, not). Depending on the statistical software, variable recoding may require hand-written code as opposed to selecting from a menu-driven interface. As before, the original variable should not be overwritten, but rather a new variable created. Appendix 2 (Code #5.6) provides a sample R code necessary to remedy the nine examples from Table 5.3.

Removing variables

Variables should generally not be removed from the research database. If the recoding operation contained an error, it will be useful to have the original data available. Pruning of the database, including omission of superfluous variables will be covered later in the book during creation of the analytic datasets.

Manipulating observations

A consequence of working with complex data sources, such as EHRs, as well as a potential byproduct of data linkage and merge operations is the need to reconcile data. Such data reconciliation may include splitting observations, removing duplicate observations, managing the record identifiers, verifying data accuracy, and so on. In short, observations may require manipulation when importing to the research database or subsetting to create the analytic dataset.

Splitting observations

As presented when reshaping the data from long-to-wide format, multiple observations were collapsed into a single observation with additional variables. It may be necessary to create new observations in the reverse case. For example, suppose the research database was derived from an obstetrical EHR, and multiple gestation offspring (i.e., twins, triplets, etc.) are stored in a single delivery record for the mother. Analyses of these data may want to consider the children as separate, distinct observations with a linking variable identifying them as siblings. This is a special case of splitting a single record into multiple records.

Table 5.3 Common examples of variables requiring recoding

Scenario	Description and example	Remedy
1. Lack of consistency within a single variable	Gender variable has some data coded as M and F and some data coded as Male and Female.	Select preferred coding & merge values together (M or Male, and F or Female).
2. Lack of consistency within multiple variables	Dichotomous Yes/No variables coded as 0 and 1 representing No and Yes respectively, while other variables coded as 1 and 2 representing No and Yes respectively.	Select single paradigm for coding variables consistently.
3. Lack of categorical paradigm	Some variables that represent categories may be coded as the value itself (marital status where possible values are Married, Not Married) while other variables contain a numeric representation of the value (employment status where 0 = Unemployed, 1 = Employed).	Select paradigm for coding variables consistently.
4. Standardization of units	Variables may be represented using English measures (body weight in pounds), but desired in Metric measures (body weight in kilograms).	Convert all units to a specific system.
5. Separation of categories into multiple variables	Variable may have too many (or inappropriate) categories to be represented by a single variable (a race/ethnicity variable with possible values of non-Hispanic Caucasian, non-Hispanic African American, non-Hispanic Asian, Hispanic Caucasian, Hispanic African American, Hispanic Asian).	Separate into multiple variables each with fewer potential categories (separate race variable for Caucasian, African American, Asian, and separate ethnicity variable for Hispanic, not Hispanic).
6. Collapsing categories within a single variable	Variable contains too many categories (an education variable with possible values grade school or below, middle school, high school no diploma, high school diploma or equivalent, college without degree, associate's degree, bachelor's degree, master's degree, doctoral degree).	Collapse into a single variable (no high school diploma, some college no degree and high school diploma or equivalent, college degree or higher).
7. Collapsing categories within multiple variables	Variable categories are presented in multiple variables (separate Yes/No variables for residency in the Northeast, South, Midwest, West).	Collapse into a single variable (a single variable with possible values Northeast, South, Midwest, West).
8. Performing calculations	Creation of a variable based on an equation (calculating body mass index from separate variables recording weight and height) or adjusting a variable for normality (to resemble a normal distribution).	Calculate and store in new variable.
9. Parsing coded data from free text	Variable contains free text and coded data (a medication variable with a list of dispensed medications with their signature and provider).	Search for occurrence of specific words or phrases in text and create appropriate indicator variables or utilize natural language processing.

In the case of twins, we will need two observations per birth, for triplets, three observations per birth, and so on. An outline for this multiple gestation splitting algorithm may look like:

1 Copy the observation to be split to a temporary location 'n' times, where 'n' is the number of new records that should be created.
2 Create a unique linking variable tying the 'n' new observations together.
3 Merge the 'n' new observations back to the original database. The original database may need a new variable corresponding to the linking variable if one does not already exist.
4 Drop the original observation.

An implementation of this algorithm using R is provided in Appendix 2 (Code#5.7). The algorithm in the appendix has assumed that the records in need of splitting have been previously identified, and exactly two records are needed per split (i.e., twins). These assumptions can be easily altered in the code.

Duplicate observations

Occasionally, as a byproduct of the EHR export or a consequence of data merging and linking, duplicate observations will occur in the research database. As used herein, duplicate observations mean that entire records – all variables – are identical. This is contrary to a situation where only the *identifiers* are duplicated, but the observations convey different information contained in the variables, as would be the case if the data are longitudinal and stored in long format. Should analysis occur on a dataset with duplicate records that are unaccounted for, the variance will be artificially inflated due to correlation between the duplicate records; as such, the duplicates need to be identified and removed.

The first step in dealing with unwanted redundancy is identifying the duplicate records. Identifying duplicate observations may be straightforward if a unique identifier is available, or quite complex if fuzzy matching is required. Many of the same considerations presented in the data linkage section apply here. In fact, identifying duplicates is similar to identifying matching records in multiple datasets, the difference being the matched records exist in a single dataset: the research database. If a unique identifier is present or can be constructed, the duplicate records can be readily identified, one or more of the other variables can be assessed for uniqueness to ensure a true duplicate, and the duplicate observations flagged for deletion or otherwise separated from the database. On the other hand, if a unique identifier is not available nor cannot be constructed, then a fuzzy matching approach is needed to identify the potential duplicate observations. If the researcher is proficient at writing code, the fuzzy matching algorithm from earlier can be readily modified to detect duplicates (see Appendix 2, Code #5.8). Many of the fuzzy matching algorithms presented in Table 5.2 can also perform record deduplication.

After the potential duplicates have been identified, they should be verified before removal. Manually inspecting the duplicates can ensure the algorithm worked as intended while also ensuring that the *entire* record is a duplicate, as opposed to only the identifiers being the same. If there were only a few duplicates detected, it would be prudent to manually inspect all of them. If there were many duplicates detected, a random sample – say 10% – can be selected for manual inspection. If no systematic errors are believed to have occurred, the redundant observations can be removed from the database, leaving only a single observation.

The choice of which redundant observations to remove is most likely an arbitrary choice. However, if the observations are date and time-stamped, then the oldest observation should be preserved as the newer one(s) created the redundancy, unless the new record contains updated data. Again, checking the entire observation instead of just the unique identifier can circumvent this occurrence. There may also be implications for failed data linkages in a relational database if observations are removed. Thus some researchers simply chose to flag observations as duplicates and not remove them until the creation of the analytic dataset. Indeed, this is the approach outlined in Appendix 2, Code #5.8. When removing duplicate records, it is customary to disclose upon research dissemination that duplicate observations were removed along with a brief description of the criteria applied.

Manipulating the database

The preceding sections have dealt with data management operations at the micro-level, including manipulating variables and observations. We conclude the chapter with macro-level data management approaches, including the consideration of unique identifiers, the identification of missing data, and the creation of a data dictionary and audit log. Finally, we will revisit some of the software solutions presented in earlier chapters, namely Microsoft Excel (Microsoft Corporation, Redmond, WA) and REDCap (Vanderbilt University, Nashville, TN), and discuss how these can be used to streamline the data management process.

Unique identifiers

The concept of a unique identifier has been introduced several times in the book, in Chapters 2 and 3, as well as earlier in this chapter. The main impetus of the unique identifier thus far has been specific to identifying source data and linking datasets. After the datasets have been merged or imported into the research database, we now need to consider a new unique identifier that will carry forward in the research database for all subsequent work. Even if the imported data have a unique identifier, such as the patient's MRN, creating a new identifier at this stage is still important to ensure absolute uniqueness among all observations. After all, an MRN could inadvertently be duplicated if the research database comprises multiple EHRs or through accidental data redundancy in a single institution EHR. This is especially true in the United States given the lack of a standardized patient identifier across healthcare systems, which has proved to be controversial (Sood et al., 2018). For our purposes, in the worst case, we have added a redundant variable into the research database. Further, an identifier may be considered protected health information (PHI; see Table 3.1 in Chapter 3) and require removal during data sharing or as dictated by the IRB, whereas a new arbitrary identifier will not be subject to removal.

The simplest unique identifier is an automatically incrementing integer that corresponds to the number of records in the database. For example, a research database with 10,000 observations could have a variable called "ID" with values from 1 to 10,000. There are any number of permutations that can be applied. For example, to ensure a consistent length of the identifier, we can pad the identifier with leading zeros: 00001, 00002, 00003, to 10,000. Or we may wish to prefix the identifier with the source of the data, for example, if the data were abstracted from an obstetrical EHR: OB00001, OB00002, OB00003, to OB10000. We can even capture multiple details in the identifier such as the source EHR and year of data abstract: OB2022_00001, OB2022_00002, OB2022_00003, to OB2022_10000. Finally, we can consider a random assignment of unique identifiers, although this requires tracking all assigned identifiers to ensure we do not, by chance alone, assign duplicates: XY12378, PL48198, QM12310, and so on.

After creating the new identifier, the original identifier should be preserved to allow the identification in the original EHR. This may be needed to retrieve additional data from the EHR, perform a manual chart review or audit of the data, or for study reproducibility purposes. As mentioned in Chapter 3, any identifier that is considered PHI should reside external to the research database, preferably with the data manager, to ensure compliance with HIPAA and IRB requirements. To do this, we can create a separate *crosswalk* spreadsheet for unique identifier matching. This spreadsheet contains a minimum of two columns (Table 5.4). The first column, "ID" in this example, is the new unique identifier that was generated as part of the research database. The second column, "MRN", is the original unique identifier that allows the record to be cross-referenced to the original secondary data. Additional columns can be created that capture other PHI as needed. To de-identify the research database, the original EHR identifier as well as additional PHI (see Table 3.1 in Chapter 3) are removed from the research database. Should the need arise to re-connect the de-identified data to the identifiable attributes, the research database identifier is crosswalked to the EHR identifier.

Table 5.4 An example ID crosswalk spreadsheet

ID	MRN	Other PHI
00001	90001001	Person name, DOB, address, etc.
00002	90001232	Person name, DOB, address, etc.
00003	90003521	Person name, DOB, address, etc.
…	…	…
10000	90123899	Person name, DOB, address, etc.

Every time the research database is updated with new data, the unique identifier must either be regenerated or preserved. Regenerating the unique identifier is straightforward but will limit the ability to track changes between datasets. Rather, the preferred approach may be to preserve the unique identifier, especially if the data are to be used longitudinally to track changes over time for the same patient. To accomplish this, we can rely on the ID crosswalk spreadsheet. After the new research database is created, the old ID crosswalk spreadsheet is checked to inherit the previous unique identifier to the current database. If records are deleted from the research database and additional (new) records are added, the unique identifier from the deleted records should not be reused. This again demonstrates the utility of the crosswalk spreadsheet that can be used to track every identifier assigned to the research database to ensure its uniqueness. As such, the crosswalk spreadsheet also serves as a running log of all entries into the research database, regardless of their final disposition. If the crosswalk spreadsheet sounds similar to the EHR's *master patient index*, they indeed serve a similar purpose: to uniquely identify patients across the enterprise with a single identifier (Carine & Parrent, 1999).

Missing data

Missing data is a complex topic that is covered in multiple places in the book. Chapter 6 discusses EHR-specific concerns about missing data, Chapter 9 focuses on how missing data may compromise study validity, and Chapter 10 presents analytic methods for handling missing data such as imputation. This section serves as a general overview of missing data in the research database and how this is handled operationally.

Depending on the database technology or statistical software in use, the actual encoding of missing data will vary. Missing data may be represented as an empty string (strings of zero length), NULL values, or via a specific missing data indicator. For example, in R it is customary to see *NA* denoting missing data, while in SAS and SPSS, a period is used. To correctly denote a data point as missing requires knowledge of what constitutes a missing value in the source data, including the EHR. As the EHR is built upon a relational database, a missing value may carry over as the representation inherent in the database technology (NULL value or empty string) or reporting software used. Given the breadth of possibilities, an exhaustive list is not possible; manually inspecting the data before import should reveal possible missing data values. Occasionally, filler values such as a "−1" or "99" are also used to denote missing data or nonresponses. Missing data may also be coded inconsistently in the source data, including combinations of any of the aforementioned missing data indicators. If the researcher has access to a codebook or data dictionary from the original data, that may reveal the missing value encoding scheme, otherwise, it may come down to a best-guess via inspection of the data.

Not all nonresponses should necessarily be coded as missing data. For example, if a question has possible responses including "Decline to answer" (e.g., coded as

Smoking history: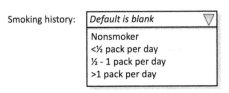

Figure 5.10 Blank entry allowable for a selection in a hypothetical EHR.

an 88), "Do not know/unsure" (e.g., coded as a 99), and the option to omit a response altogether, these three responses may all indicate unique characteristics of the respondent. Perhaps only the omitted response should be coded as a missing value and the 88 and 99 values preserved in the database. In the analytic phase, the researcher can then determine response patterns in the data and make an appropriate determination whether 88 and 99 should be analyzed separately, merged and analyzed together, or recoded as missing data.

In general, data abstracted from an EHR will have blank or NULL values that indicate missing data as opposed to filler values. However, dropdown selectors and default values that appear in some EHR user interfaces can be problematic under this assumption. Suppose a question in the EHR captured smoking history with the possible responses: no response (default selection), nonsmoker, <½ pack per day, ½ − 1 pack per day, >1 pack per day (Figure 5.10). A blank value may suggest the question was skipped or, in the interest of expedient clinical workflow, the patient was a nonsmoker, but the corresponding dropdown value was not selected.

There are three ways forward and all options are less than ideal: (1) discard this variable, (2) replace all blank values with missing data indicators, or (3) assume that a blank response is in fact a nonsmoker response. The first option may result in residual confounding or selection bias. The third option may result in information bias, unless the researcher has access to the clinicians obtaining the patients' histories and can confidently assert that a blank response is equivalent to a nonsmoker. Short of this, the best practice may be leaving all blank values as missing data in the research database and performing a quantitative bias analysis discussed in Chapter 9.

Data dictionary and audit log

The *data dictionary* (sometimes called a *codebook*) enumerates each variable in the research database along with a brief description, defines the data type and categorical variable values, and optionally, includes some descriptive variable statistics including ranges (for continuous variables), frequencies (for categorical variables), and missingness. The data dictionary should be formatted appropriately for hard copy printing and PDF creation, indicate a last updated date, and include the data owner and manager along with the IRB approval number, if applicable. It should also include a revision number that matches the version of

Immunization research data dictionary   **Created/owned by:**

Variable	Type	Values	Missing	Comment
ID	Numeric	1...1,000	n = 0 (0%)	Unique identifier
Name	Text	--	n = 20 (2%)	Person's full name
Gender	Categorical	F = Female M = Male	n = 10 (1%)	Person's gender
Address	Text	--	n = 100 (10%)	Person's mailing address
Antigen	Categorical	MMR HepB DTaP IPV	n = 0 (0%)	Antigens: MMR (Measles, Mumps, Rubella), HepB (Hepatitis B), DTaP (Diphtheria, Tetanus, acellular Pertussis), IPV (inactivated Polio vaccine)
Dose #	Numeric	1...5	n = 0 (0%)	Dose number for multidose vaccines

Last updated: September 1, 2022   *IRB Approval: 1001-2021*   *Revision: 1.0*

Figure 5.11 An example data dictionary.

the research database. This implies that any updates to the research database will correspondingly generate a revised dictionary, even if just updating the version number for consistency. Figure 5.11 depicts a data dictionary representing the hypothetical research database depicted in Figure 5.9.

An *audit log* is used to track each time a copy of the research database – or its derivative analytic datasets – is provided to a researcher. The data manager should own and update the document, and an audit log should be created even if the IRB does not require one. The audit log need not be sophisticated; a simple table will suffice (Table 5.5).

Data management software

Many of the considerations raised in this chapter can be automated and ameliorated using data management software. For a research database constructed in REDCap, the project designer allows the organization of data in wide versus long format, depending on the type of EHR research study. REDCap projects are relational in nature, thereby performing data linkage across various instruments automatically through internal identifiers obviating the need for researcher-required linkages. The instrument designer controls the data types; the variable naming convention; validation checks to ensure dates, numbers, or

Table 5.5 An example audit log

Date	Recipient & contact	Observations	Variables	Format	Intended use
1/1/2022	Person A, Address, Phone, Email	All	All, minus protected health information	R	Infant outcomes study
6/1/2022	Person B, Address, Phone, Email	Data from 2010+	All, minus protected health information	SPSS	Staff forecasting
12/1/2022	Person C, Address, Phone, Email	Data between 2010–2020	Requested variables: A, B, C, D, E, etc.	CSV file	Pre/post hand hygiene intervention study

other values fall within some prespecified range; required data points; protected health information flags; as well as automated calculations based on other data points, such as body mass index. Taking advantage of these options can minimize missing data, standardize data entry, automate and ensure unique identifiers, and avoid duplicate data entry. Further, the data import feature allows data entry, conversion, and reconciliation to occur either manually from a CSV file or on the fly through the application programming interface. By building an intermediary application that interfaces to an EHR's application programming interface, the entire data abstraction and import process can potentially be automated (Chapter 4). While REDCap is commonly used, it is not the only solution available: constructing a research database using the common data model (as described in Chapter 4) or purchasing a commercially available clinical data warehouse will also address many of the concerns raised regarding data consistency.

Regardless of the approach, the researcher will still need to recode and clean data, and although this can be done through statistical software, many commonly required tasks can be performed efficiently using Microsoft Excel. As an added benefit, using an application with a graphical user interface allows visual inspection of the data. To use Excel, the research database, or individual datasets, must be in CSV or other spreadsheet format and must not exceed 1,048,576 observations by 16,384 variables,[8] which should be sufficient for all but the largest datasets. The following Excel tools and techniques are particularly useful for data management activities[9]:

- **Filters**. Filters allow a subset of the data by selected criteria for a given variable (column). Visual inspection of the filter dropdown lists all possible values that a given variable contains, including missing data (blanks). Once criteria are selected, the observations will be subset by those criteria, with the number of selected rows visible at the bottom. Filters can be applied across multiple variables concurrently to help assess joint distributions. Filtering is useful to ascertain missingness, categorical variable conformity, data type inconsistencies, and extreme values, and can be combined with other operations for variable recoding.

- **Find/Replace**. Perhaps the simplest command to master is the find and replace operation to correct data inconsistencies or perform bulk data recoding. Find and replace operations can occur on the contents of an entire cell (data point) or within the contents of a cell. Advanced search techniques include using wildcards such as the question mark "?" to identify a single character and an asterisk "*" to identify any number of characters, as well as matching by case. Selecting a given column or column(s) before the find/replace operation will ensure only the given variable(s) are searched.

- **Formulas**. Formulas can be used to recode both numerical and categorical variables. For numerical data, they allow calculations to occur on one or more data points, such as computing body mass index from variables corresponding to weight and height. From a categorical perspective, there are string manipulation functions that can allow data parsing or concatenation. Once a formula is created it can be replicated across all observations by using the AutoFill feature. A particularly useful trick is to create a formula to "write code" that can be copied and pasted into statistical software and executed. Learning to concatenate and manipulate strings in Excel can greatly improve the efficiency of data cleaning and recoding activities.

- **Dates**. Dates are notoriously finicky to work with in statistical software unless they are in the correct format. By selecting a variable and its data (i.e., selecting the entire column), and choosing "Format cells", we can standardize the formatting of dates in a dataset. Re-exporting the data to CSV will preserve the date formatting.

- **Text to Columns**. This is perhaps one of the most useful Excel functions when working with EHR data extracts. This function will parse a single column into multiple variables using either a delimiter (more common) or a fixed width (less common). As an example, suppose an EHR extract had a single variable called "medications" that captured all medications prescribed for a patient, where one such data point was: "2/18/2022, Metformin, 500 mg PO BID; 3/30/2022, Furosemide, 40 mg PO daily; 10/20/2020, Simvastatin, 10 mg PO daily". We can use Text to Columns to parse the individual medications using a semicolon ';' delimiter, followed by parsing prescribed date, medication, and amount/route/frequency using a comma ',' delimiter. Finally, we can further separate amount, route, and frequency into distinct variables using a space "delimiter. The ability to use this function is predicated on recognizing patterns in data. If patterns are inconsistent, using filters, formulas, or find/replace can help standardize the data first.

Notes

1 Relationship files may be obtained directly from the census at: https://www.census. gov/geographies/reference-files/2000/geo/relationship-files.html. Alternatively, the Missouri Census Data Center's Geographic Correspondence Engine (Geocorr) can

produce crosswalk tables mapping from one geography to another: https://mcdc.missouri.edu/applications/geocorr2018.html.

2 https://www.census.gov/programs-surveys/surveys-programs.html.

3 https://www.census.gov/programs-surveys/geography/guidance/geo-identifiers.html.

4 https://www.census.gov/geographies.html.

5 Technically, the census uses ZIP Code Tabulation Areas instead of ZIP codes; practically, these are often the same. A crosswalk must be performed to transform ZIP codes to ZIP Code Tabulation Areas A crosswalk spreadsheet is available to download from: https://udsmapper.org/zip-code-to-zcta-crosswalk/.

6 https://geocoding.geo.census.gov.

7 In many clinical studies, the primary outcome is a composite of multiple individual variables. For example, in a cardiovascular study one may choose to operationalize a cardiovascular death, non-fatal myocardial infarction, stroke, or revascularization as a single composite variable "major adverse cardiovascular events." There may also be competing risks where the event of interest may occur from more than one cause. Composite variables are simple to create and analyze and can increase statistical power if there are few occurrences of any one event. On the other hand, the individual outcomes can have different statistical relationships with the exposure(s) and confounders may also differ. Researchers should be aware that the common practice of conducting a secondary analysis of the individual outcomes will likely be underpowered and increase the risk of a type 1 error and competing risks require a specialized modeling strategy.

8 For versions: Excel for Microsoft 365, Excel 2021, Excel 2019, Excel 2016, Excel 2013, Excel 2010, Excel 2007. A full listing of Excel's specifications and limits is available here: https://support.microsoft.com/en-us/office/excel-specifications-and-limits-1672b34d-7043-467e-8e27-269d656771c3#ID0EDBD=Newer_versions.

9 The data are assumed to be organized such that the first row contains the variable names and the second row through the end contain the observations. After any manipulation, the data should be spot-checked for errors.

References

Carine F, Parrent N. Improving patient identification data on the patient master index. Health Inf Manag. 1999 Mar–May;29(1):14–7.

Delmelle EM, Desjardins MR, Jung P, Owusu C, Lan Y, Hohl A, Dony C. Uncertainty in geospatial health: challenges and opportunities ahead. Ann Epidemiol. 2022 Jan;65:15–30.

Goldstein ND. Working with census geographies in r. Epidemiology. 2015 Mar;26(2):e22-3.

Goldstein ND, Auchincloss AH, Lee BK. A no-cost geocoding strategy using r. Epidemiology. 2014 Mar;25(2):311–3.

Rossiter K. What are census blocks? United States Census Bureau. Available at https://www.census.gov/newsroom/blogs/random-samplings/2011/07/what-are-census-blocks.html. July 11, 2011.

Sood HS, Bates DW, Halamka JD, Sheikh A. Has the time come for a unique patient identifier for the US? NEJM Catalyst 2018; 4.

UCLA: Statistical Consulting Group. How to reshape data long to wide using proc transpose. https://stats.idre.ucla.edu/sas/modules/how-to-reshape-data-long-to-wide-using-proc-transpose/ (accessed December 2, 2021), 2021a.

UCLA: Statistical Consulting Group. Reshaping data long to wide in versions 11 and up. https://stats.idre.ucla.edu/spss/modules/reshaping-data-long-to-wide-in-versions-11-and-up/ (accessed December 2, 2021), 2021b.

UCLA: Statistical Consulting Group. Reshaping data long to wide. https://stats.oarc.ucla.edu/stata/modules/reshaping-data-long-to-wide/ (accessed December 2, 2021), 2021c.

Walker K. Tidycensus: Load US Census Boundary and Attribute Data as 'tidyverse' and 'sf'-Ready Data Frames. R package version 0.9.9.2. https://cran.r-project.org/web/packages/tidycensus/index.html.

Wang JF, Li ZR, Cai CZ, Chen YZ. Assessment of approximate string matching in a biomedical text retrieval problem. Comput Biol Med. 2005 Oct;35(8):717–724.

6 Perils of Electronic Health Record Data

There is an adage in computer science, "garbage in, garbage out," which implies that regardless of the elegance of an algorithm, flawed input will result in flawed output. This sentiment certainly rings true in the analysis of EHR data: without a thorough appreciation of the perils of such data, inference from the results may lead to erroneous conclusions. It is hard not to be enamored with the possibilities of using EHR data for research purposes. As motivated in Chapter 1, the scale of data available across a breadth of patients is staggering, especially if these patients have been retained in care for many years. Yet, to borrow from the adage, more data may not equate to better research. Indeed, should the data be flawed, then by analyzing the "big data" available to us in the EHR, we have only more accurately measured a biased effect. This concept is not new to EHR research but is perhaps exemplified in it if the researcher does not consider the points raised in this chapter.

To start, we will revisit the intention of data in the EHR and the state of adoption in the field. Then, we will discuss the ever-present issues of data quality, including accuracy, completeness, and missingness. Finally, we will discuss the concept of an EHR's catchment. This is intended to allow us to vet both internal validity – whether there is a bias – as well as external validity, including the representativeness of the patient population in the EHR versus the population at large. Along the way, six vignettes are presented based on interviews conducted by the author with practicing clinicians (Boxes 6.1–6.6). These anecdotes reinforce the opportunities and challenges in EHR research, and as argued several times in the book, those who document in the EHR should be included in the research process whenever possible. Readers should also be aware that there is intentional overlap in the material presented in this chapter and Chapter 9, with the difference being the present chapter is specific to EHRs whereas Chapter 9 covers threats to validity from a more conceptual and generic perspective. For a full appreciation of the issues and remedies of these data issues, both chapters should be scrutinized.

DOI: 10.4324/9781003258872-8

Box 6.1   Interview with an Internist. Used with permission.

How do you use the EHR in your practice?

"I use the EHR in a number of ways in clinical practice. First, I use it to document what happens during patient encounters and to place orders for tests and treatments that are needed as part of the care plan. I also use the EHR to capture structured data to support billing for these encounters, including entering diagnostic and/or procedure codes that the health system can use to request reimbursement for care. I use the EHR to get a snapshot of what is going on with a patient. From this one place, I can review notes from other providers, test results, patterns of health care use, medications, and many other things. Finally, I use the EHR to communicate with my patients and with other care team members in an efficient and secure way."

What aspect(s) of the EHR works best?

"I'd guess that any aspect of the EHR that pertains to billing and coding works best. In our fee-for-service healthcare system, RVUs are paramount. EHRs were built with this idea at the forefront, in order to make them a worthwhile financial investment for large health systems. So – things like entering orders for new tests, placing referrals to specialists, adding diagnosis codes to encounters tend to work best. These processes are well-oiled machines."

What aspect(s) of the EHR is the most challenging?

"Capturing and locating health information that doesn't have a billing implication can be challenging. The context in which our patients live their lives – their social and behavioral determinants of health are poorly captured – things like their housing situation, food security, nutritional and physical activity habits. These things are all so critical for impacting the health outcomes that we care about as physicians. And yet, they're often not easily located in the EHR. Why not? Because we don't pay doctors or health systems to measure and intervene on them."

What advice would you give researchers working with EHR data?

"Don't let the messiness scare you away. These data are valuable. EHR-based research allows the more efficient study of rare conditions or treatments, and represents health services use and clinical outcomes in "real world" patient populations and care settings. However, if you're going to do research using EHR data, here are a few golden rules. First, make sure to partner with a clinician who practices in the area you're studying – learn how the data are collected and what implications this could have for measurement accuracy and completeness. Second, have a very good data cleaning plan that leverages biologic plausibility and identifies group-level outliers, but also makes use of repeated measures within an individual over time. Third, be very clear about what you're able to reliably measure in the EHR. It is easy, for example, to mistake a prevalent disease as an incident (first diagnosis in the dataset is not the same time as the first diagnosis for the patient), and easy to mistake the absence of evidence as evidence of absence (just because you don't see the ED visit for myocardial infarction in your health system doesn't mean it didn't happen). Think carefully about why certain people might be more or less likely to have certain diagnoses captured and documented. Make sure to consider whether there are systematic differences in how care is delivered between the groups you want to compare in your study – think about how this could impact the accuracy of your outcome measures. Lastly, remember that people who have data in the EHR are those who use health care more regularly – either they have better access to care, or are sicker/have a greater need for care, or both. This is important when considering the external validity of any findings – to whom do these results apply?"

EHRs as a source of research data

A paper written during the nascent stages of EHR adoption identified the merits of paper-based charts, including familiarity, portability, flexibility, and readability (Hersh, 1995). Since space was at a premium the information recorded in a paper chart tended to be concise with only the most (subjectively) relevant details recorded. Yet for the researcher, the charts were still prone to errors, lacking in completeness, and replete with narrative descriptions instead of discreet observations. Meanwhile, the electronic health record has evolved from a mere digitized copy of the patient chart to an interactive system supporting administrative (e.g., scheduling), billing, clinical decision support, and electronic order entry functions. Since space was no longer a limiting factor in collecting data, the volume of documentation in EHRs grew exponentially and researchers found access to troves of medical data through integrated query engines. Important for our purposes, the evolution of the modern EHR followed a pathway optimized from clinical and billing perspectives, not research. Thus the "troves of medical data" carry many assumptions and caveats that researchers must be cognizant of, including issues of data accuracy, data completeness, and patient representativeness. Although EHRs are a wonderful source of clinical data, they are less likely to capture traditional epidemiological risk factors or measures of public health commonly used to study health disparities or social determinants. Chapter 3 dealt with this last consideration in more detail.

Due to the rapid development of EHRs, in part spurred on by meaningful use and reimbursement incentives (U.S. Department of Health & Human Services, 2021), EHRs have become extremely complex, both to use and to understand. In fact, as a side effect of the rapid adoption, financial incentives, and requirements for government certification, healthcare fraud has occurred based on the data mined from the EHR. Several instances allege exaggerated illness and fraudulent billing codes (Rowland, 2022; Schulte, 2021). Another instance has alleged that EHR vendors delivered knowingly flawed products to qualify for incentives (Schulte & Fry, 2019a). Even if outright fraud is not suspected, the complexity of these systems introduces the possibility of errors (Schulte & Fry, 2019b) and safety concerns for patients (Schulte & Fry, 2019c).

The complexity and imperfect nature of these systems carry implications for researchers. For example, systems may be unable to retrieve the required data, retrieve data for the wrong patient, or record information in the wrong place (Schulte & Fry, 2019a, b). One study found that approximately 40% of the EHRs certified by the federal government had "nonconformities" that could lead to patient harm including dropped decimal points, missing or erroneous codes, and problems with data import and retrieval (Pacheco, Hettinger & Ratwani, 2019). Should these nonconformities carry forward to the exported data, and not be limited to an issue with data presentation, the resulting research may be compromised.

Despite widespread adoption, as of this writing EHRs are not yet ubiquitous and there may be fundamental differences in healthcare practices that have EHRs versus those that do not. For context, by 2014 nearly 75% of US-based providers had implemented EHRs (Jamoom, Yang & Hing, 2016). Independent and smaller private practices have traditionally lagged behind EHR adoption compared to larger, integrated practices (Everson, Richards & Buntin, 2019), and as such represent the healthcare settings least likely to have EHRs or least likely to allow research from the EHR. Such differences may impact the representativeness of the patient populations, discussed later. Through the year 2016 of the Medicare EHR Incentive Program, 82% of outpatient providers and 96% of hospitals had a certified EHR (ONC, 2017a, b). Figures 6.1 and 6.2 depict vendor market share for outpatient and hospital EHRs respectively, based on Medicare EHR Incentive Program participation. As of 2017, these vendors represent the EHRs most found in healthcare practices that accept Medicare insurance.

The interconnection of these systems, and the ability to mine data across multi-institutional EHRs has been described as a "sprawling, disconnected patchwork" (Schulte & Fry, 2019b). Indeed, the ability to freely share information between EHRs can be contradictory to the interest of a healthcare system to retain patients (Schulte & Fry, 2019b). Given the variety of commercial vendors (over 700 in Figures 6.1 and 6.2 in total), not to mention homegrown, self-developed software, it is no wonder accessing and obtaining EHR data is a central challenge for researchers. A safety project conducted by the Pew Charitable Trusts noted widespread problems with matching patients to their medical records: 20% of patients were not matched to their own data within an institutional EHR rising

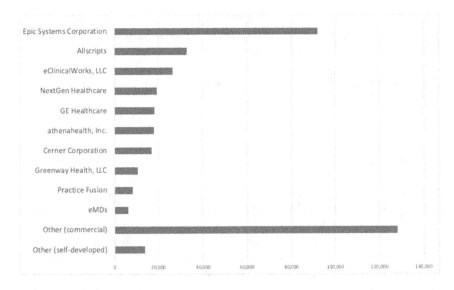

Figure 6.1 Top ten EHR vendors among ambulatory primary care physicians, medical and surgical specialists, podiatrists, optometrists, dentists, and chiropractors participating in the Medicare EHR Incentive Program.

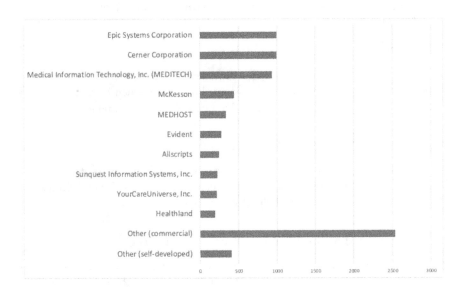

Figure 6.2 Top ten EHR vendors among hospitals participating in the Medicare EHR Incentive Program.

to 50% when data were transferred to another healthcare system (The Pew Charitable Trusts, 2017). Common reasons noted for this mismatch included typos, confusion, changes, and formatting issues. Such challenges have epidemiological implications for data linkage and longitudinal data analysis if important information goes missing or is erroneously linked to the wrong patient.

Data quality

Issues surrounding EHR data quality are well documented, and contamination of the data may occur at all steps in the research process (Verheij et al., 2018). As should be apparent, for there to be data in the EHR, the data must first have been collected and recorded (Chapter 2). Then, for secondary uses, the data must be extracted from the EHR (Chapter 4). Both steps may result in data quality issues. Assuming the data are retrievable, the data must be prepared for analysis (Chapter 5). Based on the decisions made during data cleaning and management, this can result in biased data that may impact causal inference (Tran, Lash & Goldstein, 2021). Although these steps may seem obvious at a high level, there are many subtle ways for data contamination to occur. In fact, a previous review identified 13 possible sources of bias in these steps (Verheij et al., 2018). Another analysis of EHR data found that less than half of patient records were "usable" for secondary analysis (Weiskopf et al., 2013; discussed later).

Box 6.2   Interview with a Mental Health Provider. Used with permission.

How do you use the EHR in your practice?

"I am a licensed psychologist who provides clinical services in a cancer center. I document on outpatient sessions. Previously, when I provided inpatient consults in a prior role, I also documented on those interactions."

What aspect(s) of the EHR works best?

"The ability to access all a patient's relevant records from any location permits more efficient communication and treatment planning. Beyond clinical purposes, the EHR can be a helpful source of secondary data for research."

What aspect(s) of the EHR is the most challenging?

"On the clinical side, workflow inefficiencies continue to be challenging. EHR systems appear to be optimized for billing more so than clinical care. On the research side, issues of data structure, missingness, validity, etc. are important factors to be aware of."

What advice would you give researchers working with EHR data?

"I would say that all research with EHR data should be approached with a very healthy dose of skepticism. Do not assume the accuracy or validity of data. Think about how patients came to be a part of the EHR and, perhaps more importantly, who are not in the EHR. Working closely with clinicians from the same system who use the EHR you are accessing is critical. Even if you've worked with an EHR from the same vendor at another site, the ways EHR systems are adapted and implemented to a particular health system – or even to a specific clinic within a health system – can be quite idiosyncratic. Ideally, your clinician collaborators will have good experience working in the EHR and with the same population you're studying. Even better is for your clinician collaborators to have research experience, which helps them to think through the data issues with you."

Data accuracy

The lack of accurate data in the EHR has been well documented. A Kaiser Family Foundation survey conducted in January 2019 found that 21% of patients or their family members observed an error in the EHR (Munana, Kirzinger & Brodie, 2019). The most common areas for mistakes were noted in the medical history, with 9% of participants identifying an error, and personal information, with 5% of participants identifying an error. As information tended to become more objectively collected, the error rates declined, with a 3% error rate in laboratory tests and results, a 3% error rate in medication and prescription information, and less than a 1% error rate for billing-related matters. For the epidemiologist undertaking health disparities research from the EHR, the error in personal information is problematic. Chapter 2 covered how the practice of documentation in the EHR can differ by institution, provider, or patient-level factors and Chapter 3 introduced how measures such as socioeconomic status, race, ethnicity, and gender may be incorrectly or insufficiently captured in the EHR. In one study of an EHR in New York City, 66% of patients reported race and ethnicity collected via a paper survey differently from what was captured in the EHR (Polubriaginof et al., 2019). Diagnostic accuracy has been observed to be lower when the encounter note conveys patients' behaviors (Mamede et al., 2017).

EHRs also indirectly enable inaccurate data collection. For example, the use of macros or templates to prepopulate commonly performed tasks, such as documenting the results of a physical examination, may include elements that were not assessed by the clinician either due to lack of time or irrelevance to the patient's chief complaint. Yet without manually adjusting the prepopulated values, it is quite possible that an inaccurate finding – or lack thereof – could be captured in the EHR. Medical devices that automatically synchronize with the EHR such as electronic sphygmomanometers, patient monitors, and telemetry systems may record inaccurate data if they were out of calibration, used incorrectly, or failed to capture an accurate reading. As one example, pulse oximetry devices may overestimate oxygen saturation in individuals with darker skin tone and this lack of detection of hypoxemia could negatively impact care delivery (Sudat et al., 2022). Other indirect mechanisms may lead to differential patient care and thus reduced data accuracy or completeness, such as the presence of quotes (Beach et al., 2021) or behavioral language (Mamede et al., 2017) in the clinical narrative, or symbology to depict more frequent patient encounters (Joy, Clement & Sisti, 2016).

Patient address information in the EHR presents additional challenges in terms of data accuracy and implications for geospatial analyses. For example, patients may provide addresses for billing that do not align with their residence or place(s) where they become "exposed" thereby inducing spatial misclassification (Duncan et al., 2014; Meeker, Burris & Boland, 2022). There may be multiple addresses available per patient if they have moved or otherwise provided different addresses. When multiple addresses are present, the choice of which address to select from the address history is informed by the parameters of the study and the theoretical window of time that is of greatest relevance. Linking EHR data to ecological or contextual measures, such as census data (see Chapters 4 and 5), may exacerbate these concerns. For example, assigning aggregate exposures to the individual may induce bias (Burstyn, Lavoue & Van Tongeren, 2012). Additionally, geopolitical boundaries change over time (in the United States) due to gerrymandering or redistricting based on the decennial census, which may also induce bias. For research studies that span when redistricting occurs, the researcher should consult the census temporal relationship files[1] that align the changing boundaries. Following a decennial census there are three possibilities for redistricting: (1) the census geography is unchanged, (2) the geography is divided into smaller units, such as due to population growth, or (3) the geography is aggregated from smaller units, such as due to population decline.

Although the Kaiser Family Foundation survey did not observe a high rate of "billing" errors among their respondents, this is not to say that billing codes, such as the widely used International Classification of Diseases (ICD), are unlikely to contain errors (see Chapter 2 for more details on standardized codes used in the EHR). In fact, quite the opposite has been observed. However, before discussing the accuracy of data, several terms must be defined. *Sensitivity* is the probability of a diagnostic code correctly being recorded in the EHR when a patient has the corresponding illness, whereas *specificity* is the probability that absence of a diagnostic code in the EHR correctly reflects a lack of an illness (Goldstein et al., 2022). On the other hand, *predictive values* would describe the likelihood of a patient's illness given the presence (or absence) of a diagnostic code in the EHR.

Time and again, researchers have found that ICD codes in data sources that rely on the EHR have higher specificity with correspondingly lower sensitivity. In other words, the presence of a diagnostic code is a better indicator of disease than absence of a diagnostic code. This has been demonstrated for ICD codes used inpatient EHRs (Goff et al., 2012), outpatient EHRs (Goldstein et al., 2022), clinical data warehouses (Botsis et al., 2010), ambulatory claims databases (Wilchesky, Tamblyn & Huang, 2004), and hospital discharge databases (Romano & Mark, 1994), the last three of which are EHR-derived data. A review of studies assessing the sensitivity and specificity of EHR data is provided in Williams et al. (2017) and interested readers seeking further details on the ICD coding process and how it results in errors should consult O'Malley et al. (2005). Table 2 in Schneeweiss and Avorn (2005) provides a summary of common EHR diagnoses along with corresponding measures of accuracy.

There are other complications of working with ICD codes. When retrieving a list of diagnoses via ICD codes, the date that accompanies an individual diagnosis may not reflect the actual diagnosis date but rather the last time the billing code was entered or updated. This may be especially problematic in EHRs where the problem list is separate from the encounter, and thus not updated at each visit. This also risks conflating incident versus prevalent conditions, in that a prevalent diagnosis may have already been resolved, or an incident diagnosis may not in fact be a new condition, but rather just reflect a new ICD code recorded in the EHR. The use of a washout period, such as the prior two years, may aid in delineating incident versus prevalent diagnoses. Upcoding, or the practice of recording false or exaggerated diagnoses for the purposes of inflated insurance reimbursements can create false positive diagnoses in the EHR, potentially lowering ICD code specificity. Although upcoding has been posited to occur (Hoffman & Podgurski, 2013), in at least one study, the practice was not common for Medicare reimbursements (Adler-Milstein & Jha, 2014). False positive codes may also occur based on the use of "rule out" diagnoses. One study found that among 1,453 emergency department patients with a pulmonary embolism ICD-10 code there were 257 false positives, the majority of which ($n = 193$, 75%) were "rule out" codes (Burles et al., 2017).

Box 6.3　Interview with an Intensivist. Used with permission.

How do you use the EHR in your practice?

"The EHR is used on a daily basis to chart patient progress. It provides a longitudinal record of patient care. It is used to integrate subjective clinical data along with orders, vital signs, laboratory data, imaging data, and other data points. It is not only crucial for day-to-day health care operations but for billing, benchmarking, and quality assurance."

What aspect(s) of the EHR works best?

"The EHR has been a big improvement over paper-based charting and ordering. It has eliminated issues with legibility and allows real time integration of data from multiple sources. When used for ordering, specific order sets have been developed that dramatically increase patient safety. Electronic ordering has also allowed for improved safety by providing patient alert and pop-ups. The EHR also allows a longitudinal vision of care from one hospitalization to the next or between patient care encounters."

What aspect(s) of the EHR is the most challenging?

"There are times where the use of the EHR is very time consuming. Although it can create safety alerts, clinicians develop fatigue to this alert. The sheer amount of information that needs to be documented and integrated is also growing and can be a burden on care providers. Information that is received from patients through the patient portal now puts extra demands on clinicians time."

What advice would you give researchers working with EHR data?

"Some data obtained from the EHR that are purely objective such as laboratory value or other measurements such as weight or vital signs should be accurate and robust. Other data, such as ICD-10 diagnoses or other administrative data, while easily retrieved from the EHR, are likely less accurate and limited on how they can be used and interpreted."

Data completeness

We use the terms data completeness and missing data interchangeably in this chapter. Due to the complex nature of this topic, it is covered in multiple places in the book. This section reviews the problem of data completeness in the EHR, Chapter 5 discussed how to operationalize missing data, Chapter 9 focuses on how missing data may compromise study validity, and Chapter 10 presents analytic methods for handling missing data such as imputation.

There are several mechanisms that cause missing data in EHRs as well as the data exports destined for the research database. Since our use of EHR data is for secondary research projects, the data points that are missing are likely not recoverable without supplemental data sources or prospective patient interviews. Data may be missing because of a lack of data collection in that the patient was not asked, or a lack of documentation in that the patient may have been asked but the provider did not enter the information in the EHR, or the patient declined to answer. Additionally, different EHRs capture different data points and the patient may have interacted with different healthcare systems, dubbed *EHR-continuity* (Lin et al., 2018). Further, missing data may be date dependent in that the availability of data is dependent on the characteristics of the encounter. As researchers, we should not assume that lack of documentation means that a patient did not experience some outcome. Patients who have interacted more frequently with a healthcare provider may be more likely to have a diagnosis recorded in the EHR, termed informed presence bias and discussed in Chapter 9 (Goldstein et al., 2016). Missing data in the EHR may be also problematic for the documentation of symptoms and comorbidities. For example, providers may not necessarily document "negative" values, and as such, blank values in the EHR may reflect either a negative occurrence of a symptom or comorbidity, or the lack of data collection.

Before delving further into the topic, we need to define several commonly used terms to describe missing data. Missing data may be defined as *missing completely at random* (MCAR), *missing at random* (MAR), or *missing not at random* (MNAR) (Mack, Su & Westreich, 2018). Data that are MCAR can be viewed as a random subset of the population. For example, suppose a researcher needed the variable "weight" in an outpatient EHR. If a patient's car broke down on the way to the clinic and thus weight was not recorded, the data are said to be MCAR (assuming the reason the car broke down was unrelated to a patient's weight). In data that are MAR, the probability of a data point missing depends on the observed data. As such, it is predictable (and not actually randomly missing!). Continuing with the weight example, suppose that men were less likely to be weighed than women. If we have patients' genders recorded in our EHR, we can predict patterns of missingness. On the other hand, data that are MNAR are not predictable as the probability of a data point missing now depends on unobserved data. For example, underweight individuals may be less likely to be weighed than overweight individuals in this outpatient clinic. In this case, the data are missing based on their own value. The MCAR, MAR, and MNAR designations can be confusing, and some prefer to think of missing data as ignorable/noninformative (MCAR, MAR) or nonignorable/informative (MNAR) (Figure 6.3). What matters most to the researcher is not necessarily applying

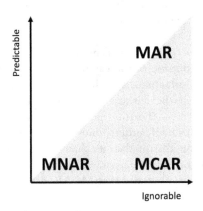

Figure 6.3 The triangle of missing data.

[Adapted from Beaulieu-Jones et al. (2018).]

the correct label, but rather attempting to understand the mechanism that led to the EHR data being missing in the first place as well as the structure of the data (Westreich, 2012).

Weiskopf et al. (2013) enumerated four elements of data completeness as applicable to the EHR: documentation, breadth, density, and predictiveness. *Documentation* means that "observations made during a clinical encounter are recorded" and is a measure of the "fidelity of the documentation process." This element is also intrinsic to the EHR: the other three elements are viewed from the perspective of the researcher working with secondary data. *Breadth* was defined as all types of data required for research are available in the patient record and its corollary *density* was defined as all types of data required for research are available in sufficient numbers. The last element, *predictiveness*, means that the data are sufficient to predict an outcome, and as such, is an analysis-based definition as opposed to a methods-based definition. Based upon these four elements, the authors studied their EHR-derived clinical data warehouse and found anywhere from 50% to 75% of records were incomplete, depending on the stringency of the definition used. In other words, only a fraction of available data was suitable for their secondary research uses. Botsis et al. (2010) also noted their clinical data warehouse had extensive missing data and concluded that data must be ascertained from multiple sources. Despite these pessimistic findings, the overall completeness of data in the EHR is markedly improved when compared to paper-based charting paradigms in a variety of settings (Bilyeu & Eastes, 2013; Hawley et al., 2014; Jang et al., 2013; Sanders et al., 2013).

The mechanisms behind missing data will vary based on patterns related to patient care practices. Haneuse, Aterburn, and Daniels (2021) demonstrated this by examining EHR-recorded measurements of hemoglobin A1C in a group of patients following bariatric surgery: some patients had rich measurement history, while others were sparse or nonexistent. What is the reason for this discrepancy? The authors proposed deconstructing the mechanisms for missingness to ultimately determine whether the data are MCAR, MAR, and MNAR, which they term modularization. This deconstruction involves examining missingness by variable type (i.e., exposure, outcome, confounders, etc.), missingness by time point, expectation of the type of clinical encounter, expectation of patients receiving care outside of the catchment area (discussed later), changes in approaches to clinical practices, and changes in patient insurance. Using this modularization approach the authors determined they had both MAR and MNAR data, depending on the time point examined, necessitating different approaches for remediation. Beaulieu-Jones et al. (2018) proposed an empiric approach for assessing the missing data mechanism in EHR-derived data. Using a machine learning algorithm on a dataset where the three types of missingness were simulated, they observed that MCAR data were not predictable (as expected, since the missing data are unrelated to any other data) while MAR data were the most predictable (again, as expected, since the missing data are contingent upon other observed data).

Box 6.4   Interview with a Nurse Practitioner. Used with permission.

How do you use the EHR in your practice?

"I use our EHR to review labs, imaging, past medical history, past surgical history, family history, social history, and previous office visits before seeing a patient. I use this info as a means of both catching myself up on a patient when it has been a while since I have seen them, reviewing any new information or changes before seeing them, and as a way of collaborating with other clinicians (i.e., if a patient needs clearance before undergoing fertility care, checking whether they have seen cardiology, endocrinology, or whichever specialist/clinician they were referred to). I also use our EHR as a way of tracking important health screenings or reminding myself to check on results/follow up with a patient in the future. For me, the EHR is an extremely important tool for every aspect of patient care."

What aspect(s) of the EHR works best?

"Each EHR I have used (currently and in the past) have had their own strengths and weaknesses. A strong EHR is one that allows a clinician to easily view data, track patient labs/imaging/plan of care, and view specific data points over time (for example, the ability to show every CBC result within a designated time frame such as the past 2 years, as an example). The best EHR I've used also had strong design strengths – it took me as a clinician through each part of the patient visit with clear tabs – Review, HPI, ROS, PE, A/P, and then sign-off. Each part of a patient visit was laid out in a clear, intuitive way that made it easy to breeze through documentation."

What aspect(s) of the EHR is the most challenging?

"The most challenging aspect of any EHR is when the shortcuts designed to make documentation easier for clinicians are too complicated or have too many steps to remember, where you need to remember a dozen or more ways to shortcut through various aspects of the patient visit. This defeats the intended purpose of making documentation easier. My least favorite EHR I've used made it almost impossible to quickly and easily access past medical information in a quick, snapshot way – I would have to pore through each previous office visit documentation to get any relevant information. It was very time consuming."

> ## What advice would you give researchers working with EHR data?
>
> "Truthfully, I think we need clinicians to be side by side with developers when an EHR is being developed. We need to have input from the beginning as to how an EHR is laid out. For researchers working with EHR data my advice would depend on the nature of the research and what the researchers are trying to do with EHR data. Each EHR system is very different, so working with multiple EHR systems would likely be challenging as one would need to become familiar with each system in order to navigate it and find the data they need."

Addressing data quality concerns

Given the concerns with data quality, approaches are required for remediation and ascertaining the impact on inference. Chapter 9 focuses on such threats to validity in a general epidemiological sense including the use of quantitative bias analysis; herein we focus on EHR-specific approaches. Schneeweiss and Avorn (2005) described a "cascade of potential biases" that may result from inaccurate EHR data, including multiple types of information bias and residual confounding, with multiple suggestions for remediation. This cascade of biases occurs as a result of moving from the clinical patient encounter to electronic research data – from the patient selection process to documentation issues to incomplete or inaccurate record linkage – and may vary by whether the data are solely EHR data or are supplemented with claims data. A review by Weiskopf and Weng (2013) identified five dimensions of EHR quality concerns with seven accompanying methods to remediate (Table 6.1). Citations that exemplify the use of a method for one or more dimensions are given in Weiskopf and Weng (2013) and can serve as a useful starting point for researchers facing similar EHR data challenges.

For researchers with access to an institutional EHR, performing an audit of the data in the research database can help identify systematic or random errors (see also Chapter 4). We can take a random sample of observations and variables from the EHR extract and compare it against chart review to calculate an error rate. With an *a priori* threshold in mind, say 10%, we can decide whether the observed error rate requires remediation. The exact number of random samples to obtain can be calculated in a traditional power analysis by specifying a given error threshold and accompanying margin of error. However, this assumes the EHR is the gold standard. If the EHR is not considered the gold standard, we must turn to external "gold standard" data sources to assess data quality.

Duda et al. (2012) demonstrated one such example of a data quality audit from an observational database, coding audited records using a 5-category paradigm:

Table 6.1 Dimensions of EHR quality concerns and remediation methods

Dimension		Method	
1. Completeness	Is the truth present in the EHR?	1. Gold standard	Use of a comparison dataset that contains "truth."
2. Correctness	Does an element capture the truth?	2. Data element agreement	Comparing against another relevant EHR element.
3. Concordance	Agreement between elements under scrutiny with internal or external data.	3. Element presence	Are required data present in EHR?
4. Plausibility	Do the data make sense in terms of scientific knowledge or context?	4. Data source agreement	Comparison against another dataset that is not the gold standard.
5. Currency	Do the data capture the right elements at the right time?	5. Distribution comparison	Descriptive analysis comparison against expectations.
		6. Validity checks	Do the data "make sense?"
		7. Log review	Use of audit logs and data entry checks.

[Adapted from Weiskopf and Weng (2013)]

(1) accurate, (2) clinically meaningful discrepancy, (3) nonclinically meaningful discrepancy, (4) missing but value exists in gold standard, (5) value exists but missing in gold standard. They noted extensive error rates driven by #2, #4, and #5, observed that dates were especially prone to errors, and provided four recommendations:

1 **Standardize the data pipeline**. This includes the way data abstraction is performed, the data entry techniques, and the personnel involved in the process.
2 **Develop structured clinical data entry**. Wherever possible, have clinicians and others who enter data in the EHR use discrete elements that exist in a common location.
3 **Retain reports**. When laboratory reports or other external services are received, they should be retained and not discarded. This motivates electronic reporting of external services in the EHR.
4 **Standardize dates**. Date entry must be flexible to allow month or year precision when days are unknown.

Once error rates are obtained, they can be incorporated into the analytic procedures to produce adjusted estimates accounting for data inaccuracies (Shepherd & Yu, 2011). This is discussed further in Chapter 9.

Acknowledging the challenges with diagnostic codes in the EHR, many researchers choose to operationalize a clinical phenotype (defined in Chapter 2) based on combinations of billing and diagnostic codes, free text notes, and other ancillary details (Pendergrass & Crawford, 2019; Richesson et al., 2013; Wei & Denny, 2015). For example, instead of operationalizing a diagnosis of diabetes solely based on the presence of an ICD code (i.e., E11.xx in ICD-10-CM), it is more prudent to define a phenotype based on a combination of ICD codes, diabetes-related medications, and a high hemoglobin A1C values. Any of these elements may or may not be present in the EHR, but as we do not rely upon an individual criterion, the chance of misclassifying diabetes is lower compared to the ICD code alone. Kaiser et al. (2022) relied on six areas in the EHR to construct a latent homeless variable: the (1) encounter note, (2) problem list, (3) patient's address, (4) social history, (5) care plan, and (6) housing status. Even in the case of missing data in the EHR combined with imperfect assessment of manifest variables, Bayesian latent class techniques can improve upon rule-based approaches to constructing a phenotype (Hubbard et al., 2019).

Before developing a phenotype definition *de novo*, which may be a time consuming process, researchers are advised to search for existing and validated clinical phenotypes; the NIH Pragmatic Trial Collaboratory has cataloged several entities[2] who have previously defined phenotypes. Once a phenotype has been defined, it should be assessed for clarity, local validity, and reproducibility, keeping in mind that each individual data element comprising the phenotype definition may be subject to the same data quality concerns raised in this chapter (Richesson et al., 2013). Pendergrass and Crawford (2019) provide a general review of phenotyping from the EHR. Relatedly, the temptation to operationalize a dichotomous predictor from continuous data, such as physiologic or laboratory measures (e.g., hypertensive, obese, neutropenic, and so on), should generally be avoided; rather the data should be analyzed using appropriate statistical methodologies (Heavner et al., 2010; Royston, Altman & Sauerbrei, 2006).

Specific to missing data, there is no single best approach for addressing issues of data completeness. In general, MCAR data lead to a loss in estimate precision whereas MAR or MNAR data may result in biased estimates (Mack, Su & Westreich, 2018). Imputation is commonly used, especially for data that are MAR, and will be discussed in Chapter 10. Readers are also directed to these references (Beaulieu-Jones et al., 2018; Li, Chen & Moore, 2019; Petersen et al., 2019; Wells et al., 2013). Data that are MNAR may require a validation study, sensitivity analysis, or other advanced approach; see Haneuse et al. (2016) and Groenwold (2020) for examples. To address the issue of missing data due to EHR-continuity, or receiving care outside of the current EHR, if claims data are available, the proportion of claims records also captured in the EHR can serve as a "continuity ratio." Restricting the data to patients with a high continuity ratio may reduce information bias (Lin et al., 2018). In the absence of claims data, one may still restrict the EHR sample based on predictors of high continuity, which have been ascertained for an outpatient oncology EHR (Merola et al., 2022).

Box 6.5   Interview with a Primary Care Physician. Used with permission.

How do you use the EHR in your practice?

"Our EHR is the foundation of our practice. We use the EHR to write notes, maintain a medical record for our patients, track preventive care and vaccines and order imaging/labs. As a practice owner, it helps me run reports on the growth of the practice, provides a billing platform for our patients and manages our in-house pharmacy inventory. We can communicate with patients through a portal which they can also use to look up their medical history within the practice."

What aspect(s) of the EHR works best?

"The best part of our EHR design is the medication inventory system as well as the patient portal. Both are very accurate and easy to use."

What aspect(s) of the EHR is the most challenging?

"The largest challenge we experience with our EHR is the CPT and ICD-10 codes. They occasionally will not match up with the lab we use which can cause issues. The second downside of our EHR is in the receipt of labs/imaging. As we are an independent practice with a small EHR, we do not have automatic integration with the large systems in our area which can result in delays."

What advice would you Give researchers working with EHR data?

"Be mindful that some information/data may be embedded in a note or the previous handwritten record and thus may be needed to fully interpret the data."

Understanding catchment

The catchment area of a healthcare system, also known as the referral network or service area, defines the expected characteristics of current and future patients and is a complex process driven by geographic, demographic, economic, and medical factors (Institute of Medicine, 2003). More specifically, we define catchment as a patient being present in the EHR although it is possible that the catchment of a healthcare facility and its EHR do not align if there are systematic differences in who has an EHR entry. Regardless, these two types of catchment definitions will be used interchangeably.

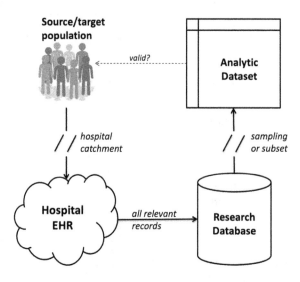

Figure 6.4 Selection of patients into a research study from the EHR.

Catchment is important to understand in terms of hospital services offered, referral patterns, resource allocation, staffing needs, emergent and nonemergent transportation, public health surveillance (if measures are derived from the EHR), and, of course, research.

The EHR's catchment has implications for researchers in terms of the representativeness of the patients as well as potential for bias. Internal and external validity may both be threatened due to the catchment process. As implied, selection forces drive patient encounters (Figure 6.4) and it is important to be able to identify how the catchment may relate to the source and target populations for an EHR-based study. These concepts are discussed in more detail in Chapter 9, but briefly, the source population are those eligible to be in the study, while the target population are those who the inference from the study results applies. The source and target population may or may not be the same.

By identifying the source and target populations, we can then evaluate whether the catchment of the EHR is representative. This evaluation can be objective, if data are available for comparison between the EHR and source or target population, but more likely this will need to be a subjective comparison using expert opinion or familiarity with the composition of the populations. Indeed, the catchment area can be nebulous: it may be delineated by geopolitical or administrative boundaries or arise organically based on natural processes. Catchment for a single healthcare system can also vary by sociodemographic strata, limiting the use of a single, global definition. Nevertheless, several geographic information system approaches to defining catchment are commonly used including distance radii from the healthcare location and road and transportation network models (Schuurman et al., 2006). Extant patient records can also provide insight into the catchment area (Peters & Hall, 1999). Researchers may choose to use census data (see Chapters 4 and 5) as the basis for the comparison between the EHR and source or target populations, but this will mainly be limited to sociodemographic and economic factors as the census includes limited information for assessing health states[3], namely disability, fertility, and insurance and payments. Census comparisons are most useful when catchment is driven primarily by geography; when catchment is driven by other factors, such as the breadth and depth of specialty care provided by a large academic medical center, the source and target populations may not align geographically with the area of the institution. As such, the results from a study of patients in the EHR of an academic medical center situated in an urban, impoverished area may not be applicable to the local community.

Alternative to the census is the use of population representative health surveys for comparison with the EHR. In the United States, well-known national surveys include the National Health and Nutrition Examination Survey (NHANES)[4], the National Health Interview Survey (NHIS)[5], the Behavioral Risk Factor Surveillance System (BRFSS)[6], and the National Longitudinal Study of Adolescent to Adult Health (Add Health)[7]. There are myriad other state and local health surveys available to researchers. In contrast to census data, these health surveys allow for the comparison of health-related risk factors or disease prevalence to a given EHR or aggregation of EHRs. Researchers have demonstrated EHRs to be representative of obesity rates in NHANES – for adults and children – with respect to most demographic strata (Flood et al., 2015; Funk et al., 2017). However, this does not guarantee these studies will be free from selection bias (see Chapter 9). In fact, the EHR itself can be conceived as a complex survey, analogous to NHANES, where patients are unintentionally over- or under-sampled with respect to the catchment strata. Viewing the EHR through this lens introduces the use of weighting techniques to account for this nonrandom sampling when the target of inference is the community (Bower et al., 2017).

Representativeness is also not the only criterion for consideration in evaluating catchment. In fact, in certain cases we may want to avoid an overly representative sample, for example, if we wish to understand subgroup differences (Rothman, Gallacher & Hatch, 2013). As such, just because the EHR may not be representative of some catchment area does not mean the study cannot proceed. Catchment can also result in a selection bias, if individuals who select into the healthcare system are systematically different from those in the community on their exposure and outcome (Goldstein et al., 2021), or informed presence bias, which may induce a selection bias or information bias (Goldstein et al., 2016; McGee et al., 2022). Again, these concepts are further discussed in Chapter 9.

Up to this point, catchment has been described as a uniform process impacting the entire EHR; however, catchment can differ in nuanced ways. Inpatient and outpatient catchment for a healthcare system may differ. Even within a given type of encounter, say inpatient, if a healthcare system has a national reputation in terms of a clinical specialty, such as transplant surgery, this can impact the types of hospitalized patients in the EHR for transplant surgeries compared to other inpatient services, such as emergency department admissions. As such, the considerations from above should be specific to the research study at hand, and not necessarily the entire healthcare system. In short, catchment influences patient selection forces both at a population level and an individual study level and must be evaluated on a per-study basis (Björk et al., 2020).

Box 6.6   Interview with an Emergency Medicine Physician. Used with permission.

How do you use the EHR in your practice?

"The EHR is needed to properly care for patients. As an Emergency Medicine Physician, I need to collect as much data about a patient as necessary in a short time period and use this information to provide the best possible care for the patients. I use the EHR to look up patients' past surgeries, past medications that have been attempted on the patients, and the success of these intervention or unfortunately failures. I use this information to prevent mistakes that have happened in the past including allergies or medications that have not worked prior. It is easy to see my colleagues' workups on these patients in the past and what they are dealing with. It provides a good picture of the personality and type of patient I am dealing with."

What aspect(s) of the EHR works best?

"Paper charts could be time consuming in that you need to have written permission from patient to gather the information from their other physicians. The physicians' office may need to fax the correct documents over and documents could be missed. The EHR keeps track of every aspect of what has been going on with the patient and little chance of that information being lost. Speed of access to a large portion of medical data about patients is helpful."

What aspect(s) of the EHR is the most challenging?

"The EHR is still evolving. There have been massive strides in improving the system. The part that is still challenging is if you have patients from other states or even in state but in other cities, and their physicians use an EHR that is not connected or related to our EHR, there is no way to access the information unless signed permission and faxes have to be done. The EHR is a great resource for research but from a clinical standpoint, when research is being done or administrators are seeing things that are being missed, they put in more 'clicks' causing me to have to spend more time in front of a computer rather than caring for patients. This is becoming an increasingly problematic thing."

What advice would you give researchers working with EHR data?

"Researchers should find a way to gather data without adding 'clicks' for the end user. Also, when the EHR says someone meets criteria for a health event you may be researching, look into the patient's chart to see if the criteria being met relates to the presenting issue. For example, a kid who broke his leg with a high white count and tachycardia is not septic despite meeting our EHR criteria as there is no sign or suspicion for infection. I would look at how the EHR defines the criteria you are looking for. From an Emergency standpoint, some EHR input is not always correct. For example, if you are researching people who are vaccinated against COVID-19 who presented to the ED for respiratory symptoms, oftentimes in the process of getting the patient to the rooms, healthcare workers do not always inquire about vaccination status and may record 'unknown'."

Notes

1 https://www.census.gov/geographies/reference-files/2000/geo/relationship-files.html.
2 https://rethinkingclinicaltrials.org/chapters/conduct/electronic-health-records-based-phenotyping/finding-existing-phenotype-definitions/.
3 https://www.census.gov/topics/health.html.
4 https://www.cdc.gov/nchs/nhanes/index.htm.
5 https://www.cdc.gov/nchs/nhis/index.htm.
6 https://www.cdc.gov/brfss/index.html.
7 https://addhealth.cpc.unc.edu.

References

Adler-Milstein J, Jha AK. Electronic health records: The authors reply. Health Aff (Millwood). 2014 Oct;33(10):1877.

Beach MC, Saha S, Park J, Taylor J, Drew P, Plank E, Cooper LA, Chee B. Testimonial injustice: Linguistic bias in the medical records of black patients and women. J Gen Intern Med. 2021 Jun;36(6):1708–1714.

Beaulieu-Jones BK, Lavage DR, Snyder JW, Moore JH, Pendergrass SA, Bauer CR. Characterizing and managing missing structured data in electronic health records: data analysis. JMIR Med Inform. 2018 Feb 23;6(1):e11.

Bilyeu P, Eastes L. Use of the electronic medical record for trauma resuscitations: How does this impact documentation completeness? J Trauma Nurs. 2013 Jul–Sep;20(3):166–168.

Björk J, Nilsson A, Bonander C, Strömberg U. A novel framework for classification of selection processes in epidemiological research. BMC Med Res Methodol. 2020 Jun 15;20(1):155.

Botsis T, Hartvigsen G, Chen F, Weng C. Secondary use of EHR: Data quality issues and informatics opportunities. Summit Transl Bioinform. 2010 Mar 1;2010:1–5.

Bower JK, Patel S, Rudy JE, Felix AS. Addressing bias in electronic health record-based surveillance of cardiovascular disease risk: Finding the signal through the noise. Curr Epidemiol Rep. 2017 Dec;4(4):346–352.

Burles K, Innes G, Senior K, Lang E, McRae A. Limitations of pulmonary embolism ICD-10 codes in emergency department administrative data: Let the buyer beware. BMC Med Res Methodol. 2017 Jun 8;17(1):89. doi: 10.1186/s12874-017-0361-1.

Burstyn I, Lavoué J, Van Tongeren M. Aggregation of exposure level and probability into a single metric in job-exposure matrices creates bias. Ann Occup Hyg. 2012 Nov;56(9):1038–1050.

Duda SN, Shepherd BE, Gadd CS, Masys DR, McGowan CC. Measuring the quality of observational study data in an international HIV research network. PLoS One. 2012;7(4):e33908.

Duncan DT, Kawachi I, Subramanian SV, Aldstadt J, Melly SJ, Williams DR. Examination of how neighborhood definition influences measurements of youths' access to tobacco retailers: A methodological note on spatial misclassification. Am J Epidemiol. 2014 Feb 1;179(3):373–381.

Everson J, Richards MR, Buntin MB. Horizontal and vertical integration's role in meaningful use attestation over time. Health Serv Res. 2019 Oct;54(5):1075–1083.

Flood TL, Zhao YQ, Tomayko EJ, Tandias A, Carrel AL, Hanrahan LP. Electronic health records and community health surveillance of childhood obesity. Am J Prev Med. 2015 Feb;48(2):234–240.

Funk LM, Shan Y, Voils CI, Kloke J, Hanrahan LP. Electronic health record data versus the national health and nutrition examination survey (NHANES): A comparison of overweight and obesity rates. Med Care. 2017 Jun;55(6):598–605.

Goff SL, Pekow PS, Markenson G, Knee A, Chasan-Taber L, Lindenauer PK. Validity of using ICD-9-CM codes to identify selected categories of obstetric complications, procedures and co-morbidities. Paediatr Perinat Epidemiol. 2012 Sep;26(5):421–429.

Goldstein BA, Bhavsar NA, Phelan M, Pencina MJ. Controlling for informed presence bias due to the number of health encounters in an electronic health record. Am J Epidemiol. 2016 Dec 1;184(11):847–855.

Goldstein ND, Kahal D, Testa K, Burstyn I. Inverse probability weighting for selection bias in a Delaware community health center electronic medical record study of community deprivation and hepatitis c prevalence. Ann Epidemiol. 2021 Aug;60:1–7.

Goldstein ND, Kahal D, Testa K, Gracely EJ, Burstyn I. Data quality in electronic health record research: An approach for validation And quantitative bias Analysis for imperfectly ascertained health outcomes via diagnostic codes. Harv Data Sci Rev. 2022 Spring;4(2). doi:10.1162/99608f92.cbe67e91.

Groenwold RHH. Informative missingness in electronic health record systems: the curse of knowing. Diagn Progn Res. 2020 Jul 2;4:8.

Haneuse S, Arterburn D, Daniels MJ. Assessing missing data assumptions in EHR-based studies: A complex and underappreciated task. JAMA Netw Open. 2021 Feb 1;4(2):e210184.

Haneuse S, Bogart A, Jazic I, Westbrook EO, Boudreau D, Theis MK, Simon GE, Arterburn D. Learning about missing data mechanisms in electronic health records-based research: A survey-based approach. Epidemiology. 2016 Jan;27(1):82–90.

Hawley G, Jackson C, Hepworth J, Wilkinson SA. Sharing of clinical data in a maternity setting: How do paper hand-held records and electronic health records compare for completeness? BMC Health Serv Res. 2014 Dec 21;14:650.

Heavner KK, Phillips CV, Burstyn I, Hare W. Dichotomization: 2 × 2 (× 2 × 2 × 2...) categories: Infinite possibilities. BMC Med Res Methodol. 2010 Jun 23;10:59.

Hersh WR. The electronic medical record: Promises and problems. J Am Soc Inform Sci 1995;46(10):772–776.

Hoffman S, Podgurski A. Big bad data: Law, public health, and biomedical databases. J Law Med Ethics. 2013 Mar;41(1):56–60.

Hubbard RA, Huang J, Harton J, Oganisian A, Choi G, Utidjian L, Eneli I, Bailey LC, Chen Y. A Bayesian latent class approach for EHR-based phenotyping. Stat Med. 2019 Jan 15;38(1):74–87.

Institute of Medicine. 2003. Unequal Treatment: Confronting Racial and Ethnic Disparities in Health Care. Washington, DC: The National Academies Press. doi: 10.17226/12875.

Jamoom EW, Yang N, Hing E. Adoption of certified electronic health record systems and electronic information sharing in physician offices: United States, 2013 and 2014. NCHS Data Brief. 2016 Jan;(236):1–8.

Jang J, Yu SH, Kim CB, Moon Y, Kim S. The effects of an electronic medical record on the completeness of documentation in the anesthesia record. Int J Med Inform. 2013;82(8):702–707.

Joy M, Clement T, Sisti D. The ethics of behavioral health information technology: Frequent flyer icons and implicit bias. JAMA. 2016 Oct 18;316(15):1539–1540.

Kaiser P, Pipitone O, Earl A, Miller M. Identifying homelessness from EMRs: Standard and custom approaches. Society for Epidemiologic Research Annual Meeting, Chicago, IL, 2022.

Li R, Chen Y, Moore JH. Integration of genetic and clinical information to improve imputation of data missing from electronic health records. J Am Med Inform Assoc. 2019 Oct 1;26(10):1056–1063.

Lin KJ, Singer DE, Glynn RJ, Murphy SN, Lii J, Schneeweiss S. Identifying patients with high data completeness to improve validity of comparative effectiveness research in electronic health records data. Clin Pharmacol Ther. 2018 May;103(5):899–905.

Mack C, Su Z, Westreich D. Managing Missing Data in Patient Registries: Addendum to Registries for EvaluAting Patient Outcomes: A User's Guide, Third Edition [Internet]. Rockville, MD: Agency for Healthcare Research and Quality (US); 2018 Feb. Types of Missing Data. Available from: https://www.ncbi.nlm.nih.gov/books/NBK493614/

Mamede S, Van Gog T, Schuit SC, Van den Berge K, Van Daele PL, Bueving H, Van der Zee T, Van den Broek WW, Van Saase JL, Schmidt HG. Why patients' disruptive behaviours impair diagnostic reasoning: A randomised experiment. BMJ Qual Saf. 2017 Jan;26(1):13–18.

McGee G, Haneuse S, Coull BA, Weisskopf MG, Rotem RS. On the nature of informative presence bias in analyses of electronic health records. Epidemiology. 2022 Jan 1;33(1):105–113.

Meeker JR, Burris H, Boland MR. An algorithm to identify residential mobility from electronic health-record data. Int J Epidemiol. 2022 Jan 6;50(6):2048–2057.

Merola D, Schneeweiss S, Schrag D, Lii J, Lin KJ. An algorithm to predict data completeness in oncology electronic medical records for comparative effectiveness research. Ann Epidemiol. 2022 Jul 22;S1047-2797(22):00150–00158.

Munana C, Kirzinger A, Brodie M. Data Note: Public's Experiences With Electronic Health Records. https://www.kff.org/other/poll-finding/data-note-publics-experiences-with-electronic-health-records/ (accessed March 8, 2022), 2019.

O'Malley KJ, Cook KF, Price MD, Wildes KR, Hurdle JF, Ashton CM. Measuring diagnoses: ICD code accuracy. Health Serv Res. 2005 Oct;40(5 Pt 2):1620–1639.

Office of the National Coordinator for Health Information Technology. ONC. 'Certified Health IT Developers and Editions Reported by Health Care Professionals Participating in the Medicare EHR Incentive Program,' Health IT Quick-Stat #30. 2017a. https://www.healthit.gov/data/quickstats/health-care-professional-health-it-developers. July 2017.

Office of the National Coordinator for Health Information Technology. ONC. 'Certified Health IT Developers and Editions Reported by Hospitals Participating in the Medicare EHR Incentive Program,' Health IT Quick-Stat #29. 2017b. https://www.healthit.gov/data/quickstats/hospital-health-it-developers. July 2017.

Pacheco TB, Hettinger AZ, Ratwani RM. Identifying potential patient safety issues from the federal electronic health record surveillance program. JAMA. 2019 Dec 17;322(23):2339–2340.

Pendergrass SA, Crawford DC. Using electronic health records to generate phenotypes for research. Curr Protoc Hum Genet. 2019 Jan;100(1):e80.

Peters J, Hall GB. Assessment of ambulance response performance using a geographic information system. Soc Sci Med. 1999 Dec;49(11):1551–1566.

Petersen I, Welch CA, Nazareth I, Walters K, Marston L, Morris RW, Carpenter JR, Morris TP, Pham TM. Health indicator recording in UK primary care electronic health records: Key implications for handling missing data. Clin Epidemiol. 2019 Feb 11;11:157–167.

Polubriaginof FCG, Ryan P, Salmasian H, Shapiro AW, Perotte A, Safford MM, Hripcsak G, Smith S, Tatonetti NP, Vawdrey DK. Challenges with quality of race and ethnicity data in observational databases. J Am Med Inform Assoc. 2019 Aug 1;26(8–9):730–736.

Richesson RL, Hammond WE, Nahm M, Wixted D, Simon GE, Robinson JG, Bauck AE, Cifelli D, Smerek MM, Dickerson J, Laws RL, Madigan RA, Rusincovitch SA, Kluchar C, Califf RM. Electronic health records based phenotyping in next-generation clinical trials: A perspective from the NIH health care systems collaboratory. J Am Med Inform Assoc. 2013 Dec;20(e2):e226–e231.

Romano PS, Mark DH. Bias in the coding of hospital discharge data and its implications for quality assessment. Med Care. 1994 Jan;32(1):81–90.

Rothman KJ, Gallacher JE, Hatch EE. Why representativeness should be avoided. Int J Epidemiol. 2013 Aug;42(4):1012–1014.

Rowland C. Beat cancer? Your Medicare Advantage plan might still be billing for it. https://www.washingtonpost.com/business/2022/06/05/medicare-advantage-records-fraud/ (accessed June 7, 2022), 2022.

Royston P, Altman DG, Sauerbrei W. Dichotomizing continuous predictors in multiple regression: A bad idea. Stat Med. 2006 Jan 15;25(1):127–1241.

Sanders DS, Lattin DJ, Read-Brown S, Tu DC, Wilson DJ, Hwang TS, Morrison JC, Yackel TR, Chiang MF. Electronic health record systems in ophthalmology: Impact on clinical documentation. Ophthalmology. 2013 Sep;120(9):1745–1755.

Schneeweiss S, Avorn J. A review of uses of health care utilization databases for epidemiologic research on therapeutics. J Clin Epidemiol. 2005 Apr;58(4):323–337.

Schulte F. Justice Department Targets Data Mining in Medicare Advantage Fraud Case. https://khn.org/news/article/justice-department-targets-data-mining-in-medicare-advantage-fraud-case/ (accessed March 3, 2022), 2021.

Schulte F, Fry E. Electronic Health Records Creating A 'New Era' Of Health Care Fraud. https://khn.org/news/electronic-health-records-creating-a-new-era-of-health-care-fraud-officials-say/ (accessed March 3, 2022), 2019a.

Schulte F, Fry E. Electronic Health Records Creating A 'New Era' Of Health Care Fraud. https://khn.org/news/death-by-a-thousand-clicks/ (accessed March 3, 2022), 2019b.

Schulte F, Fry E. No Safety Switch: How Lax Oversight Of Electronic Health Records Puts Patients At Risk. https://khn.org/news/no-safety-switch-how-lax-oversight-of-electronic-health-records-puts-patients-at-risk/ (accessed March 3, 2022), 2019c.

Schuurman N, Fiedler RS, Grzybowski SC, Grund D. Defining rational hospital catchments for non-urban areas based on travel-time. Int J Health Geogr. 2006 Oct 3;5:43.

Shepherd BE, Yu C. Accounting for data errors discovered from an audit in multiple linear regression. Biometrics. 2011 Sep;67(3):1083–1091.

Sudat SEK, Wesson P, Rhoads KF, Brown S, Aboelata N, Pressman AR, Mani A, Azar KMJ. Racial disparities in pulse oximeter device inaccuracy and estimated clinical impact on COVID-19 treatment course. Am J Epidemiol. 2022 Sep 29:kwac164.

The Pew Charitable Trusts. Patient Matching Errors Risk Safety Issues, Raise Health Care Costs. https://www.pewtrusts.org/en/research-and-analysis/data-visualizations/2017/patient-matching-errors-risk-safety-issues-raise-health-care-costs (accessed March 8, 2022), 2017.

Tran NK, Lash TL, Goldstein ND. Practical data considerations for the modern epidemiology student. Global Epidemiol 2021;3:100066.

U.S. Department of Health & Human Services. Meaningful Use. https://www.healthit.gov/topic/meaningful-use-and-macra/meaningful-use (accessed December 1, 2020), 2021.

Verheij RA, Curcin V, Delaney BC, McGilchrist MM. Possible sources of bias in primary care electronic health record data use and reuse. J Med Internet Res. 2018 May 29;20(5):e185.

Wei WQ, Denny JC. Extracting research-quality phenotypes from electronic health records to support precision medicine. Genome Med. 2015 Apr 30;7(1):41.

Weiskopf NG, Hripcsak G, Swaminathan S, Weng C. Defining and measuring completeness of electronic health records for secondary use. J Biomed Inform. 2013 Oct;46(5):830–836.

Weiskopf NG, Weng C. Methods and dimensions of electronic health record data quality assessment: Enabling reuse for clinical research. J Am Med Inform Assoc. 2013 Jan 1;20(1):144–1451.

Wells BJ, Chagin KM, Nowacki AS, Kattan MW. Strategies for handling missing data in electronic health record derived data. EGEMS. 2013 Dec 17;1(3):1035.

Westreich D. Berkson's bias, selection bias, and missing data. Epidemiology. 2012 Jan;23(1):159–164.

Wilchesky M, Tamblyn RM, Huang A. Validation of diagnostic codes within medical services claims. J Clin Epidemiol. 2004 Feb;57(2):131–141. doi: 10.1016/S0895-4356(03)00246-4.

Williams R, Kontopantelis E, Buchan I, Peek N. Clinical code set engineering for reusing EHR data for research: A review. J Biomed Inform. 2017 Jun;70:1–13.

Section II

Epidemiology and Data Analysis

7 Study Design and Sampling Strategies

This chapter begins section II of the text covering epidemiological methods useful for EHR data analysis. As a recap, section I of the book was focused on designing a research database from the EHR, along with understanding the accompanying EHR data strengths and limitations. At this point, this research database may be in a format that is directly analyzable or be an intermediate step on the path between the EHR and the final analytic datasets (Figure 7.1). For example, a clinical data warehouse will likely require further data exports to create the final analytic dataset, whereas a research database stored in Microsoft Excel (Microsoft Corporation, Redmond, WA) or the statistical software can be directly analyzed. As necessary, we may apply sampling methodologies to the research database to create the analytic datasets that will be used to test specific hypotheses. On the other hand, the research database itself may have already been "sampled" from the underlying EHR and thus represent an analytic subset of patients. Understanding these differences and creating the analytic dataset is the goal of this chapter.

Why is an analytic dataset needed?

While it is tempting to perform the analysis on the entire research database, this is not desirable for several reasons. First, there are many extraneous data points in the research database that could convolute the analysis, and possibly introduce data errors that could otherwise have been avoided. Second, the exclusion of superfluous variables will prevent "fishing" through the data for statistical associations. Instead, we want to take a directed approach to the analysis based on an *a priori* research question. Third, due to size considerations and software limitations, having an analytic dataset containing all the data may be impractical. Last, the analysis needs to be reproducible and including only the relevant data in the analytic dataset enables reproducibility.

A motivating example

Chapter 3 introduced an EHR research planner and included a hypothetical example to assess neonatal outcomes associated with very low birth weight in the neonatal intensive care unit (NICU) (see Table 3.2 for the completed planner).

DOI: 10.4324/9781003258872-10

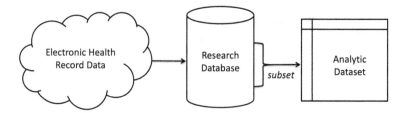

Figure 7.1 Relationship of the EHR to the research database and analytic dataset.

These data were derived from an inpatient EHR. We will build on this example in this chapter to create the analytic datasets by using various study designs and sampling strategies. Analytic data for this example will come from the *birthwt* dataset available in the *MASS* package (Venables & Ripley, 2002) in the R statistical software (R Core Team, 2020).

Which observations?

The "Data description" section of the researcher planner depicted in Table 3.2 tells us which observations are available for analysis. The "Years of data" question indicates that data are available as far back as 2001 and continue to the present day, or at least the date of the last EHR export. As such, we can expect approximately 12,000 observations representing 10,000 neonates. Details on the desired study design including the inclusion and exclusion criteria are found in the "Epidemiology" section of the planner. The inclusion criteria specify only NICU admissions between 2001 through 2020, and to exclude any neonates that were not born within the local hospital. Based on this planner, we have a clearer understanding of which observations are needed for analysis.

Which variables?

A typical research database abstracted from the EHR may contain hundreds, if not thousands, of variables. However, according to the "Variables" section in the research planner, only a subset is needed for this research question, which was informed based on our prior knowledge and literature review. For this analysis, several variables are exactly enumerated (MRN, birthweight, staph infection, delivery method, sex, race, ethnicity, and maternal marital status and age) while other variables are more generally defined (maternal and pregnancy risk factors, maternal infections, infant comorbidities, NICU procedures). We can also see from the research planner that maternal infection was identified as a potential confounder but is not available in the data. For the other variables that were only generally defined at the time the planner was completed, they now need to be appropriately operationalized for inclusion in the analytic dataset, although the specifics of this are irrelevant for this chapter.

As discussed in Chapter 4, ideally the analytic dataset does not contain any protected health information. If identifiable data were needed to create the research database, they should be removed from the analytic dataset and captured via the crosswalk spreadsheet should the original medical record require consultation. See Chapter 5 for details on this process.

Which study design?

This final question leads us into the methods for designing an epidemiologic study from EHR data, the focus of this chapter. In the "Epidemiology" section of the research planner, we can see that incidence of staph infection is the desired outcome measure, and more specifically, a risk comparison is needed to measure the association between the exposure groups based on infant birthweight (<1500 grams versus ≥1500 grams, termed very low birthweight). As incidence is the desired disease measure, this implies a cohort study design. While a cohort study was specifically identified in the planner, we will also consider other study designs based on these data as didactic examples. What follows in this chapter is a presentation of each study design with the applicable methodology to move from EHR data to an analytic dataset, but we begin with a general overview of observational study design.

Study design overview

Study design and sampling are one of the core tenets of epidemiology. The study designs covered herein focus on secondary data obtained from the EHR as there is no expectation of primary data collection. As a preview of the next few chapters, Chapter 8 introduces commonly used epidemiological measures, including measures of disease frequency – prevalence and incidence – and measures of disease risk – relative risks and odds ratios. These measures are presented within the context of the epidemiological study. Chapter 9 covers sources of bias and confounding, which both threaten the validity of the study, followed by Chapters 10 and 11 dealing with epidemiological analysis. These chapters are not meant to be an exhaustive review of epidemiology and epidemiological methods; there are many excellent textbooks on the market that cover these topics in detail ranging from introductory to advanced (see, e.g., Celentano & Szklo's *Gordis Epidemiology*, Aschengrau & Seage's *Essentials of Epidemiology in Public Health*, Szklo & Nieto's *Epidemiology: Beyond the Basics*, and Lash, VanderWeele, Haneuse & Rothman's *Modern Epidemiology*). Rather, these chapters are a review of relevant materials for the clinical researcher working with EHR data.

In traditional etiologic research, when a putative exposure is believed to be associated with a health outcome, an analytic study is undertaken, known as analytic epidemiology. A study defines the population and sampling methodology with the goal of hypothesis testing and can either be experimental or observational. As opposed to experimental studies, where the researcher manipulates an exposure and tracks differences in people over time such as is routinely done in a randomized controlled trial, an observational study does not explicitly involve the researcher intervening. Secondary data analyzed from the EHR is an example of an observational study. The exposure occurs naturally in the population through people self-selecting (e.g., cigarette smoking), by chance (e.g., genetics), or by some process otherwise external to the study. Depending on the perspective of the researcher, the exposure and outcome may have been in the past or may develop in the future. The specific type of study design can be viewed through this "researcher perspective" lens, and the choice of which study design to use is often driven by practical considerations. While there are only a few core study designs, there are numerous permutations of them, as well as general gray areas that may not clearly delineate one design from another. Didactically the various study designs are presented as separate entities, yet it is important for the researcher to keep in mind these designs are not rigid.

As a contrast to etiologic research, some researchers may engage in purely descriptive work. In descriptive epidemiology, we aim to measure and quantify some characteristics present in the EHR, such as the proportion of patients in the oncology service who are neutropenic. Descriptive analyses can occur based on characteristics measured through a cross-sectional snapshot or a longitudinal cohort. Many of the principles of epidemiologic study design apply whether the research question is descriptive or etiologic (Lesko, Fox & Edwards, 2022).

Designing an epidemiological study requires the researcher to identify a population that the study participants represent. This can either be a well-defined group of people, such as patients admitted to a hospital, or a more nebulous group, such as people living with HIV in a city. The population can either be *retrospective* having occurred in the past or *prospective* and followed into the future. Secondary data analyzed from the EHR is an example of a retrospective study. It is the perspective of the investigator during the collection of study data that determines the temporality of the research (Figure 7.2). Using the EHR, the researcher may be able to assemble a cohort representing a subgroup of individuals in the EHR and follow them through time, either prospectively or retrospectively. In this context, a *cohort* represents a group of people with some common characteristic, such as being within the catchment of this EHR. If a population cannot be recruited into a cohort, or the outcome to be studied is rare and thus an extremely large population would be needed, a *sample* of the population can be drawn, such as a sample of people living with HIV in a city. In the absence of a well-defined and enumerated cohort, a sample is still derived from a population. The ability to articulate characteristics of the population will be important when assessing how well the sample represents the population.

Distinguishing between a sample and a population is important when working with secondary data, as the secondary data will fall into one of these two

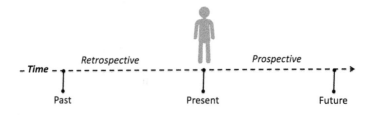

Figure 7.2 The researcher's perspective on time.

categories. A research database that has been derived from an institutional EHR likely consists of a well-defined population of individuals that shared some common characteristic, such as being a patient at that hospital. On the other hand, if the research database is obtained from elsewhere, it may consist of a sample of individuals. It is quite rare that we have access to the original population, but rather we have access to some subset or sample of this population. For example, if studying HIV outcomes from an outpatient EHR in New York City, all patients living with HIV in New York City will not be captured in this EHR. It needs to be determined whether this subset or sample of individuals is representative of the original population they were drawn from, which may require comparison with survey data, census data, or even other EHRs.

When working with secondary data the choice of study design is limited by the data, and thus accessibility of the underlying population. In other words, the data are driving the study type. This is in direct contrast to primary data, where the study type drives the collection of data. This inherent difference is important because it limits the type of study that can be conducted. In fact, secondary data derived from a sample greatly restricts the ability to design a new study from these data since the researcher does not have access to the source population. Fortunately, secondary data derived from the EHR allows for more flexibility in study design as the source population is likely available to form a cohort or allow sampling.

In general, the most efficient study designs are those based on existing records in the EHR including cross-sectional or prevalence studies, retrospective cohort studies, repeated measures or longitudinal studies, and case–control studies. These study designs are "take what you get" in that the data are already recorded in the EHR, and we are analyzing what is available. Recall that EHRs are great at capturing clinical data but less so for epidemiological data (Chapter 3). This is not to say that we are entirely limited to the data at hand: one can design a prospective clinical study based on existing patients in the EHR or link to external data (Chapter 4). EHR-based studies of hospitalized patients are useful for studying hospital-based events, severe diseases, or conditions that require inpatient treatment. Loss to follow-up (the notion of *follow-up* time is defined later) is generally not an issue for inpatient studies, although follow-up time tends to be right skewed in that sicker patients will be hospitalized for longer periods of time. Outpatient studies are useful for community-based events or diseases and treatments that can be managed in an office setting. Loss to follow-up is a concern, especially if those lost are materially different from those retained. Whereas longitudinal data in the inpatient realm tend to be balanced and complete, longitudinal data in outpatient EHRs are often unbalanced and incomplete, in that measurements are not recorded on a recurring basis and may be missing altogether.

To make this more concrete, consider the hypothetical research study motivated earlier to assess the relationship between very low birthweight and neonatal staph infection in the NICU. Primary data collection is not an option in this scenario, and we must therefore work with secondary data, namely the linked obstetrical and neonatal records abstracted from the institutional EHR (Figure 7.3). The EHR can be conceptualized as a cohort of maternal-neonatal dyads who delivered at

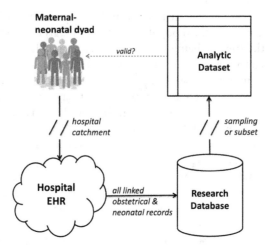

Figure 7.3 Selection of patients into a research study from the EHR.

this institution and were admitted to the NICU. How laboring women naturally select into this cohort is a function of the catchment area of the hospital, including its reputation for obstetrical and neonatal care, costs, ability to care for high-risk pregnancies, and other factors that may not be describable. Furthermore, suppose that we have access to multiple NICUs across disparate geographies that care for varying acuity of babies: would we expect consistent findings across these EHRs? These points motivate the need to understand EHR catchment and the representativeness of the cohort to a target population. These important concepts were introduced in Chapter 6 and are discussed in further detail in Chapter 9. For now, we will assume the hospital EHR represents a source of people eligible for inclusion in an epidemiological study.

We now turn to defining the individual study types. The study designs are framed within the context of an etiologic analysis of EHR data to understand the relationship between a hypothesized exposure(s) and some health outcome(s). Even though the research question is etiologic, descriptive analyses also apply. All the presented study designs are conducted on an individual, patient level. We will not consider group-level designs, also known as ecological studies, although study designs that employ both group- and patient-level data (i.e., multilevel or hierarchical studies) are discussed briefly in Chapter 11. Again, this material is presented as an overview and is not intended to be an exhaustive treatment of each study type.

Cross-sectional study

The most basic individual-level epidemiological study is the cross-sectional study, also termed a prevalence study. As its name implies, a cross-sectional study is a snapshot of a population at a specific point in time. From the researcher's

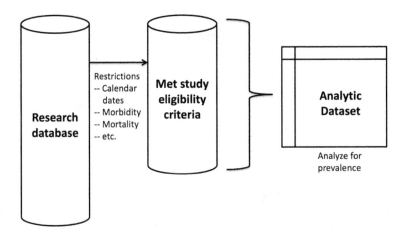

Figure 7.4 A cross-sectional analytic dataset.

perspective, all observations have occurred at one point in time, and the exposure or health outcomes have been assessed simultaneously. The researcher can then readily calculate the frequency of certain characteristics in the population, such as the prevalence of an exposure or an outcome. Applying the neonatal example from earlier, the exposure is very low birthweight and the outcome is staph infection in the NICU. *Prevalence of the exposure* is simply the total number, expressed as a proportion, of very low birthweight infants, and *prevalence of the outcome* is the total number, again expressed as a proportion, of infants who had a staph infection while in the NICU. To sample the cross-section from the research database will require subsetting the patients based on the years 2001 through 2020 that were admitted to the NICU and not outborn, while keeping only the core variables needed for the analysis (Figure 7.4).[1] See Code #7.1 in Appendix 2 for an example code.

In addition to overall prevalence, the prevalence of an exposure in diseased – very low birthweight among infants with a staph infection – or the prevalence of exposure in nondiseased – very low birthweight among infants without a staph infection – can also be calculated. However, since cross-sectional data do not have an inherent time component, the ability to infer that very low birthweight was the ascribable reason infants had a staph infection is severely limited, and therefore cross-sectional studies are often viewed as providing the lowest quality of evidence for causality among observational studies (Sackett et al., 1997) (Figure 7.5). Nevertheless, these types of studies are often used to provide data on putative exposure to outcome associations and are thus termed hypothesis-generating studies. The hypotheses can then be further explored in cohort or case–control studies.

What fundamentally distinguishes the cross-sectional design from the other designs is a lack of follow-up (Figure 7.6). *Follow-up* means that for each individual there is a time component suggesting one event has preceded (or followed) another event. Sometimes follow-up is explicitly available and can be calculated, as in a cohort study, and other times follow-up is only implicit and cannot be

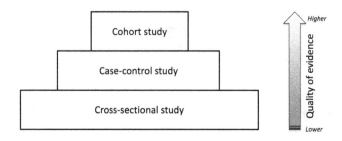

Figure 7.5 Hierarchy of evidence for observational epidemiology.

calculated, as in a case-control study. Follow-up is particularly useful in epide-miological analyses as it helps to establish temporality; that is, the exposure has preceded the outcome and therefore provides greater evidence of *causality*.

Suppose we extract a cross-section of data from the EHR and that this cross-section occurred on a random sample of patients on a given day. The dotted rec-tangular box in Figure 7.6 depicts how our knowledge of events will be limited to what is documented in the EHR at this point in time. Although this type of study design corresponds to a specific point in time when the data were extracted from the EHR, this does not mean that we cannot assess other time points: we have access to historic data documented in the EHR, and if we wish to recruit the patients into a study, we can interview them about possible future events. In fact, the vast majority of cross-sectional surveys ask the respondent to recall a point in

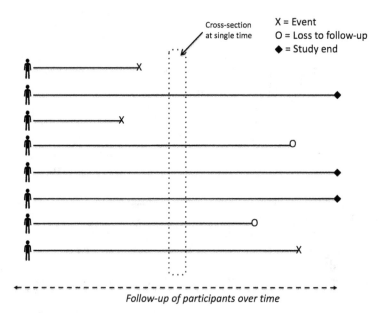

Figure 7.6 Lack of follow-up in a cross-sectional study design.

time in the past when assessing exposures. The challenge in these types of surveys is accurate recall of past exposures, which to some degree is obviated by the historic data in the EHR.

Occasionally cross-sectional samples may be obtained serially, in that they are obtained at multiple points in time. Suppose we formed a cross-section of patients seen at an outpatient clinic every six months (Figure 7.7). Such serial cross-sectional samples allow for trend estimation, such as measuring the change in prevalence, however as the potential patients *differ* at each time point, this study design is still subject to the same limitation of attributing causality. The notion of a serial cross-sectional design should not be conflated with a longitudinal design where multiple measures are obtained at future time points among the *same* group of patients. In longitudinal studies, the data have repeated measures and require a specialized analysis, discussed later in this chapter. As opposed to obtaining a new sample of outpatients every six months, in a longitudinal study, we would have identified a group of patients to follow over time, while still taking measurements every six months (Figure 7.7).

If the EHR is in a setting with mostly acute patient encounters, such as an urgent care facility, then the data on each patient resembles that of a cross-section conducted at the point in time of the encounter. Exposure and disease information were collected concurrently at that encounter. However, if the EHR is in a setting with health maintenance visits, chronic patient encounters, or represents inpatient records with multiple measures during the stay, the data are not cross-sectional as there is follow-up time available for each person. However, if the follow-up time is ignored, then the data can be treated as a cross-sectional study for estimating prevalence. Our example earlier used a cross-section based on a random sample of patients on a given day; however, we need not limit ourselves to only a single day when forming the cross-section. Indeed, estimates of prevalence can be calculated across the entire research database if we treat these data as

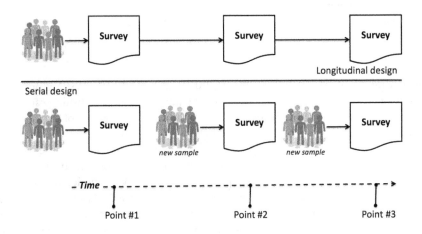

Figure 7.7 Longitudinal versus serial cross-section study design.

a cross-section for a period instead of a point (i.e., period prevalence versus point prevalence; see chapter 8).

Cross-sectional studies have many advantages. First, they are efficient. They are quick and easy to conduct, especially with secondary data from the EHR. Second, they are useful for estimating the burden of some conditions, particularly chronic conditions, and are often used for resource planning. Third, they provide initial clues as to the nature of exposures and can motivate performing more costly epidemiological studies. Unfortunately, cross-sectional studies suffer from several important limiting factors. They cannot be used to estimate incidence, only prevalence. Without a temporal component, the researcher cannot be certain that the exposure preceded the outcome, as opposed to vice versa, and therefore disease etiology cannot be revealed. Furthermore, any exposure and outcome relationship has to be interpreted as pure correlation, not as an actual measure of the risk of the outcome due to the exposure. Finally, in the presence of rare characteristics, prevalence studies need substantial numbers of individuals to truly estimate the burden, as opposed to a study design that samples based on a rare characteristic.

Returning to the neonatal example presented earlier, if the data on each neonate were collected in a way that ignored the time component, the study design can be considered cross-sectional. We can estimate the prevalence of either the exposure or outcome among the neonates in the study. However, as the secondary data were derived from the hospital's EHR, and infants are hospitalized in the NICU for varying periods of time, as researchers we could employ several study types if we consider this follow-up time (i.e., length of stay) acknowledging that risk for staph infection may change over time. The choice to analyze the data as cross-sectional implies that the entire NICU stay has essentially been collapsed into a single time point for each infant, thereby losing the concept of follow-up, and allowing the calculation of a cross-sectional prevalence. Pragmatically, this might not be necessary since we have a follow-up on these patients during their hospitalization. While this is a straightforward way to analyze the data, the loss of the time component means we can no longer look at the potentially important factor of time, which would have been possible with another study design: the cohort study.

Cohort study

According to the study design hierarchy in Figure 7.5, a cohort study provides the strongest evidence among observational study types for establishing causality, the goal of etiologic research. In a cohort study, a *cohort*, or group of people with a shared characteristic, is recruited and followed over time. Depending on the perspective of the researcher (Figure 7.2) a cohort can be recruited in the present time and followed up into the future, termed a prospective or concurrent design, or could have occurred in the past, termed a retrospective or nonconcurrent design. An ambidirectional cohort utilizes both retrospective and prospective data collection. Cohorts assembled from EHRs tend to be retrospective in nature, as they rely on existing patient records for exposure and outcome, although it is not infrequent to draw a prospective cohort population from a clinic and supplement with EHR data (see Chapter 12 for further discussion of ambidirectional cohorts). Aside from EHR-based studies, studies of diseases with long incubation periods tend to be retrospective in nature. Consider workers at a concrete factory where asbestos was used several decades ago, and among those workers, there have been a large number of rare cancers – mesotheliomas – recently diagnosed. In this instance, the researcher may recruit an occupational cohort defined by the presence of a historic exposure – asbestos – and assess its relationship to cases of mesothelioma that have already been diagnosed. As the outcome has already occurred, the cohort is retrospective. This should not be confused with the case-control study that specifically recruits participants by the outcome; in this case, we are still recruiting by the presence of the exposure, asbestos; it just so happens that the outcome is already known to the investigators. In addition to the temporal directionality of a cohort, a cohort may be *open* or dynamic, meaning people can enter or leave the cohort at any time, or *closed*, meaning the people who formed the original cohort are fixed and do not change (Figure 7.8). An open cohort typically involves births, deaths, and migrations as mechanisms to entering and leaving the cohort and can span many years.

Formation of a cohort typically starts with identifying an exposed and unexposed group. In a prospective study, an exposure is hypothesized to lead to an outcome, and participants are selected based on their exposure status. Occasionally a cohort will be recruited without a specific exposure of interest, but rather a need to elucidate risk factors associated with an outcome. In such cases, one or more exposures are then determined post-enrollment based on observed differences in the study group. Recruiting a cohort from the EHR without an *a priori* exposure is an example of this strategy. Regardless of how recruited, if the exposure truly

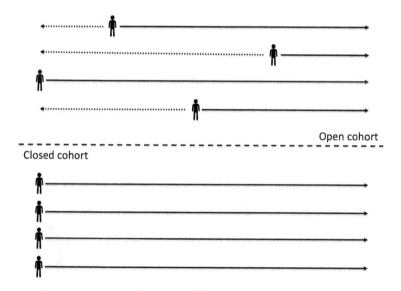

Figure 7.8 An open versus closed cohort.

caused the outcome, then the investigator would expect to see a greater incidence of the outcome in the exposed group. Alternatively, if the exposure were protective of the outcome, the investigator would expect to see greater incidence of the outcome in the unexposed group (Figure 7.9). Unlike an experimental study, the researcher did not introduce or manipulate the exposure; it occurred naturally or through nonintervening means. For example, if the exposure was very low birthweight and the outcome was a staph infection, the study design could include an exposed group of neonates who were very low birthweight and an unexposed group who were not. Importantly, the researcher did not "cause" very low birthweight; this was a preexisting phenomenon. On the other hand, if the researcher had somehow caused a very low birthweight, ignoring the ethical implications, this would constitute an experimental study since the researcher is manipulating the exposure. This distinction is the foundation of observational epidemiology.

In a cohort study, follow-up of participants lends itself to studying disease incidence. Calculating follow-up can be tricky when the number of people in the cohort is large and have entered or left the cohort at various times. In studies of disease incidence, a cohort member can have one of two outcomes: they develop an outcome or they do not. Unfortunately, while it is relatively straightforward to assess who develops an outcome, especially mortality, assessing who does not develop an outcome is not as clear, especially for diseases of insidious onset, long latent periods, or loss to follow-up. At the conclusion of the follow-up, we can say that participants have either developed the outcome or are censored. *Censoring* means that at the end of the study the participant did not experience the outcome

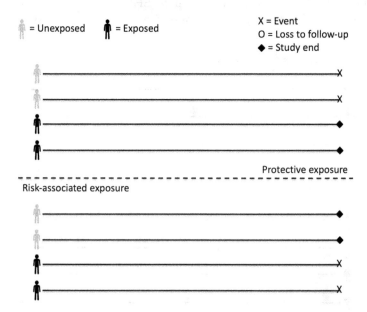

Figure 7.9 Relationship of a 100% effective exposure to disease in an ideal cohort study to demonstrate the difference between protective and risk-associated exposures.

or the participant was lost to follow-up. Lost to follow-up may mean the study personnel could not get in touch with the research subject or the participant withdrew from the study. In both instances, we do not know whether they might have developed the outcome after they were lost to follow-up, but if censoring was independent of the outcome, the analysis will not be biased. It is not always clear whether the loss was indeed independent of the outcome but examining the measured and available characteristics of the participants who were lost to follow-up may reveal important differences from those who remained in the study. When considering the outcome of a participant in a study, this type of censoring is known as right censoring, as depicted in Figure 7.10. In an open cohort, there may be left censoring, where the history of the participant is unknown before entering the cohort (Figure 7.8, dotted lines). Nuances of operationalizing cohort measures, including the exposure and follow-up time, are discussed in Chapter 8.

The EHR itself can be conceived as an open cohort as inpatient or outpatient encounters with providers stagger over long periods of time and people move in to and out of the area served by the hospital. This important observation allows us to consider hybrid study designs (discussed later) from the EHR since the underlying population is well enumerated. Viewed through this open cohort lens, data in EHR may be left-censored if we lack information on patients' health states before they entered care, and data may be right-censored if we lack complete follow-up on these patients. The implication of censoring is that there is potential for selection bias and missing data, discussed further in Chapter 9.

Cohort studies have many strengths. First, if the recruitment process occurred via the presence or absence of an exposure, the study design becomes efficient

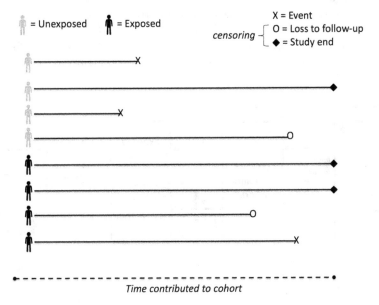

Figure 7.10 Right censoring in a closed cohort.

when the exposure is rare. Additionally, once an exposure is identified, multiple outcomes can be assessed for the duration of the cohort. Second, the follow-up component of a cohort strengthens temporality. In other words, the exposure likely preceded the outcome, particularly for acute outcomes and outcomes without long latent periods or insidious onset. Third, cohorts can be used to directly measure disease incidence. They are particularly useful for "before and after" comparisons to infer success or failure of interventions. Finally, cohort studies tend to be robust in terms of typical biases that affect observational studies, discussed further in Chapter 9.

Despite the many strengths of the cohort study, there are some weaknesses to acknowledge. First, the outcome must be observable during follow-up. This requires potentially not only a long study period but also a relatively frequent outcome to ensure statistical power. For rare outcomes, the cohort may fail to produce adequate numbers for analysis, unless the cohort recruited an extremely large number of individuals. During the study period, the researchers must be diligent about minimizing loss to follow-up, as a systematic pattern to study dropout for many participants can invalidate the study. Finally, cohort studies are expensive to conduct. For these reasons, retrospective cohorts are frequently conducted and are an added benefit to using a research database mined from an EHR.

To conclude the overview of a cohort study, let us revisit the neonatal example. In the cross-sectional study section, we saw how to use the data derived from an EHR to estimate the prevalence of very low birthweight neonates as well as staph infections. Suppose we now wish to assess whether very low birthweight is a risk factor for developing staph infection in the NICU. For simplicity, we will assume that all pregnancies resulted in a singleton birth (no twins or triplets), complete follow-up of study participants has already occurred, and the cohort has sufficient statistical power. The population of mother–infant dyads derived from the obstetrical and neonatal records form a retrospective cohort. The framework for creating this cohort from the research database is depicted in Figure 7.11.

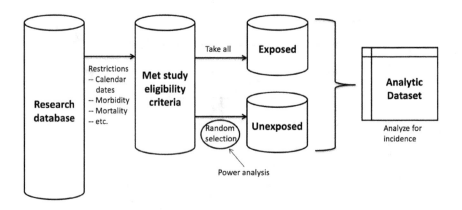

Figure 7.11 A cohort analytic dataset.

From our previous example, the neonates can be grouped into exposed or unexposed based on their birthweight, where a birthweight <1500 grams defines an exposed infant. As a heuristic, we can "recruit" all infants in the exposed group and then recruit a random sampling of infants in the unexposed group (≥1500 grams), forming the cohort's population. A power analysis determines the exact number of unexposed infants needed, although recruiting all unexposed individuals is not unusual. In such cases, the researcher will need to be cognizant of overpowering the study and use caution when interpreting differences in groups, discussed later. While these differences may be statistically significant, they may not be clinically meaningful. Follow-up occurs in the cohort until the outcome occurs or the study period ends. Depending upon the type of data, the study conclusion may be a specific date, or, in this example, when the infants were discharged, transferred, or expired. Follow-up is then calculated based on the amount of time contributed to the cohort, in this case, the length of stay in the unit. In the ideal cohort, all infants have one of two outcomes: (1) they do not develop the outcome, and their length of stay is used for the follow-up time, or (2) they develop the outcome, and their length of stay to the time they develop the outcome is used for the follow-up time. As this is a retrospective cohort, all data necessary for determining exposure status, outcome status, and follow-up are already available. The rate of staph infections can be computed for each group of infants based on their birthweight exposure, and the risk of infection can be compared between exposure groups.

Code #7.2 in Appendix 2 provides sample code for assembling a cohort from the research database for two options: (1) including all exposed and unexposed individuals, and (2) a random selection of unexposed individuals at a 1:1 ratio for all exposed individuals. The second option is a subset of the first option, and depending on the results of the power analysis, may have the necessary statistical power for hypothesis testing.

Case-control study

A case-control study is one of the more elegant epidemiological study designs that are frequently encountered in the literature. A well-conducted case-control study can closely mirror the validity of a cohort study, yet a poorly conducted case-control study will be subject to a host of biases that will undermine the study, possibly producing spurious associations or failing to detect real ones. For secondary data where the outcome is infrequent, a case–control design may be the preferred design for estimating disease associations.

As opposed to the cohort, which is often formed based on the exposure being present or absent, the case-control study, as its name implies, is formed based on the outcome being present or absent. A case need not be a disease in a traditional sense, but any phenomenon that can be measured and dichotomized. A control, therefore, is absence of this phenomenon. By recruiting based on the outcome, the case-control study is retrospective in that the investigator "looks back" through time to assess the exposure status of the cases and of the controls. If the exposure was more frequent among the cases, we can say the exposure was a risk factor for the development of the outcome. Alternatively, if the exposure was more frequent among the controls, we can say the exposure was protective against the development of the outcome (Figure 7.12).

Selection of the cases and controls, and the implied assessment of the exposure, is the greatest challenge in case-control study design, as by definition the exposure has occurred in the past and can unknowingly influence the selection. We do not want to select into case–control on basis of the exposure (and outcome) lest we induce a selection bias. In other words, the putative exposure(s) for cases must be unrelated to controls. Miettinen (1985) enumerated the following criteria that are still relevant to selecting a control series in an EHR study:

1   Controls should be derived from the same data source as the cases, such as the same EHR.
2   The referent disease or health state used for control sampling should:

   a   Be unrelated to the putative exposure(s); and
   b   Be similar in terms of the selection forces at play to the cases to appear in the same data source, such as the EHR.

Often assessment of exposure is achieved by participant recall: the participant is self-reporting whether they had a particular experience at some point in the past.

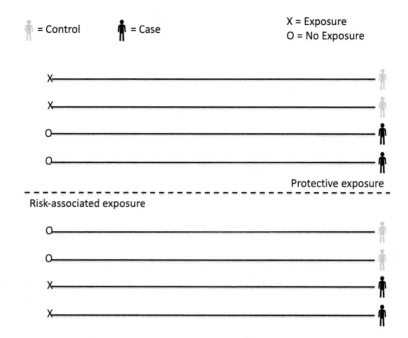

Figure 7.12 Relationship of a 100% effective exposure to disease in an ideal case-control study.

As may be deduced, people that have experienced a potentially harmful outcome may be more likely to recall (or suspect) they had an exposure, a phenomenon known as recall bias. Therefore, a case-control study does not explicitly state the exposure of interest, but rather tries to conceal it in the interview process by asking about many past exposures. In the case of secondary data derived from the EHR, an exposure may have been objectively recorded in the patient chart by the clinician thereby minimizing the potential for recall bias. On the other hand, if the exposure is based on subjective patient interviewing, the bias may be possible.

In further contrast to the cohort design where follow-up time can be explicitly measured, in a case-control study follow-up time is implicitly assumed. When assessing a past exposure, some hypothetical amount of time has elapsed between the exposure and the outcome. Yet, without actual knowledge of this elapsed time, incidence cannot be directly calculated, and the assumption of the exposure preceding the outcome can only be inferred. In fact, the incidence is "fixed" in a case-control study by the ratio of cases to controls. Establishing temporality is but one of a host of challenges in the case-control study.

Similar to the cohort study being able to assess multiple outcomes from a single exposure, the case-control study allows the researcher to assess multiple exposures from a single outcome. This is a useful feature when the exact etiology of an outcome is unknown and investigators can only speculate on possible causes. Once a putative cause is identified in the case-control study, an observational cohort or an interventional study (if the exposure can readily and ethically be changed) can be created to establish temporality and provide stronger evidence toward a causal role for that exposure.

One of the main features of overcoming some of the inherent validity issues with case–control studies is the notion of matching. In a case-control study, the controls can be *matched* to the cases on one or more characteristics. This allows for tighter control over potential confounding, discussed further in Chapter 9. For example, for an inpatient study where the length of stay is right skewed, matching on length of stay can help control this confounding effect. Matching can be done on a specific characteristic, such as the exact age of a patient, or can be done on a range over a specific characteristic, such as age by decade of a patient (Figure 7.13). When the matching is on the exact characteristic, it is termed individual or *exact matching*, and when the matching is done on the distribution of a characteristic, it is termed *frequency matching*. The specific type of matching comes back into focus during the analysis of a case-control study. The type of matching is also dictated by the availability of controls. Matching on too many characteristics can greatly reduce the pool of potential controls as well as result in a phenomenon known as overmatching. In overmatching, the characteristics matched between cases and controls were also associated with the exposure of interest, thereby balancing the exposure between groups, and potentially nullifying the ability to detect its effects.

The goal of matching is to make the cases and controls similar on some set of characteristics. At the end of the day, if the cases and controls were similar in all other respects, but only differed based on an exposure, there is greater evidence of

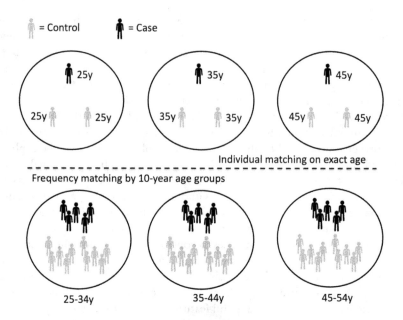

Figure 7.13 Examples of matching in a case-control study by age of the participant. Each circle contains a 2:1 control-to-case matching ratio.

a causal relationship leading to the differences in the groups, namely becoming a case or not. Without matching, the characteristics that differ between the groups must be controlled for in the analysis phase of the research. A question may naturally arise, "How many controls do I select per case?" This is the goal of the power analysis, but the general rule of thumb is to not have more than four controls for any given case. People may also be eligible to serve as controls for multiple cases, depending on the pool of controls and the random selection process.

Recruitment into a case-control study is done by sampling. As opposed to a cohort where recruitment occurs directly from the source population, a case-control study represents a sample of this population. This is an important distinction, as the representativeness of that sample to the underlying source population is of primary concern for the study to be valid. Typically, all available cases are selected and then a random sample of controls are chosen. For each potential control, if they fulfill the preestablished criteria (e.g., matching criteria) they are selected. If not, they are returned to the potential pool of controls to possibly be chosen for a subsequent match. This process is repeated until each case has the predetermined number of controls. Figure 7.13 depicts a hypothetical case-control study where each case was matched to two controls.

In practice, matching, especially frequency matching, can be a difficult concept to grasp. Suppose we have two hypothetical scenarios that we would like to compare matching approaches for a hospital-based case-control study. In scenario #1, we match on the variable "age" and in scenario #2 we match on the variables "age" and "length of stay." We are sampling from the inpatient EHR and based on the results of the power analysis, we need three controls for each case. In the individual matching approach, we may proceed as follows for scenario #1:

1 For each case...
2 Select a potential control from the pool of controls available.

   a If the potential control matches on age (could be the exact age or within some range, such as ±5 years), consider the matching successful and remove the control from the eligible pool. Make a record of the matched case and control, for example, by setting a variable for the case called "matched" to the unique record identifier.
   b If the potential control fails to match, leave the control in the eligible pool and repeat step #2 until successful.

3 Repeat step #2 until three successful matches occur.
4 Repeat step #1 until all cases have been matched.

Scenario #2 just requires a slight modification to the first scenario; in step 1a we attempt to match on "age" and "length of stay." If we run out of potential controls then we cannot match on both characteristics. Lack of comparable controls is a limitation of matching on too many variables, as is the phenomenon of overmatching, previously discussed.

In the frequency matching approach, we must proceed differently. First, we need an idea of the distribution of the matching characteristics among the cases. To make this easy, let's consider categorizing the two characteristics as follows:

- *Age*: <40 years, 41–60 years, >60 years
- *Length of stay*: <5 days, 5–10 days, >10 days

Then, we calculate frequency tables for each scenario. This is hypothetical data; in practice, this will be informed by the known distribution of the cases. Under scenario #1, Table 7.1 is a frequency table for the variable "age" as categorized above. To achieve the frequency matching, we draw three controls for each cell. Implementation of this approach may proceed as follows:

1 For each category of the matching characteristic (3 in total)...
2 Select a potential control from the pool of controls available.

   a If the potential control matches on the age category, consider the matching successful and remove the control from the eligible pool.
   b If the potential control fails to match, leave the control in the eligible pool and repeat step #2 until successful.

3 Repeat step #2 until three times the number of cases are matched.
4 Repeat step #1 until all categories have been matched.

Table 7.1 Frequency matching in a hypothetical case-control study by "age"

	Age	
<40 years	*41–60 years*	*>60 years*
25 cases	45 cases	40 cases
75 controls	135 controls	120 controls

Case data are hypothetical and matched 1:3 to controls.

Note three important differences from the individual matching approach. First, we do not loop through each case, but rather each category of the matching characteristics; that is, each cell in the contingency table: <40 years, 41–60 years, >60 years. Second, we do not record matching identifiers because there is no exact match occurring. Third, rather than needing three successes in step 3, we now need three times the number of cases in that cell to achieve the 3:1 ratio.

Under scenario #2, Table 7.2 is a frequency table for the variables "age" and "length of stay" as categorized previously. Again, to achieve the frequency matching, we draw three controls for each cell. Our frequently matched algorithm is slightly modified from scenario #1 to now include the additional categories, 9 in total now (=3 age categories ★ 3 length of stay categories), which require matching. Adding additional characteristics can get unwieldy quite quickly as we then need additional tables stratifying on the characteristics. For example, adding a third characteristic with 3 levels would require 27 cells in the contingency tables to match on (=3★3★3).

Case–control studies have important advantages, especially when compared to the other epidemiological study designs. Of primary importance, the studies are quick, inexpensive, and straightforward to conduct. In other words, they are efficient studies. They can be conducted with smaller samples than their counterpart cross-sectional or cohort studies, as well as allow the examination of multiple risk factors concurrently. When the outcome is rare, or has a long latency, case–control studies are particularly advantageous.

Table 7.2 Frequency matching in a hypothetical case-control study by "age" and "length of stay"

Length of stay	Age		
	<40 years	*41–60 years*	*>60 years*
<5 days	5 cases	10 cases	5 cases
	15 controls	30 controls	15 controls
5–10 days	15 cases	20 cases	5 cases
	45 controls	60 controls	15 controls
>10 days	5 cases	15 cases	20 cases
	15 controls	45 controls	60 controls

Case data are hypothetical and matched 1:3 to controls.

On the other hand, the drawbacks to a case-control study may offset the advantages. Despite being straightforward to assemble, careful consideration of the study design is required to mitigate biases. Unlike a cohort study that can assess *de novo* occurrence of many outcomes, case–control studies by their sampling nature, can only study a single outcome at a time. Combined with the historic assessment of exposure (risk), they are particularly prone to bias that may affect validity. Additionally, while there is an implied timeframe to the study, this cannot be explicitly measured, therefore incidence cannot be calculated and estimates of risk are indirect. Finally, the representativeness of the sample to the source population must ensure that both cases and controls do not differ with respect to the exposure from the source population.

In the case of secondary data derived from an EHR, the underlying population represents a cohort; therefore a cohort design will often be preferable. However, if a case-control study is the only option, for example, because there is a cost involved with abstracting the medical records for each subject, the study may fall under a nested case–control or a case–cohort design (discussed later) and is dependent upon the availability of control sampling from the entire EHR.

As an example of a case-control study, we will build upon the neonatal example used already in this chapter. The research question remains the same: how does very low birthweight impact the risk of staph infection in the NICU? In the cohort study, we recruited neonates admitted to the NICU identified from the EHR and followed them through their stay. The cohort study was able to obtain a measure of incidence – specifically staph infection – necessary to form a conclusion about how the risk of infection may be attributed to birthweight. Suppose in this population staph infection was rare and there was a cost involved to medical record abstraction precluding a cohort design. In this case, a case-control study will be more efficient. The study begins by sampling infants who had a staph infection in the NICU, where the outcome has either occurred, deemed a case, or not occurred, deemed a control (Figure 7.14). All cases can be included in the analytic dataset as the outcome is presumed to be rare and a random sampling of controls

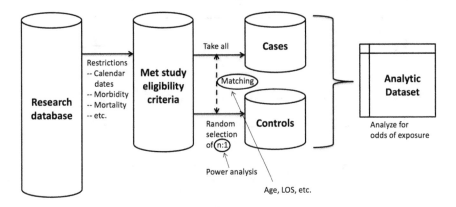

Figure 7.14 A case–control analytic dataset.

is subsequently obtained. The exact ratio of controls to cases (n:1) is determined *a priori* by the power analysis. Additionally, during the sampling phase, common confounders, such as gestational age, can also be matched, although matching on many confounders may severely limit the pool of controls and result in over-matching. Once our sample is obtained, and we can assess for a diagnosis of very low birthweight by "looking back" in the obstetrical or neonatal EHR for such documentation. With the exposure assessed, the groups can be compared with the expectation of lower birthweight in the case group and greater birthweight in the control group. Code #7.3 in Appendix 2 depicts example code for assembling a case–control sample from the research database with the potential for matching.

Other observational study types

Cross-sectional, cohort, and case–control studies are the cornerstones of analytic observational epidemiology, and the sampling strategies are compared visually in Figure 7.15. The cross-sectional study can only ascertain what has occurred at a given snapshot in time, whereas the cohort follows participants until some pre-specified point in the time occurs. The case–control is sampled by the outcome at a single point in time, although the outcomes may have occurred at any point historically. There are other study designs relevant to EHR research that the researcher should be familiar with.

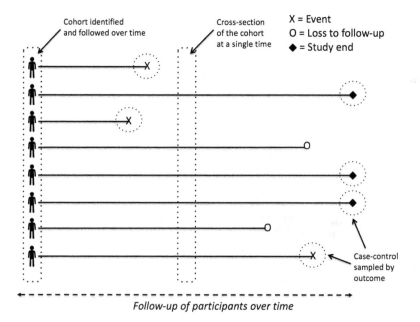

Figure 7.15 Recruiting a population of patients by exposure (cohort), outcome (case–control), or a single point in time (cross-sectional).

In a *case-crossover* study, also known as a case-only study, only cases are re-cruited. This study is useful when the exposure immediately precedes the out-come, such as an inpatient "coding" and the subsequent risk of mortality. The case serves as his or her control until the event happens. When a defined cohort is available, but the entire population is not needed or accessible, an embedded case-control study can be conducted that samples cases and controls from within the cohort. Indeed, this is the premise behind conceiving the EHR as an open cohort. If the controls are selected at the time each case occurs in the cohort, the embedded study is referred to as a *nested case-control* study using incidence-density sampling. Mechanically, this entails sampling a control within a date range from when the case is diagnosed with an outcome. Code #7.3 in Appendix 2 can be adapted for incidence-density sampling by including the diagnosis date in the "matching characteristics" section, thereby matching controls that had hospital visit dates overlapping with the case. If desired, the control can be further matched to the case on potential confounding characteristics, such as age or length of stay, however, the pool of available controls may shrink drastically using incidence-density sampling. If the controls are selected at baseline within a cohort, as op-posed to when the cases arise, the embedded study is referred to as a *case–cohort study*. Mechanically, this entails sampling all the controls at once from the start of the cohort, essentially creating a subcohort of noncases. In a case–cohort study, some of the controls may go on to become cases over time and are handled by analyzing those controls as cases, which suggests that the power calculations need to account for this potentiality.

Occasionally, the researcher may be interested in contextual attributes in ad-dition to individual attributes. A contextual attribute defines a characteristic that links individuals together, such as inpatients who share a room or outpatients who live in the same neighborhood. If these contextual units are related to the measure of risk, for example, if the risk of a healthcare-associated infection is influenced by nonsterile surfaces in a hospital room, then the contextual units must be accounted for statistically as the observations may no longer be independent of one another. Contextual attributes may be aggregates of individuals or truly ecological. Study-ing contextual attributes allows the researcher to ask questions such as "Do patient rooms impact the risk of infection," "Are there individual differences in patient risk after accounting for room-to-room differences," and "Do patient room differences modify individual differences" (Hox, 2002). When only the contextual attributes are studied, the study design is referred to as *ecological*. When contextual and individ-ual attributes are studied together, the design is referred to as *multilevel* or *hierarchical*.

Lastly, a patient may provide multiple measurements during the study period, termed a *repeated measures*, or *longitudinal*, design (Figure 7.16). There are three different longitudinal data-generating processes. In a traditional repeated meas-ures study, the outcome may occur more than once and is referred to as a *repeated outcome measures* study. For example, an inpatient hospital study examining blood pressure as the outcome will have many measurements over the duration of the stay. In other cases, the outcome may occur only once, but the exposure (or other covariates) may have multiple measurements. This may be the case if inpatient

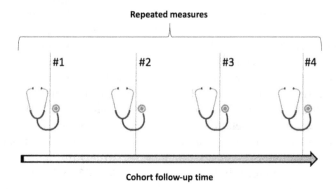

Figure 7.16 An example of repeated outcome measures by study visit.

mortality is the outcome with blood pressure serving now as the exposure. Finally, there could be a situation where both the exposure (or other covariates) and the outcome are measured repeatedly. Often repeated measures occur within the context of a cohort or longitudinal survey (Figure 7.7).

Visits in a prospectively recruited longitudinal study typically occur at defined time points, for example, every three months or semi-annually. In contrast, when working with secondary data derived from an EHR, a patient encounter may occur at irregular times or there may be missing visits as discussed in Chapter 6. This presents a complication for the analysis of the repeated outcome measures, as they have not been occurring on the same basis for all subjects: they are not *balanced* measurements. This is especially likely in outpatient studies or if examining multiple hospitalizations over time, as these events may occur at arbitrary times. On the other hand, repeated measurement studies within a single inpatient admission may have regularly recurring measurements that are balanced. All these other observational study types require special techniques for analysis and are not covered in detail in this book, although longitudinal and multilevel data are briefly discussed in Chapter 11.

When assembling a repeated measure analytic dataset, the data need to be in long format for analytic purposes. This is opposed to the wide format used thus far in the book. In long format, each outcome measure is treated as a separate observation, and thus one patient contributes multiple observations to the dataset. If the cohort analytic dataset is currently in wide format, Code #7.4 in Appendix 2 may be used to transform the data to long format.

Study sample size and power analysis

A study is powered to detect a difference between groups that is not attributable due to chance alone. The ability of a study to detect a difference when in fact there is one is known as the *power* of the study. For no specific reason other than historic precedent, power has become standardized as a *de facto* 80%. This means on average, 80% of the time if there is a true difference in the groups with relation to some measure, the hypothesis testing will yield a correct conclusion. The converse to detecting a true difference when there is one is not detecting a difference in the absence of one. This is a by-product of the significance level of the hypothesis test, and again, for historic reasons, has generally been set to 95%. On average 95% of the time, if there is no difference, the hypothesis testing will not erroneously conclude there is one. As can be seen, studies tend to err on the conservative side of not detecting a difference.

The 80% and 95% levels are defined by the two types of errors than can occur in hypothesis testing: false negatives and false positives. A false negative, also known as a type II error defined by the Greek letter β, suggests that there was in fact a difference in the population, but the study failed to detect it. If an acceptable type II error rate is 20%, then the power of the study is one minus beta or 80%. A false positive, also known as a type I error defined by the Greek letter α, suggests that there was not a difference in the population but the study erroneously concluded there was. If an acceptable type I error rate is 5%, then the ability to not detect a difference in the absence of one is one minus alpha, or 95%.

Lowering α or β, and thus lowering the risk of type I or II error rates, means you are asking for greater confidence in your answer. Requesting greater confidence by increasing the precision in your answer translates to more data points, which often means more people or more measurements of those people. For example, going from a standard $\alpha = 0.05$ to $\alpha = 0.01$ will increase sample size demands as will going from a $\beta = 0.20$ (80% power) to $\beta = 0.10$ (90% power). Likewise, a weaker effect will also require a larger sample. Figures 7.17a and b depict the relationship between varying sample sizes and values of α and β, respectively, calculated for Pearson correlations of two continuous variables across a range of effect sizes.

With these definitions in mind, it is possible to calculate the size of a study based on α, β, and some information about the expected outcome and study population. If the outcome is continuous and the researcher is interested in exploring the mean difference between groups, a sample size based on a *t*-test can be calculated. The researcher would need to specify the mean difference in outcome based on the hypothesized exposure effect and the standard deviation of the population. In the presence of a case-control study or cohort with a dichotomous (incident) outcome, the sample size may be calculated based on a proportion test. The researcher would need to specify the proportion with each outcome based on the hypothesized exposure effect, and perhaps the difference in group sizes: the ratio of cases to controls. Calculating the sample size does not require purchasing specialized software; it can be done by hand, using the integrated power calculators in the researchers' statistical software, or from one of the freely available calculators on the Internet (Dupont & Plummer, 2014). As always, when in doubt consult a bio(statistician) or epidemiologist.

Sample size should be calculated in advance when conducting a clinical trial. When calculating sample size under an observational study design, the calculations mentioned earlier presume an unbiased effect: that is, the study is free of confounding, measurement error, and selection bias (see Chapter 9). This is to

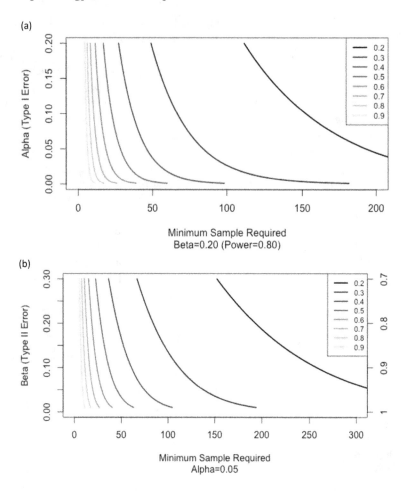

Figure 7.17(a & b) The relationship between varying sample sizes and values of alpha (a) and beta (b), calculated for Pearson correlations of two continuous variables across A range of effect sizes.

make the calculation simple and tractable but rarely matches the reality of observational studies. In secondary data analysis of the EHR, the patient population already exists in a database. Thus, the utility of these calculations is even more questionable (Hernan, 2022).

The EHR as a secondary data source may contain many thousands, if not millions, of records. Consequently, the issue is one of the precision of the estimates obtained. For exceedingly rare outcomes – such as an incidence of one per million – the precision of the corresponding disease measure will be quite poor in a single institution EHR. This study should still be undertaken, however, as subsequent meta-analyses will improve the precision should additional EHR databases become available (Hernan, 2022). More commonly the issue in large observational databases is one of an overpowered study, rather than an underpowered one. This suggests that even minor differences between groups will result in a statistically significant test result because of the large number of people in the study and assuming a somewhat more common outcome. This is not to suggest that the error rates in the study change – they are fixed – rather the hypothesis testing has the potential to discover small differences between groups that may not have clinical relevance. It is up to the researcher therefore to determine if these small differences are meaningful. For example, consider a finding of a 1 mm of Hg difference in blood pressure between groups. While this may be a true statistical difference, this is not clinically relevant. The magnitude, or size, of the estimate and its accompanying error is more important than the presence of statistical significance. Yet despite the large number of observations typical in an EHR, sample size can dwindle rapidly if the outcome is rare, there are complex study inclusion and exclusion criteria, or the study is a multilevel or longitudinal design. Rather than calculate a sample size, we can use the data at hand to calculate the power of the study by essentially reversing the sample size calculations if desired. In fact, sample size calculators often have accompanying power calculators. However, the decision to undertake an EHR study should not be based on sample size or power calculations alone.

Note

1 A cohort can also be recruited in this manner, but importantly for a cross-sectional study, we ignore any time component, viewing the entire hospitalization as a single event in time. In other words, while the data may be the same, our analytic perspective and goals help to define the study type.

References

Dupont WD, Plummer WD. PS: Power and Sample Size Calculation. Vanderbilt University Department of Biostatistics. https://biostat.app.vumc.org/wiki/Main/PowerSampleSize (accessed December 2, 2021), 2014.

Hernán MA. Causal analyses of existing databases: no power calculations required. J Clin Epidemiol. 2022 Apr;144:203–205.

Hox J. Multilevel Analysis: Techniques and Applications. Mahwah, NJ: Lawrence Erlbaum Associates, Inc., 2002.

Lesko CR, Fox MP, Edwards JK. A framework for descriptive epidemiology. Am J Epidemiol. 2022 Nov 19;191(12):2063–2070.

Miettinen O. Theoretical Epidemiology. New York, NY: John Wiley & Sons, Inc., 1985. p. 79.

R Core Team. R: A Language and Environment for Statistical Computing. Vienna,: R Foundation for Statistical Computing, 2020. https://www.R-project.org/

Sackett DL, Richardson WS, Rosenberg WM, Haynes RB. Evidence Based Medicine: How to Practice and Teach EBM. New York, NY: Churchill Livingstone, 1997.

Venables WN, Ripley BD.. Modern Applied Statistics with S. 4th ed. New York, NY: Springer, 2002.

8 Epidemiologic Measures

If proper study design is one of the tenets of epidemiology, another is the metrics used to understand disease burden and risk. Epidemiological measures of disease can broadly be categorized into two classes: measures of disease frequency, or occurrence, and measures of disease association, or risk. Measures of disease frequency include incidence, survival (the inverse of incidence), and prevalence. Respectively, these terms refer to developing disease *de novo*, not developing disease, and presence of disease. Measures of disease association include ratio–based measures and difference–based measures. A ratio–based measure relates developing disease to not developing disease, whereas a difference–based measure quantifies the excess cases of a disease.

Before discussing each of these measures in detail, we need to define several terms used throughout this chapter. When studying disease, or any health state for that matter, the most basic measure is a *count* of the number of cases of the health state. This serves as the numerator in many *proportion* measures, where the denominator is the number of people in a population. For example, if 1% of the population carries a disease, this means that the count is one person with the disease (numerator) for every 100 people at risk of having the disease (denominator). Note how the numerator is a component of the denominator, as the cases arise from the population who are at risk for the health state. The count may also be used in *ratio* measures, where the numerator is not a subset of the denominator. For example, in a population of 100, if a disease affects 10 people and leaves 90 healthy, a ratio measure would be 1:9, or about 11%.

When the denominator in a proportion is not the number of people in a population but incorporates a measure of time that people are in this population, the measure is referred to as a *rate*. For example, if instead of 100 people in the denominator, we know that 100 people were followed for 5 years each (meaning the denominator is 100 people × 5 years = 500 person-years) and 10 cases of a disease developed, the proportion measure becomes 5 cases per 500 person-years (equivalent to 1 case per 100 person-years). Person-time is more thoroughly discussed later in the chapter.

In many measures of disease morbidity and mortality, the formulas include a multiplier to present the rates per 1,000 or per 100,000 people. For example, infant mortality rates are "the number of infant deaths that occur for every 1,000

DOI: 10.4324/9781003258872-11

live births" (CDC, 2021). We calculate the infant mortality rate by dividing the number of infant deaths by the number of live births, then multiplying by 1,000. The use of a multiplier, such as 1,000, is to present the statistic in a consistent, meaningful, and intuitive way. Suppose we have a disease that causes mortality in 100 individuals in a population of 20,000. The crude death rate would equal $100/20,000 = 0.005$ deaths per person. This is not an intuitive number as it is difficult to appreciate 0.005 people. In such cases, it is common to apply a multiplier to make the number more meaningful. This multiplier is in some sense arbitrary, although common multipliers include 1,000 and 100,000. Mortality is often presented as per 1,000 people, so in our example, we can multiply $0.005 \times 1,000$ to arrive at five deaths per 1,000 people. That statistic is more interpretable because we can intuitively grasp five people.

Measures of frequency

Prevalence

Prevalence is the count of all existing cases of a disease or condition and may be determined for a specific point in time, known as the *point prevalence*, or for a period of time, known as the *period prevalence*. The difference between point prevalence and period prevalence depends on how the data were ascertained. For example, if a researcher inquired about current cases of the disease on a given day, this would be a point estimate. On the other hand, if the researcher inquired about historic cases of the disease, the estimate would represent a period prevalence. Period prevalence may include current cases as well, dependent upon the period, and often the word prevalence is used without the timeframe descriptor to avoid this potential ambiguity. The prevalence of a condition is frequently ascertained through a cross-sectional study, such as the prevalence of very low birthweight infants in a neonatal intensive care unit (NICU) on a given day. As the cross-sectional study by nature assesses the current state of health at a specific time point, prevalence is inherently measured. The point versus period delineation in the definition also aligns with that of a cross-sectional study that sampled at either a single time point or for a historic time period.

The numerator in a prevalence calculation is the count of existing cases of some disease or condition and the denominator is the population at that point in time. Although prevalence is a common and useful measure for determining the burden of a disease in a population, it does little to address the etiology of the disease. Importantly, the type of outcome studied affects prevalence calculations. Diseases that are acute and have a short course will lead to lower prevalence estimates as compared to diseases that are chronic and have a long duration. For example, influenza often has a shorter, self-limiting course and therefore any survey of prevalent flu cases in the population will tend to underestimate the burden of the disease, whereas surveying for a chronic disease, such as HIV infection will indicate a greater number of prevalent cases as individuals are living near full lives due to highly effective antiretroviral therapy.

As a didactic example, suppose we are interested in assessing maternal vaccination during pregnancy and have access to an obstetrical EHR that contains prenatal records through delivery (Figure 8.1). In this small population of eight women, six received prenatal vaccination, corresponding to a 75% prevalence of vaccination at delivery.

Incidence

Incidence is the count of new cases of disease over some time and is estimated through a cohort study. There are two types of incidence measures: cumulative incidence and incidence rate. The most basic measure of incidence is a proportion, termed the *cumulative incidence*, and defines the proportion of new events in the population. An example of cumulative incidence is the percentage of new cases of disease in a given population during the past year. The corollary to cumulative incidence is *survival*. If incidence defines the probability of an event occurring, survival represents its inverse, namely the probability of an event not occurring. Stated another way, survival equals one minus the cumulative incidence.

Although the cumulative incidence is straightforward to interpret, it does not readily consider the timing of when the case arose or the occurrence of censoring: the follow-up time. A more robust measure of incidence considers time contributed by each person in the cohort and is termed the *incidence rate*. An example of

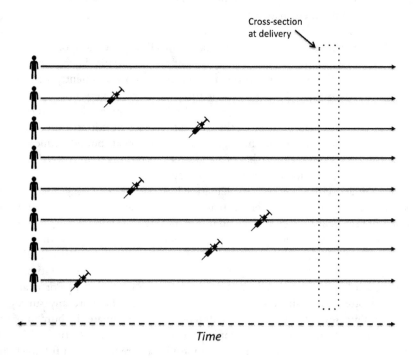

Figure 8.1 Calculating prevalence of maternal vaccination at delivery.

incidence rate is the count of new cases of disease per person-time contributed to the study. Since an explicit measure of follow-up time is needed, incidence rates are often presented within the context of a cohort study.

When calculating incidence, we exclude prevalent cases as well as persons who are not at risk for disease. For example, consider a hypothetical population of 1,000,000 people where 50% are cisgender men and 50% are cisgender women. If we were calculating the cumulative incidence of cervical cancer during the past calendar year, we would not include the 500,000 cisgender men in the denominator. We would further exclude any women who already have cervical cancer or do not have a cervix in the calculation.

Both measures of incidence – cumulative incidence and incidence rate – start with a count of new cases as the numerator, but they differ in the denominators. The denominator in cumulative incidence is based on the size of the initial at-risk population, whereas in an incidence rate (sometimes called an *incidence density*), the denominator is based on person-time. Person-time is calculated from the time to an event – disease occurrence – or the follow-up time to a nonevent – loss to follow-up or study conclusion. As each person contributes a varying amount of time to the cohort due to developing the outcome or censoring, follow-up time needs to be calculated for everyone in the study and then tallied to arrive at the total observation time among the population. Figure 8.2 is a hypothetical cohort of eight infants followed for one-year postpartum with a total follow-up time of 73 months.

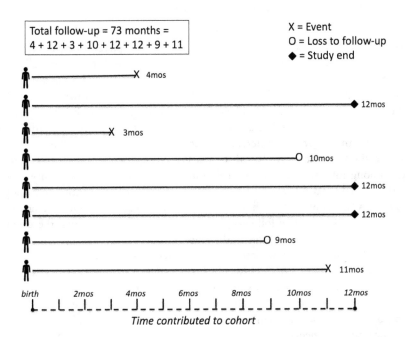

Figure 8.2 Calculating follow-up time.

Incidence need not focus on new cases of disease. The incidence can focus on new events of any type. When the new event is death the measure of incidence is known as the *mortality rate.*[1] When the outcome is an acute health state such as a food-borne illness, an *attack rate* can be specified. The calculation of these measures is the same as for cumulative incidence if person-time is not a component of the denominator or is the same as for incidence rate if person-time is a component of the denominator.

The example cohort study presented in the last chapter examined very low birth-weight infants in the NICU and their relationship to incident cases of staph infection during hospitalization. Suppose we now follow these infants post-discharge for one year until some new event occurs (Figure 8.2). These data are abstracted from the inpatient obstetrical EHR and then linked to an outpatient pediatric EHR for follow-up. The study commences at delivery, and we follow all infants through one-year of age, which concludes the study. The cumulative incidence proportion equals the number of new cases of the event divided by the total population = 3/8 = 0.38, or 38 per 100 infants (38%). Survival, or the cumulative probability of not having the event under study = 1 − 0.38 = 0.62, or 62 per 100 infants (62%). The incidence rate equals the number of new cases of the event divided by the follow-up time contributed by each infant = 3/73 = 0.04 cases per person-month. To express this in the more common person-years, we can divide the incidence rate denominator by 12 months in a year = 3/(73/12) = 0.48 events per person-year.

Choice of cumulative incidence versus incidence rate

Research preferences as well as characteristics of the cohort often drive which measure of incidence to calculate. If follow-up is complete, a cumulative incidence proportion is an intuitive way to present incidence. If follow-up is incomplete or time-to-event is of importance, an incidence rate will be the least biased measure. In general, the incidence rate is the more flexible measure.

Since both the cumulative incidence and incidence rate have the same numerator − counts of an event − they are related to one another; it is the denominator of the measure that drives the difference. Generally, the cumulative incidence will be less than the incidence rate. Recall the earlier example of incident cases of some event among infants where the annual cumulative incidence proportion was 0.38 and the annual incidence rate was 0.48. This relationship is most intuitively grasped by a contrived example of a cohort study that follows eight individuals over a one-year period with complete follow-up (Figure 8.3). If we assume that the event of interest occurs at the conclusion of the study (event Y), the absolute value (while ignoring the units of the cumulative incidence) will equal the incidence rate, as the denominators are both equal. However, if the event of interest occurs at any time before the conclusion of the study (event X), the incorporation of the time-to-event will shrink the denominator, thereby increasing the calculated value of the rate. The incorporation of censoring will further shrink the denominator. While cumulative incidence can also incorporate time-to-event and censoring, this requires methods such as survival analysis that are not covered in this text.

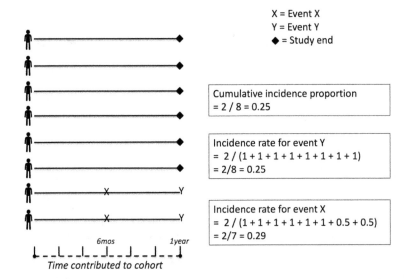

Figure 8.3 Relationship of cumulative incidence to the incidence rate in a contrived cohort.

When calculating any measure of incidence that involves censoring, there is a core assumption of the independence of censoring and survival. For example, in Figure 8.2, assume that that the two "loss to follow-up" participants withdrew from the study because they were ill, presumably from the event of interest. Our measure of incidence would be underestimated; the opposite would be true if the participants who withdrew were healthier. An additional assumption is the cohort was not subject to secular trends, such as recent developments in effective treatments at some point during the cohort.

Relationship of prevalence and incidence

Prevalence and incidence are closely related, and in fact can be represented mathematically by the formula shown in Figure 8.4. The left-hand side of the formula simplifies to only "prevalence" when the outcome is rare, about 10% or less. This relationship can be visually demonstrated. Assume that the incidence of some condition is 1% and the mean duration of the condition to cure or death is 5 of the same time units (the units of time are irrelevant for this exercise). After some time has elapsed to stabilize the population, the prevalence will be approximately 5% (Figure 8.5).

$$\frac{\text{Prevalence}}{1 - \text{Prevalence}} = \text{Incidence} * \text{Duration}$$

Figure 8.4 Mathematical relationship of prevalence to incidence.

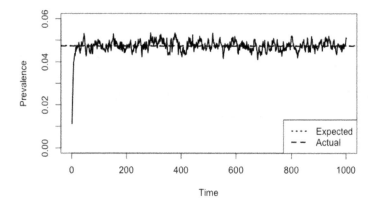

Figure 8.5 Simulation of a hypothetical population with a 1% incident disease and mean duration of five time-steps to resolution. Expected prevalence = 0.01 × 5 = 0.05, or 5%.

Another way to think about the balance between incidence and prevalence is through analogy (Figure 8.6). The container represents all individuals that have some condition (A; the prevalence). The people being added into the container represent new cases (B; the incidence), and people leaving represent the termination of the condition (C). The balance of people will be determined by changes to incidence and prevalence (D). More people in the container, and thus a higher prevalence, can be attributed to an increased incidence or increased survival (B). Fewer people in the container, and thus a lower prevalence, can be attributed to a decrease in incidence (for example, due to prophylactic measures), decreased survival (a particularly severe disease), or cure (C). Infection with HIV is a historic example of a disease with increasing prevalence with approximately steady incidence, mainly due to antiretroviral therapy and more individuals living longer with infection (CDC, 2022).

Lastly, as mentioned in Chapter 6, it may be easy to conflate incident versus prevalent health conditions in the EHR. The date that accompanies an individual diagnosis may not reflect the actual date of disease onset but rather a diagnosis date or the last time the diagnostic code was modified. This central challenge has been observed with notifiable disease surveillance in public health (Goldstein, Quick & Burstyn, 2021). Stale diagnoses are quite possible, and a condition deemed prevalent when the EHR data were retrieved may have already been resolved. Likewise, a new or incident diagnosis may not in fact be a new condition, but rather just reflect a new EHR entry recorded by the clinician. The use of a wash-out period, such as the prior two years, may aid in delineating incident versus prevalent diagnoses in the EHR.

Standardization

The measures presented in this chapter are all unadjusted for potential confounding factors: this will be treated in detail in Chapter 11. However, suppose we are

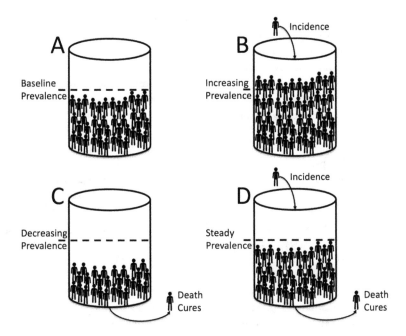

Figure 8.6 Relationship between incidence and prevalence.

Adapted from Gordis Epidemiology, 6th edition, Celantano DD, Szklo M, The Occurrence of Disease: I. Disease Surveillance and Measures of Morbidity, Copyright © 2020, with permission from Elsevier.

measuring the mortality rate in the NICU, and in this setting, mortality is highly dependent upon gestational age. A crude mortality rate might be misleading, not just for understanding mortality in the studied NICU, but especially if we wish to compare across multiple NICUs where the distribution of gestational ages could vary substantially depending on the level of care provided. As such, we may wish to stratify or standardize the measures of disease frequency by a second variable, such as gestational age. Stratification is used when we would like to describe how mortality differs by gestational age and standardization is used when we would like to control for the effects of the gestational age on mortality, thereby treating gestational age as a nuisance variable. Mortality, incidence, and prevalence measures can all be standardized, most commonly by age. The techniques to perform direct and indirect standardization can be found in most intermediate epidemiology textbooks.

Measures of association

Although descriptive epidemiology is valuable for many reasons (Fox et al., 2022), as clinical researchers, we may wish to describe attributes of the population that lead to these conditions, in other words, the search for causes. Measures of association are primarily used in outcome etiology research as they allow the researcher to make claims about risk or protective factors that can ultimately improve patient health through intervention. The type of study influences the type of measure of association, and therefore this section is presented within the study design context. As an aside, uses of EHR data for other purposes, such as quality improvement activities and health services delivery, are presented in Chapter 12.

The terminology used in this section will be specific to classical epidemiology, where there is a dichotomous exposure, either present or absent, and a dichotomous outcome, either diseased or healthy. Continuing with the very low birthweight example from the last chapter, our exposure is very low birthweight and our outcome is staph infection in the NICU. For the purposes of the equations shown, let "E" represent the exposure, "D" represent the outcome, "+" represent presence of the exposure or outcome, and "−" represent absence of the exposure or outcome. The notation "|" means *given*, such that the expression "D+ | E+" corresponds to the presence of disease given the presence of the exposure.

All ratio measures are interpreted relative to the value of 1.0. If the numerator is the same as the denominator the fraction equates to 1.0, corresponding to no difference between the groups. If the ratio is greater than 1.0, this means the group comprising the numerator has a larger effect than the group comprising the denominator. Vice versa, if the ratio is less than 1.0, the group comprising the denominator has a larger effect than the group comprising the numerator. The interpretation of these effect estimates depends on the ratio measure itself.

Cross-sectional measures

The basis of the cross-sectional study is a measure of prevalence; therefore, the measure of association is the *prevalence ratio*. This measure can establish whether some state or condition is more prevalent in one group versus another. For example, in the neonatal study, suppose the cross-section of the NICU was taken on a given month in the year 2022. At this time, we know which infants were very low birthweight as well as which infants had a staph infection during this period. Overall prevalence of infection in the NICU can readily be calculated and we can stratify prevalence estimates by birthweight. The prevalence ratio is thus the ratio between these two measures (Figure 8.7).

Suppose the one-month cross-section obtained the following sample. Among 1,000 neonates admitted to the NICU, 800 were ≥1,500 grams (not very low birthweight). Among these 800 neonates, 25 developed a staph infection. Of the 200 very low birthweight neonates (<1,500 grams), 35 developed a staph infection. The prevalence of disease given the absence of exposure was 25/800 = 0.03 (or 3%), and the prevalence of disease given exposure was 35/200 = 0.18 (or 18%).

Depending on how we wish to set up our comparison, we can calculate a prevalence ratio comparing infants ≥1,500 grams to infants <1,500 grams or

$$\text{Prevalence Ratio} = \frac{\text{Prevalence}(D+ \mid E+)}{\text{Prevalence}(D+ \mid E-)}$$

Figure 8.7 Prevalence ratio formula.

comparing infants <1,500 grams to infants ≥1,500 grams. Assuming the former, the prevalence ratio equals $(25/800)/(35/200) = 0.03/0.18 = 0.17$. Assuming the latter, the prevalence ratio equals $(35/200)/(25/800) = 0.18/0.03 = 6.00$. It should be noted that $6.00 = 1/0.17$, allowing for rounding. In other words, to switch the reference group, we can simply take the inverse of the calculation.

There is a qualitative and a quantitative interpretation of these measures. Focusing on comparing not very low birthweight to very low birthweight infants, as the fraction is less than 1.0, this suggests that the prevalence of disease was greater in the denominator, which corresponds to the exposed, very low birthweight neonates. The specific value of 0.17 means that infants ≥1,500 grams were on average 0.17 times as likely to also have the prevalent infection during this one-month cross-section, compared to infants <1,500 grams. This can also be stated as a percentage by subtracting the estimate from $1 = 1.00 - 0.17 = 0.83$, or 83%. Not very low birthweight neonates had an average 83% reduction for staph infection in the one-month cross-section, compared to the very low birthweight group.

While prevalence ratios are easy to calculate, their utility in identifying causal effects is limited. Essentially, we are positing that the prevalence represents the incidence because we are trying to make a connection between very low birthweight and the development of new cases of infection among neonates in the NICU. By revisiting the definition of prevalence, we must satisfy two conditions for this to be true: (1) the disease must be relatively rare (~5% or less) and (2) the duration of the disease must not vary by exposure (i.e., among those with a staph infection, the disease course is unlikely to be different by birthweight). Additionally, prevalence underrepresents diseases of acute duration, such as many acute infectious conditions, and temporality in cross-sectional studies cannot be assured. Therefore, the potential for this *incidence–prevalence bias* is large since the prevalence poorly approximates the incidence. Consequently, prevalence ratios are not frequently used.

Cohort measures

As the basis of the cohort study is a measure of incidence, the measure of association is a ratio of the incidences between the exposed and unexposed groups. Conceptually, if the exposure was unrelated to the outcome, the incidence, or number of new cases of the outcome, in the exposed group will approximately equal the incidence in the unexposed group allowing for some margin of random variability. This ratio measure can directly estimate the risk of new disease between the exposed and unexposed groups, and therefore is known as the *relative risk*. Unlike the prevalence ratio which only approximates the incidence, the relative risk is a direct measure of incidence and consequently is less subject to the biases present in other measures of association that examine causal effects. As the basis of the relative risk is a comparison of incidence between exposure groups, this relative risk can either be measured as a cumulative incidence proportion if we assume complete follow-up, termed the *risk ratio*, or an incidence rate if incidence cannot be approximated by a simple proportion, termed the *rate ratio*. In either case, the interpretation of the relative risk is similar.

Table 8.1 A cohort study contingency table

Independent variable	Dependent variable		Totals
	Disease (D+)	No disease (D−)	
Exposed (E+)	a	b	$a + b$
Unexposed (E−)	c	d	$c + d$
Totals	$a + c$	$b + d$	$a + b + c + d$

Calculating cumulative incidence by group can readily be accomplished by using a contingency table (also known as a 2 × 2 table) when the exposure and outcome are categorical. Table 8.1 depicts a standard setup for a cohort study contingency table[2] where we let *a* represent the number of exposed individuals who developed disease, *b* represent the number of exposed individuals who did not develop disease, *c* represent the number of unexposed individuals who developed disease, and *d* represent the number of unexposed individuals who did not develop disease. Note the marginal totals define the total numbers exposed $(a + b)$, unexposed $(c + d)$, diseased $(a + c)$, not diseased $(b + d)$, and the entire population $(a + b + c + d)$.

As a reminder, the cumulative incidence proportion is calculated as disease count divided by the at-risk population. If we calculate the cumulative incidence measures relative to exposure, the calculations become incidence(D+ | E+) and incidence(D+ | E−), where "D+ | E+" is presence of disease given presence of the exposure, and "D+ | E− "is presence of disease absent the exposure. The relative risk is the ratio of these two measures (Figure 8.8).

Now suppose the results of the neonatal cohort are as follows (Table 8.2; these data are intentionally different from the cross-sectional study). Among 1,000 neonates recruited to the cohort, 150 were very low birthweight. Among these infants, 30 infants were diagnosed with an infection before the study ended. Among the 850 not very low birthweight infants, 65 were diagnosed with an infection. The cumulative incidence in the exposed group is 30/150 = 0.20 (or 20%), and in the unexposed group is. 65/785 = 0.08 (or 8%). The ratio of these two measures corresponding to the cumulative incidence relative risk equals (30/150)/(65/785) = 0.20/0.08 = 2.5.

As before, there is a qualitative and a quantitative interpretation of the measure. As the fraction is greater than 1.0, this suggests that the incidence of disease was greater in the exposed, very low birthweight group. The specific value of 2.5 means that infants with a birthweight <1,500 grams were on average 2.5 times as likely to have a staph infection during their NICU stay compared to infants with

$$\text{Relative Risk} = \frac{\text{Incidence(D+ | E+)}}{\text{Incidence(D+ | E-)}} = \frac{a / (a+b)}{c / (c+d)}$$

Figure 8.8 Cumulative incidence relative risk formula for calculating a risk ratio.

Table 8.2 The very low birthweight and staph infection cohort contingency table

Independent variable	Dependent variable		Totals	Follow-up
	Infection (D+)	No Infection (D−)		
<1,500 grams (E+)	30	120	150	4,280 days
≥1,500 grams (E−)	65	785	850	17,020 days
Totals	95	905	1,000	21,300 days

a birthweight ≥1,500 grams. This can also be stated as a percentage by subtracting 1.0 from the estimate = 2.5 − 1.0 = 1.5, or 150%: the very low birthweight group had an averaged 150% increase in incident disease during their NICU stay, compared to the not very low birthweight group. While the interpretation may sound similar to the prevalence ratio, they are inherently different measures.

Calculating a rate ratio based on the incidence rates for the exposed and unexposed groups requires follow-up time information on time-to-event and time-to-censoring for the neonates in the cohort. Conceptually, if the exposure was not associated with the outcome, the time-to-event will be approximately equal between the exposure groups. From Table 8.2, we have assumed a certain distribution of incident cases of disease contingent upon exposure. Suppose we have information that includes the day of infection relative to their admission date (time-to-event among those with the outcome) or the day of discharge, transfer, or death relative to their admission date (time-to-censoring among those without the outcome). Assuming no loss to follow-up, follow-up would conclude at the study end for infants that did not have an infection; however, for children that developed an infection, the amount of follow-up time is their day of hospitalization upon diagnosis. Instead of the marginal total for exposed and unexposed serving as the denominator for each of the incidence measures, we now would have a measure of person-time serving as the denominators for each of the incidence measures.

Adding to the information we have from Table 8.2, suppose the follow-up time of the neonatal cohort was as follows. Among the 150 infants in the very low birthweight group, we had 4,280 person-days of follow-up, and among the 850 infants in the not very low birthweight group, we had 17,020 person-days of follow-up. The incidence rate in the exposed group is 30/4,280 = 0.007 cases per person-day, and in the unexposed group is 65/17,020 = 0.004 cases per person-day. The ratio of these two measures (i.e., the incidence rate ratio) equals (30/4,280)/(65/17,020) = 0.007/0.004 = 1.75, again a strong risk factor for staph infection among those with a birthweight <1,500 grams. The overall incidence was 95 cases for 21,300 person-days = 0.004 cases per person-day. To express per 1,000 person-days, we can multiply by 1,000 = 0.004 × 1,000 = 4 cases per 1,000 NICU days. Other units of time are calculated in the same manner.

Regardless of the type of incidence relative risk calculated, it is a powerful tool for comparing risks between groups. Yet it does not answer the question of how much risk can be removed from the population by some intervention, such as

$$\textbf{Attributable Risk Difference} = \text{Incidence}(D+ \mid E+) - \text{Incidence}(D+ \mid E-)$$

$$= (a/(a+b)) - (c/(c+d))$$

$$\textbf{Attributable Risk Proportion} = \frac{\text{Incidence}(D+ \mid E+) - \text{Incidence}(D+ \mid E-)}{\text{Incidence}(D+ \mid E+)}$$

$$= \frac{(a/(a+b)) - (c/(c+d))}{(a/(a+b))} = \frac{RR - 1.0}{RR}$$

Figure 8.9 Cumulative incidence attributable risk formula. RR, relative risk.

minimizing preterm birth (assuming this was the driver of very low birthweight and is achievable). If we wish to answer the question of the excess risk attributable to the exposure (i.e., very low birthweight), we may calculate the *attributable risk*. The attributable risk is the incidence of disease due to the exposure with the background risk of the incidence of disease not due to exposure removed. It can be calculated as an absolute difference or a proportional difference (Figure 8.9). It can be used for both cumulative incidence proportions and incidence rates. When the exposure is a protective factor as opposed to a risk factor, the exposures can be flipped from absent to present in the formulas to avoid negative numbers in the calculations.

Applying these formulas to the results from the earlier cohort study yields an attributable risk difference of $(30/150) - (65/850) = 0.20 - 0.08 = 0.12$, and an attributable risk proportion of $((30/150) - (65/850))/(30/150) = (0.20 - 0.08)/0.20 = 0.60$, or 60%. If we believe very low birthweight was the cause of staph infection, the attributable risk difference suggests that each very low birthweight infant leads to 0.12 extra cases of staph infection. The attributable risk proportion suggests that overall, 60% of staph infections are attributed to very low birthweight. The proportion is the more intuitive measure to comprehend, as it does not consider fractions of people, although we can adjust the multiplier for this measure if desired. For all attributable risk calculations, there is an inherent assumption of the exposure as causally related to the outcome. Suppose it was not very low birthweight that led to a staph infection, but cross-contamination via the healthcare worker. The attributable risk becomes misleading when causality is unclear, therefore it should only be presented if there is substantiating evidence of causality.

Cohort measures: follow-up time

We now take a brief tangent to discuss follow-up time in more detail in cohort studies and its appropriate calculation. A main feature of the cohort study is enforcing temporality of the exposure and outcome. A prospective cohort recruited based on exposure provides stronger evidence that the exposure preceded the

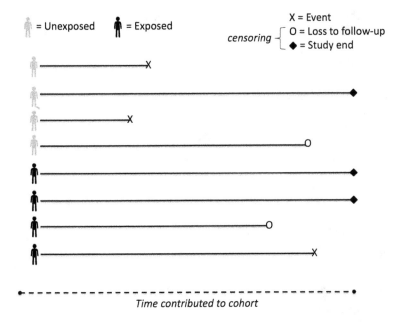

Figure 8.10 Right censoring in a closed cohort.

outcome, especially in the cases of acute diseases. Outcomes with long incubation or latent periods are less clear as there could be reverse causality. In a retrospective cohort derived from the EHR, ensuring temporality becomes more of a challenge and greater care needs to be given when operationalizing the exposure.

Figure 8.10 is a reprint of Figure 7.10 from Chapter 7 and serves as a hypothetical cohort. In a prospective study, the cohort is recruited based on the exposure, hopefully ensuring some degree of temporality, but in a retrospective study, we already have knowledge of the outcome. As such, we must operationalize the exposure correctly to ensure the "at-risk" follow-up period is analyzed correctly. To make this more concrete, assume a cohort is formed to assess new cases of healthcare-acquired infections in a hospital and the exposure is the average number of occupied beds during the patient's length of stay. For simplicity, let us further assume the exposure is dichotomized, split by the upper quartile, where we hypothesize that a higher average number of occupied beds will confer a greater risk for infection. The outcome is straightforward to operationalize in that the patients will either have a diagnosed infection or be right censored.

Naively, the exposure can be operationalized by simply counting the number of occupied beds for each person's length of stay and then performing the dichotomization as previously described once all cohort members' data are collected. However, doing so is problematic because the exposure must precede the outcome. We will need to define the "at-risk" period more accurately for each patient in the cohort. For those that do not experience the outcome and are censored, the "at-risk" period is truly the entire length of follow-up. But for those that have the outcome, the "at-risk" period is not the entire length of stay, but the follow-up period until they were diagnosed with the outcome[3]. This should make intuitive sense, as this is exactly what one does in a prospective study: patients stop contributing to cohort time when they either experience the outcome or are censored. In this example, failure to consider the outcome will result in an information bias; more specifically, a differential misclassification of the exposure. That is, we incorrectly classified the exposure variable based on the outcome. Not only do we need to calculate the exposure with this caveat in mind, but any covariate or part of the analysis that considers follow-up.

In the data management and recoding portion of the analysis we can use an if-then-else statement to define follow-up as follows:

1   For each person in the cohort…

   a   Set cohort_start to the date of cohort enrollment
   b   Set cohort_end to…

       i Date of outcome if they experienced the outcome
       ii Date of censor if they were censored

   c   Calculate follow-up as cohort_end minus cohort_start

2   Repeat step #1 until all cohort members have their follow-up operationalized

To further complicate this, when operationalizing the exposure, one must equally guard against incorporating person-time *prior* to the exposure. This is known as immortal person-time. Immortal time means that a cohort member cannot be considered "at risk" of the outcome prior to receiving the exposure. While this seemingly minor detail may appear obvious, it is not always so in the confines of the retrospective cohort obtained from EHR data because of sometimes ambiguous notion of the start period in a cohort study. This can be contrasted with a randomized controlled trial that has an explicit start date for the intervention.[4]

For example, consider Figure 8.11 which is an adaption of Figure 8.10. This retrospective cohort may have been operationalized based on the admission date to the hospital, where the admission date is used as the date of cohort inception. A given exposure, such as a medication, may not start at the date the cohort was assembled, especially if the medication relied upon a diagnosis that was not made at or immediately after admission. Incorporating the period prior to exposure in the follow-up calculation results in a misclassification of person-time. If this misclassification is dependent upon the patient's outcome (as in the earlier case), then it becomes differential misclassification. On the other hand, discarding this information altogether and starting the cohort follow-up time upon exposure also has the potential to misclassify this individual. This type of information bias is more specifically known as *immortal time bias* (Suissa, 2008). There are several ways to remediate this issue. One can consider a window of time to define the exposed group, say within 48 hours of hospital admission. In this case, even those exposed at a later point in time are still analyzed as

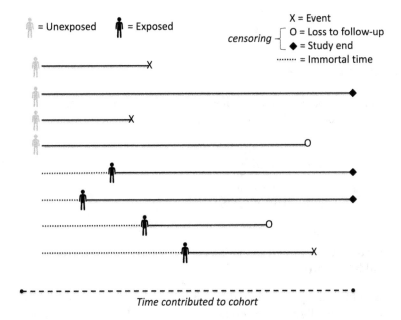

Figure 8.11 Immortal time in a cohort.

unexposed. This is easy to implement and analyze, but unfortunately now those unexposed may be misclassified if they receive treatment later in their hospitalization. The best solution is where exposure becomes time-varying for each day during the hospitalization, requiring a corresponding daily exposure variable. Renoux, Azoulay and Suissa (2021) illustrate several examples of drug effectiveness studies during COVID-19 and how immortal time bias may have impacted the validity of the study findings.

Case-control measures

Incidence cannot be directly estimated in a case-control study since the sampling fixes the incidence at a predetermined level corresponding to the ratio of cases to controls. Therefore, we must infer incidence another way. The case-control study uses the *odds ratio* to approximate the relative risk; the limits of this approximation are discussed later in this section. To understand the odds ratio, we will first revisit the concept of odds.

Odds are the ratio of the probability of an event occurring to the probability of an event not occurring, defined by the equation in Figure 8.12. If the event is the incidence of a disease, the odds can represent cumulative incidence. For this approximation to hold true, the probability of an event must be small. This is well suited to case-control studies as we often employ them when outcomes are rare, and the sampling must be done on the outcome to achieve sufficient numbers for the study.

$$\text{Odds} = \frac{\text{Probability(event)}}{1 - (\text{Probability(event)})}$$

Figure 8.12 Calculating odds.

Consider the following two examples of odds and probability. Example one is a case where the outcome has a lower prevalence while example two is a case where the outcome has a higher prevalence.

Example #1.   Lower prevalence

a   Probability(event) = 0.07, or 7%
b   Odds = 0.07/(1 − 0.07) = 0.075.

Example #2.   Higher prevalence

a   Probability(event) = 0.55, or 55%.
b   Odds = 0.55/(1 − 0.55) = 1.22.

The odds differ substantially from the probability when the event is more frequent, while only minimally when the event is less frequent. Thus, odds of incidence can approximate probability of incidence when the outcome is not common (a rule of thumb is ~10%). However, as mentioned, the case–control study cannot estimate incidence directly. Instead, we can estimate the odds of the exposure given the presence and absence of disease: Odds(E+ | D+) and Odds(E+ | D−), respectively. The ratio of these two odds estimates becomes the *odds ratio* and defines the odds of exposure in the case-control sample (Figure 8.13).

With a dichotomous exposure, we can again set up the data from a case-control study in a contingency table replacing the terms "disease" and "no disease" with "case" and "control," respectively. Using these data, we may calculate the odds of exposure relative to no exposure and then infer the odds of the outcome relevant to no outcome. In other words, the odds ratio can approximate the relative risk of disease given exposure.

To make this more concrete, assume the very low birthweight and staph infection study was recruited based on the outcome of staph infection with the resultant contingency table in Table 8.3. Note that these data are intentionally different data from the cohort study and show a sampling ratio of cases to controls of 1:4. The odds of exposure in the case group equals 45/55 = 0.82, and the odds of exposure in the control group equals 60/340 = 0.18. The odds ratio is (45/55)/(60/340) = 0.82/0.18 = 4.56.

We again have a qualitative and a quantitative interpretation of the measure. As the odds ratio is greater than 1.0, this suggests that the odds of the very low

$$\frac{\text{Odds}}{\text{Ratio}} = \frac{\text{Odds(E+ | D+)}}{\text{Odds(E+ | D−)}} = \frac{a/c}{b/d} = \frac{a*d}{b*c}$$

Figure 8.13 Odds ratio formula.

birthweight exposure was greater among the cases than the controls. The specific value of 4.56 means that neonates with a diagnosed staph infection in the NICU had on average 4.56 times the odds of also being very low birthweight compared to neonates that did not have a staph infection. Recall that we can also make this claim about the odds of disease in the presence of exposure: on average, very low birthweight neonates had 4.56 times the odds of also being diagnosed with a staph infection in the NICU compared to not very low birthweight neonates. This can again be stated as a percentage by subtracting 1.0 from the estimate = 4.56 – 1.00 = 3.56, or 356%: the very low birthweight group had an averaged 356% increased odds for staph infection in the NICU compared to the not very low birthweight group.

Returning to an earlier topic, when does the odds ratio approximate the relative risk to allow inference about incidence? First, the case-control sample needs to have been obtained, or sampled, without bias. That is, it needs to be a population-based sample and representative of all diseased and non-diseased individuals with respect to the exposure (see Chapter 9). Second, the outcome must not be prevalent, also known as the rare disease assumption. The prevalence of the outcome is sometimes termed the "built-in bias" of the odds ratio estimate (Szklo & Nieto, 2006). When the prevalence is low, the bias is minimal. In this case, we can also apply the attributable risk proportion equation to quantify excess risk attributable to the exposure substituting the odds ratio for the relative risk (Figure 8.9). Doing so does not imply that both relative risks and odds ratios should be calculated and compared within the same study, but rather the odds ratio may approximate relative risk under certain conditions. However, according to modern epidemiology theory, the rare disease assumption is unnecessary in most case-control studies where the control sampling occurs based on case diagnosis date (incidence-density sampling) or from an open cohort (Vandenbroucke & Pearce, 2012). As discussed in Chapter 7, EHRs can be conceived as an open cohort, potentially obviating the need for the rare disease assumption in EHR-based case-control studies.

Concluding differences between groups

In all the ratio measures comparing groups in this chapter, the measures were interpreted based on their effect sizes – also called point estimates – alone, and further that these were meaningful differences between groups. However, to conclude that the effect sizes are in fact statistically different between groups requires a measure of error for each ratio measure to account for random variation. This measure of

Table 8.3 The very low birthweight and staph infection case-control contingency table

Independent variable	Dependent variable		Totals
	Case (D+)	Control (D−)	
Exposed (E+)	45	60	105
Unexposed (E−)	55	340	395
Totals	100	400	500

error is presented commonly as the confidence interval around the point estimate. Quantifying random error allows for hypothesis testing. The results of hypothesis testing allow us to conclude that either we should fail to reject the null hypothesis and conclude there is no statistical difference between groups, or that we should accept the alternate hypothesis and conclude there is a statistical difference between groups beyond chance alone. Rather than hand calculate confidence intervals and the test statistics needed for the hypothesis testing, we will use software to do this. This will be discussed further in the Chapters 10 and 11. The measure of precision we will use is the 95% confidence interval, and if the interval contains the value of 1.0, we say the ratio measure of association was not statistically significant.

Notes

1 The use of the word "rate" in its purest sense suggests person-time is included in the denominator, however rates are often presented as synonymous with proportion measures. Unless the researcher is calculating incidence based on person-time, the word rate should be avoided in deference to the word proportion, unless it is convention to do otherwise.

2 We can also create contingency tables for other study designs so long as the dependent and independent variables are categorical. In practice, these tables become quite unwieldy for variables that have >2 levels.

3 To capture the "at risk" time more accurately, we should further consider the incubation period of the pathogen.

4 This is also discussed in Chapter 12 as part of the target trial paradigm of designing observational studies; see Hernán and Robins (2016).

References

Centers for Disease Control and Prevention (CDC). Infant Mortality. https://www.cdc.gov/reproductivehealth/MaternalInfantHealth/InfantMortality.htm (accessed April 5, 2022), 2021.

Centers for Disease Control and Prevention (CDC). Statistics Overview. https://www.cdc.gov/hiv/statistics/overview/index.html (accessed April 5, 2022), 2022.

Fox MP, Murray EJ, Lesko CR, Sealy-Jefferson S. On the need to revitalize descriptive epidemiology. Am J Epidemiol. 2022 Jun 27;191(7):1174–1179.

Goldstein ND, Quick H, Burstyn I. Effect of adjustment for case misclassification and infection Date uncertainty on estimates of COVID-19 effective reproduction number. Epidemiology. 2021;32(6):800–806.

Hernán MA, Robins JM. Using big data to emulate a target trial when a randomized trial is not available. Am J Epidemiol. 2016 Apr 15;183(8):758–764.

Renoux C, Azoulay L, Suissa S. Biases in evaluating the safety and effectiveness of drugs for the treatment of COVID-19: Designing real-world evidence studies. Am J Epidemiol. 2021;190(8):1452–1456.

Suissa S. Immortal time bias in pharmaco-epidemiology. Am J Epidemiol. 2008;167(4):492–499.

Szklo M, Nieto J. 2006. Epidemiology Beyond the Basics. Burlington: Jones and Bartlett Publishers.

Vandenbroucke JP, Pearce N. Case-control studies: basic concepts. Int J Epidemiol. 2012 Oct;41(5):1480–1489.

9 Bias and Validity in Observational Research

With the foundation of study design and measurement of frequency and risk de-fined, we next turn our attention to the question, "When and under what condi-tions are the results of an EHR-based epidemiological analysis valid?" Statistical associations between independent and dependent variables – the exposures and the outcomes – under study can be caused by one or more combinations of five mechanisms: (1) true causation between the exposure and the outcome, (2) *bias*, or an artificial association due to systematic errors in measurement or selection, (3) *confounding*, or a real association caused by an extraneous variable, (4) *reverse causation* where the outcome caused the exposure unbeknownst to the researcher, and (5) *random error*. In etiologic research, our goal as researchers is to appreciate and thereby minimize mechanisms #2–#5, so the strongest explanation for an association between the exposure and the outcome is a causal one. While it may never be possible to eliminate all threats to validity, an in-depth examination of each threat can help determine the extent of its potential impact on study findings. Indeed, the field of *quantitative bias analysis* that concludes chapter is predicated on conducting sensitivity analyses to assess the impact of bias.

Mechanisms #2–#5 are considered threats to *internal* validity: did the study measure the exposure and outcome relationship correctly? Was it free from sys-tematic errors in the design, implementation, or analysis, on average? There is also the question of whether the results from a particular study are applicable to other target populations than the one studied. This is termed *external* validity and may be decomposed into *generalizability* and *transportability*. Before continuing, the distinction between populations in EHR-based analyses is essential to understand (Figure 9.1).

The target population represents the target of inference from the study; in other words, to whom do the study results apply? The target population may be defined by geography, such as the local community, or patients who share similar attributes, such as sex, gender, age, or illness regardless of geography. The source population may or may not be a subset of the target population and represents the mechanism for appearing in the EHR: the catchment. The study popula-tion is derived from the source population (EHR) and now includes only those under analysis. Occasionally the study and source populations will be the same,

DOI: 10.4324/9781003258872-12

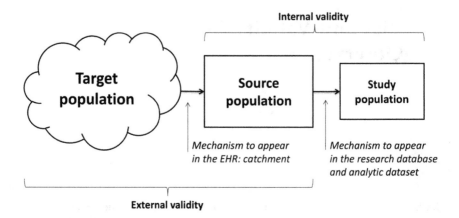

Figure 9.1 Selecting the study population from an EHR.

as in a retrospective cohort drawn from the EHR where all eligible people were included, but often, the study population is only a subset or a sample.

The threats to validity are presented separately in this chapter, but it is important to recognize they are not mutually exclusive and can operate in concert. For example, bias can induce confounding, and any or all mechanisms can be present at a given time. Incremental errors can accrue based on researcher decisions made when undertaking an EHR study, inducing selection bias, information bias, and residual confounding (Rassen, Murk & Schneeweiss, 2021). Didactically, confounding is treated separately from bias in this chapter, although some epidemiologists consider confounding to be a type of bias. This is more a theoretical distinction than a practical one. Additionally, some epidemiologists prefer to think about validity issues as forms of missing data. For example, confounding is the result of data missing on a key variable related to the exposure and outcome, information bias is data missing on a variable's true value, and selection bias is data missing on participants (Edwards, Cole & Westreich, 2015; Howe, Cain & Hogan, 2015). Viewing these issues through a missing data lens allows us to consider imputation approaches to mitigate the threats to validity. Practically speaking, errors in data management or analysis can also threaten validity. For example, assumptions made about missing data, duplicate records, variable selection and operationalization, study design, and model specification can all impact statistical or causal inference (Tran, Lash & Goldstein, 2021).

For readers seeking a concise summary of validity issues germane to EHR-based research, Gianfrancesco and Goldstein (2021) identified four central challenges: (1) the representativeness of patients in the EHR, (2) data types, consistency, and interpretation, (3) missing measurements, and (4) missing visits. These four concepts have already been introduced piecemeal in various places in the book and are now collated in this chapter into a cohesive view of the validity of EHR research.

Bias

Bias in an epidemiological analysis is the creation of an artificial association because of some systematic error in the design, implementation, or analytic phase of the study. There are numerous types of biases encountered in the epidemiological literature: recall bias, incidence-prevalence bias, healthy worker bias, surveillance bias, immortal time bias, informed presence bias, and so on. An exhaustive description of all of them would merit an encyclopedia of biases (Porta, 2014). Rather than focusing on individual biases, we will approach them from the broadest conceptual level, classifying them as either a selection bias or an information bias. A selection bias relates to participation in the study, whereas an information bias is a deficiency in the measurement of variables.

Selection bias

A *selection bias* is present when the participants under study systematically differ from the population the study was recruited or sampled from. It is essentially a flaw in the composition of the analytic groups due to inappropriate exclusion of participants, whether implicit or explicit. In classical epidemiology, selection bias arises when participants are selected into a study based on their exposure *and* outcome status, thereby impacting the measures of association: the measure of association in the study differs from that in the population. Outside of epidemiology, the term selection bias may be used when the assessment of a single characteristics does not reflect the source population, such as measures of incidence or prevalence. Epidemiologists would likely refer to this occurrence not as a selection bias but rather a *sampling error*. Björk et al. (2020) proposed a framework attempting to reconcile these differences, viewing selection bias as both a threat to internal and external validity. This unified view may help researchers identify the specific catchment mechanisms that lead to biased populations and samples without getting mired down in the differences between terminologies.

In classical epidemiology, the terms selection bias, sampling error, and representativeness are related but distinct. In a strict sense, any deviation from randomness when selecting the study participants from a target population may result in a non-representative sample and potentially impact inference. If this deviation is patterned on the exposure and outcome, then this can be termed a selection bias (Richiardi, Pizzi & Pearce, 2013). If the study sample is a true random sample from the target population, then we have avoided both sampling error and selection bias and achieved representativeness. If the study sample is not a random sample from the target population, which is most likely the case in EHR-based studies, yet not conditional on exposure and outcome, then sampling error and representativeness are of greater concern than selection bias. This could impact the estimates of prevalence of various attributes in the sample but would not be expected to alter the correlation between the exposure and outcome, unless stratified by a third variable that differs across populations (Björk et al., 2020). On the other hand, some have argued that true representativeness is undesirable in scientific study in that inference may be limited to only the participants in the study and lack any external validity (Rothman, Gallacher & Hatch, 2013).[1] This is a criticism lobbed at clinical trials, where strict inclusion and exclusion criteria are present (Greenhouse et al., 2008).

As mentioned, when the study population does not accurately represent the source population with respect to both the exposure and outcome, a selection bias may ensue. This is especially true in a case–control study where the study sample is being selected by their outcome status. In this case, if the exposure status is also implicitly selected in this process, a selection bias can be created. For example, consider a case–control study drawn from the inpatient EHR where the exposure is coffee consumption, and the outcome is pancreatic cancer. In reality and unbeknownst to the investigators, there is no causal relation. The cases are drawn from the oncology service, while the controls are drawn from the gastroenterology service. It is quite possible that gastroenterology patients have modified, most likely reduced, their coffee consumption habits based on their morbidities; therefore, an artificial coffee and pancreatic cancer relationship will occur. This would occur because non-coffee drinking control patients were more likely to participate in this study because of choosing controls from the gastroenterology service. Some readers may have recognized that this is in fact a classic example of selection bias that occurred in a hospital setting in the early 1980s (MacMahon et al., 1981). As we now know, hospital-based case–control studies are particularly prone to this type of bias as controls may have altered risk factors (Feinstein et al., 1981).

As another example of a case–control study susceptible to selection bias, consider oral contraceptive use as the exposure and diabetes as the outcome. As opposed to the previous example using inpatient EHR data, this sample is drawn from the outpatient EHR. Being on oral contraceptives likely results in more physician visits compared to someone not on oral contraceptives. Therefore, the likelihood of detecting subclinical diabetes is increased. As a result of the case–control sampling, the exposure may be overrepresented thereby exaggerating the exposure and outcome relation. In short, cases on oral contraceptives are more likely to participate in this study because of their increased likelihood to have subclinical diabetes detected relative to cases drawn from another source. To minimize the chance of selection bias invalidating a case–control study, the researcher may sample directly from the target population, if possible, or randomly sample from the source population as opposed to systematically sampling.

Cohort studies can also be subject to selection bias based on the future probability of disease. For example, if loss to follow-up affects the exposed group more than the unexposed group due to sicker people withdrawing from the study, a selection bias can occur. This is known as differential loss to follow-up and is minimized by ensuring as complete follow-up as possible. As another example, selection into the study population from the source population may be the result of being healthy, known as the healthy worker effect, and thus participants are less likely to experience the outcome. In both examples, while the outcome was not known at the formation of the cohort, there was a differing propensity for the outcome in the study population compared to the source population.

Diving deeper into the use of EHRs as a data source reveals additional complications that can manifest as a selection bias: these are related to healthcare access and utilization. As discussed in Chapter 6, catchment is the process by which patients select into a healthcare system and this process may induce a selection bias. Figure 6.4 in Chapter 6 is a schematic representation of this process. If the target of inference is the local community, it is quite possible that an EHR-based study could be biased. Goldstein et al. (2021) utilized an outpatient EHR to assess how community deprivation may relate to a diagnosis of hepatitis C. They observed that being in the catchment of the outpatient clinic was related to both greater deprivation and a higher likelihood of hepatitis C diagnosis. In other words, selection into this clinic was predicated on both the exposure and outcome. The authors applied a methodology known as inverse probability of selection weighting that was able to account for this systematic error and concluded that "researchers working with [EHR-based] outpatient data [...] consider the patient selection process and how that may relate to [the] exposure and outcome under study." On the other hand, researchers have found that sampling error was minimal when studying the prevalence of obesity from their EHRs as compared to the population-based U.S. National Health and Nutrition Examination Survey (Flood et al., 2015; Funk et al., 2017). In short, catchment influences patient selection forces at a population level and an individual study level and must be evaluated on a per-study basis (Björk et al., 2020).

Chapter 6 also introduced the notion of *informed presence bias* where patients who have interacted more frequently with a healthcare provider may be more likely to have a diagnosis recorded in the EHR (Goldstein et al., 2016). This may be true if patients have more frequent visits, or among patients who have an equivalent number of visits, if some patients receive more scrutiny (McGee et al., 2022). In other words, data are missing either from lack of a healthcare encounter or lack of a measurement. Decisions made about these missing data could induce selection bias, for example, if the participants excluded from the analytic sample systematically differ from those retained. Indeed, applying study exclusion criteria from the EHR can theoretically induce multiple biases (Chubak et al., 2022). There is also an interplay between informed presence bias and catchment: patients outside of the catchment have fewer opportunities to have a condition captured in the EHR, while patients inside of the catchment may have inaccurate or missing data on the condition. Haneuse and Daniels (2016) proposed a framework for considering selection bias in EHR-based studies that can help investigators think through the various mechanisms that may lead to this bias.

Theoretically, informed presence bias is a threat to validity; however, the literature is conflicting as to the impact of this bias: some have noted an overall smaller effect under controlled conditions (Goldstein et al., 2019), while others have noted a more extreme impact (McGee et al., 2022). Approaches for informed presence bias include conditioning on the number of visits, imputing data for the missing visits, or reweighting patients in the analytic sample using inverse probability weighting (Gianfrancesco et al., 2020; Sayon-Orea et al., 2020). There is no single best solution. For example, while controlling for the number of visits is straightforward, it may induce selection bias (Goldstein et al., 2016). Imputing missing visits will depend on whether the patterns of missingness among those with fewer visits are nonignorable: the reasons for missing visits may not be captured in the observed data. On the other hand, conceiving of informed presence bias as an information bias, where patients who are sicker have more information than those who are not, brings into play misclassification approaches that are well established in epidemiology (McGee et al., 2022; discussed later). Prospectively collecting additional validation data on those with fewer healthcare visits or lacking recent healthcare visits can help to identify meaningful differences in patient characteristics associated with the variables under study (Chubak et al., 2022).

Information bias

Information bias arises from measurement error and can affect the exposure, outcome, or any of the covariates under study, although the exposure and outcome typically receive the most scrutiny in the literature. Measurement error suggests that there was an imperfect definition of continuous or categorical variables under study or a systematic error in collecting the data. If the variable under study is categorical, the measurement error may result in *misclassification*, where the incorrect category is assigned. As with selection bias, didactically it is easiest to examine the phenomenon of information bias using a dichotomous exposure and outcome, thus representing misclassification. However, generally the common clinical research practice of dichotomizing continuous predictors (e.g., hypertensive, obese, neutropenic, and so on) should be avoided as it may further compound measurement error or induce residual confounding (Flegal, Keyl & Nieto, 1991; Royston, Altman & Sauerbrei, 2006; Gustafson & Le Nhu, 2002).

There are several well-known mechanisms for measurement error in observational epidemiology, especially in case–control studies. *Recall bias* occurs when knowledge of the outcome affects participant recall of the exposure. When the knowledge of the outcome affects the interviewer's propensity to inquire about exposure, this is known as *interviewer bias*. If the outcome is subject to measurement error by either the participant through self-report or the observer through interview, similar biases may arise and are termed *respondent bias* and *observer bias*, respectively.

When the misclassification affects only the exposure or outcome, irrespective of the other, it is said to be *nondifferential* misclassification. When measurement error affects the exposure or outcome and is contingent upon the value of the other, it is said to be *differential* misclassification; recall bias can be considered a form of differential misclassification (Raphael, 1987). An oft-quoted heuristic states that nondifferential misclassification of a binary exposure will bias the results toward the null hypothesis of no observed effect, although this claim is true in only a specific set of circumstances (Yland et al., 2022). Differential misclassification can bias in either direction and is therefore more difficult to predict its impact on the observed effect. A related type of misclassification that is also equally difficult to predict is known as *dependent* misclassification. In dependent misclassification, if one variable is misclassified, such as the exposure, then another variable, such as the outcome or a covariate, may also be misclassified at a given level (Brooks et al., 2018). In other words, the errors are correlated. Dependent misclassification should not be conflated with differential misclassification: *differential* impacts one variable (albeit conditional on the value of another), whereas *dependent* impacts multiple variables concurrently. Dependent misclassification may be especially pernicious in EHR data as often the same assessment methods, such as a physical examination performed by the clinician, are used to collect multiple, concurrent observations; unfortunately, guidance is limited to remediate this occurrence analytically (Brooks et al., 2018). Multiple types of misclassification can be present in the same study.

Several hypothetical examples can help demonstrate the differences between measurement error and misclassification. In the EHR, a patient's weight may be mismeasured if, for example, the scale needed calibration or the patient was wearing heavy clothes. Importantly, we, as researchers, are unaware of this issue. This type of measurement error is likely to be distributed randomly in the data and therefore will have a similar impact across all mismeasured participants in our study, attenuating or exaggerating the true statistic. On the other hand, perhaps women are weighed less often than men, and thus their weights are not contemporary. This non-random, systematic error is particularly troublesome, as it could bias any gender-specific results, again without our knowledge.

As an example of a categorical variable subject to misclassification, suppose we wished to determine someone's tobacco smoking status from the EHR. If the healthcare worker simply does not ask this question, then any residual information in the EHR may be inaccurate, albeit similarly across all participants under the care of this clinician. However, it is quite conceivable that there are patterns among patients who were asked their smoking history: perhaps men who are known to smoke more on average, or those with certain other "risk factors" such as being in a lower socioeconomic position, having medical comorbidities, or substance use disorders. Accuracy of reporting of smoking may also depend on whether there is a rapport between the healthcare provider and the patient such that the patient may be more likely to divulge sensitive information about a socially undesirable behavior with a more trusted physician. Again, this systematic error is particularly concerning as we likely lack information as to why this variable was misclassified, and thus may not appreciate the type of bias that may ensue.

A categorical variable may also be misclassified based on decisions about underlying continuous data, such as the cut point used in operationalizing a positive diagnosis or condition based on laboratory assay results. When categorical reports of underlying continuous traits are collected, complex patterns of errors with respect to the true category are virtually assured. Again it bears repeating that dichotomizing continuous predictors should be avoided as it may further compound measurement error or induce residual confounding (Flegal, Keyl & Nieto, 1991; Royston, Altman & Sauerbrei, 2006; Gustafson & Le Nhu, 2002).

As one final example, suppose we are conducting an observational study from an obstetrical EHR where the outcome is a diagnosis of a birth defect and the exposure is prenatal vitamin supplementation. If all the women in the study accurately recalled taking vitamins, no exposure misclassification is present. If some women did not remember taking vitamins, but these women occurred in equal proportions among those with offspring that had birth defects and those without, the exposure misclassification is nondifferential. If mothers of children with birth defects specifically thought it was the absence of vitamins that led to the birth defects, and therefore more accurately recalled not taking them, the exposure misclassification is now differential with respect to the outcome. If the assessment methods elicited the same degree of over- or underreporting in the exposure and outcome, then the misclassification may have dependent errors. If the birth defects diagnosis was inaccurate, then outcome misclassification arises which may be nondifferential or differential to the exposure, for example, if knowledge of the lack of prenatal care led to closer scrutiny of the offspring. Nondifferential nondependent misclassification is probably more of a theoretical distinction and differential misclassification, whether dependent or nondependent, is the more frequent type encountered.

As mentioned, the effects of differential and/or dependent misclassification are not readily apparent without the investigator undertaking a sensitivity analysis, whereby the suspected errors in measurements are adjusted in a hypothetical what-if scenario and the analysis is re-run (discussed later in the chapter). In all these examples, discarding these variables from analysis may simply not be possible if these variables were of critical importance to the analysis: the exposure, the outcome, or an important confounder.

The magnitude of misclassification can be assessed through measures of variable accuracy. The most common measures include sensitivity and specificity, and positive and negative predictive values. Let us discuss each of these measures within the context of a potentially misclassified health outcome in the EHR. As discussed in Chapter 6, the use of International Classification of Diseases (ICD) codes to identify health outcomes is subject to misclassification. *Sensitivity* is the probability of a diagnostic code correctly being recorded in the EHR when a patient has the corresponding illness, whereas *specificity* is the probability that absence of a diagnostic code in the EHR correctly reflects a lack of an illness (Goldstein et al., 2022). As an aside, outcome misclassification is especially relevant for EHR-based case–control studies; specificity should be maximized to minimize bias (Jurek, Maldonado & Greenland, 2013). *Positive predictive value* describes the likelihood of a patient's illness given the presence of a diagnostic code in the EHR, whereas *negative predictive value* describes the likelihood of the absence of a patient's illness given the lack of a diagnostic code in the EHR (Goldstein et al., 2022). These definitions and their calculations are visually depicted in Figure 9.2.

The interplay between sensitivity and specificity can be readily appreciated via analogy: when setting the threshold for a car alarm we need to balance both measures. Suppose we want a car alarm that never goes off unintentionally. In such a case, there will be almost no "false positive" alarms; therefore, the specificity will be excellent. On the other hand, we expect there will be a lot of "false negatives" in that the alarm did not sound when it should have, so the *sensitivity* will be poor

True Diagnostic Status

EHR ICD Code	Positive (+)	Negative (-)	Totals
Positive (+)	a	b	a+b
Negative (-)	c	d	c+d
Totals	a+c	b+d	a+b+c+d

$$\text{Sensitivity} = \frac{a}{a+c} \qquad \text{Specificity} = \frac{d}{b+d}$$

$$\text{Positive Predictive Value} = \frac{a}{a+b} \qquad \text{Negative Predictive Value} = \frac{d}{c+d}$$

Figure 9.2 Measures of variable accuracy. ICD, International Classification of Diseases.

and the car will be stolen. We tend to see this relation of near perfect specificity and inferior sensitivity when assessing potentially stigmatizing behaviors or
conditions, as people may prevaricate to obscure the truth. Continuing with the
analogy, suppose we want a car alarm that never misses a potential criminal. This
alarm will go off incessantly with great sensitivity and no false negatives but will
annoy all people within earshot, so the specificity will be poor with many false
positives. This is akin to the "car alarm who cried wolf" and therefore the car will
be stolen anyway because people will ignore the alarm!

   In the simple case of nondifferential, nondependent misclassification, sensitivity and specificity (or predictive values) capture the accuracy of the classifier. We
only need to calculate a single set of values given the classifier under examination.
However, under differential misclassification, we must now stratify our calculations by levels of the second variable. In a dichotomous exposure and outcome
setting, this will equate to two sets of sensitivity and specificity measures (or
predictive values); as the number of categories increases, the number of strata increases as well. In the case of dependent misclassification, the values of sensitivity
and specificity (or predictive values) are correlated. As one variable gets better or
worse in its accuracy, so too does a second variable. For dependent misclassification, we would need an idea of the amount of correlated error, although this
information is rarely available in practice.

   Accuracy of a classifier may be determined from a validation study, literature
review, expert opinion, or even intuition. A validation study measures both the
potentially misclassified variable as well as a gold standard. The gold standard
may reflect the truth or may just be an improvement in the accuracy but itself

not perfect. The validation study may be internal on a subset of the data at hand or external using new data, provided the patients are exchangeable between the original study and the validation study. Researchers have additionally explored data accuracy by comparing claims data to EHR data (Lin et al., 2018; Merola et al., 2022). Not only can this be used to confirm agreement between the two data sources, but it can also be used to measure EHR continuity, defined as receiving care outside of the current EHR. Restricting the study population to high continuity patients may reduce information bias (Lin et al., 2018).

The epidemiologic literature is rich with examples and procedures for handling different types of health data misclassification (Bodnar et al., 2010; Brennan et al., 2021; Brooks et al., 2018; Desai et al., 2020; Edwards et al., 2013; Funk & Landi, 2014; Goldstein et al., 2022; Keogh et al., 2020; Srugo et al., 2021). In fact, there is even a textbook devoted to the topic (Gustafson, 2003). Bodnar et al. (2010) explored how self-reported weight captured in the EHR was inaccurate, impacting the calculation of body mass index, and thus biasing the association between weight and several adverse pregnancy outcomes. Srugo et al. (2021) proposed a study to examine maternal pre-pregnancy weight and incident allergic disease in their offspring using administrative databases, and, as with Bodnar et al., suspected that self-reported weight will be misclassified. Goldstein et al. (2022) presented a case study on how the accuracy of an ICD classifier for chronic hepatitis C diagnosis may be determined in an EHR and provided guidance for researchers faced with a similar challenge of misclassified health outcome data. Tying these examples together is the application of quantitative bias analysis to assess the impact of misclassification in an epidemiological investigation. Quantitative bias analysis is discussed at the end of this chapter.

Confounding

If bias is an artificial relationship between the exposure and the outcome created by a systematic error in study design, implementation, or analysis, *confounding* is a real – albeit unwanted – relationship between the exposure and outcome created by an extraneous variable. It is this extraneous variable – or variables – that explains part of or all the observed relationship under study. By not accounting for this extraneous variable in the study design or analysis, the researcher may be under the false impression the exposure is the causal mechanism. Confounding is classified as a threat to internal validity, as it represents a systematic error in the study. It may be wholly responsible for the exposure to outcome relation, or more likely than not, partially responsible for the exposure to outcome relation. Keep in mind that the threats to validity are not mutually exclusive; they all work together in concert affecting the observed statistical associations between variables.

Under the classical definition of confounding, for one or more variables to be a confounding variable (or more simply, a confounder), it must fulfill these criteria:

1 The confounder is causally related to the outcome. That is, it can cause the outcome on its own.

2   The confounder is related to the exposure. It does not have to necessarily cause the exposure, but it must be associated with the exposure's presence. Implicit in this criterion is that the confounder is differentially distributed by exposure groups. As it is related to the exposure, presence of the exposure means presence of the confounder, unless the confounder is associated with lack of exposure, then vice-versa is true.

3   The confounder cannot be on the causal pathway between the exposure and outcome. In other words, the exposure cannot cause the confounder that will then cause the outcome. This type of variable is known as a *mediator*.

Even if these three criteria are satisfied, it is up to the researcher to decide whether the variable should be accounted for analytically. Some confounders may satisfy these criteria, but have a negligible confounding impact (e.g., statistical vs. clinical importance), while other confounders may not satisfy these criteria but be important for the analysis (e.g., age or sex). One common approach for assessing confounding is via statistical tests for the above criteria, but we should also consider a theoretical or conceptual basis for confounding. Ideally, consideration for confounding variables will be done at the study outset, and not during the data analysis phase. However, given our focus on EHR data, the list of potential confounders is driven by the available variables collected in and abstracted from the medical record, or those which can be readily linked to the EHR. It is quite possible that a confounder exists but is not measured. Techniques are available for assessing the impact of unmeasured (residual) confounding and are presented later in the quantitative bias analysis section in this chapter.

Many find it helpful to depict confounding using schematic diagrams.[2] In the diagram depicted in Figure 9.3, there is a direct link between the exposure and the outcome, but there is also an indirect link between the exposure and outcome through the confounder (known as a backdoor pathway using the directed acyclic graph framework). Using the conceptual diagram framework, the bidirectional arrow between the exposure and confounder suggests a relationship, although not necessarily causal, whereas the unidirectional arrow between the confounder and outcome represents a causal relationship. Visualizing these relationships not only helps to identify potential confounders, but also to identify other types of mechanisms at play in the study.

A confounder can either exaggerate or attenuate a relationship, respectively known as *positive* or *negative* confounding. Positive confounding is more frequently

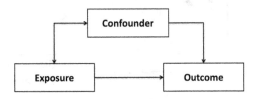

Figure 9.3 A causal diagram depicting confounding.

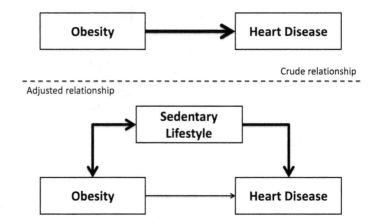

Figure 9.4 A positive confounder. The arrow weight depicts the strength of the relationship.

observed in the literature, as well as being a more intuitive concept. An example of positive confounding can be seen with the example relationship between obesity and heart disease, with sedentary lifestyle as a confounder (Figure 9.4). In the crude relationship without the confounder, the researcher may detect a strong, positive association between obesity and heart disease. However, once the sedentary lifestyle confounder is accounted for, the relationship may be attenuated, although not completely since there may be other mechanisms at play. In this example, the confounder exaggerated the true relationship between obesity and heart disease.

An example of negative confounding can be seen in the example relationship between mercury exposure and cardiovascular disease, with mercury-containing fish as a confounder (Figure 9.5). In the crude relationship, the researcher may fail to detect an association between mercury exposure and cardiovascular disease,

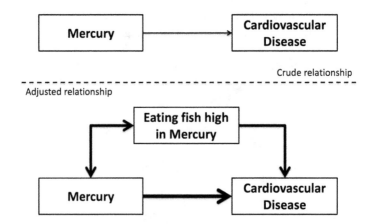

Figure 9.5 A negative confounder. The arrow weight depicts the strength of the relationship.

because the protective benefits of seafood consumption are offsetting the harmful exposure of mercury in the fish (Choi et al., 2008). However, once we adjust for mercury-containing fish in the diet, the relationship becomes quite apparent in that mercury exposures lead to cardiovascular disease. In this example, the confounder attenuated the true relationship. This example also demonstrates that failure to detect a crude relationship in the data should not suggest that a relationship does not exist. Rather than stopping the analysis at this point, a prudent researcher will see the study to conclusion.

One approach to assessing confounding is through stratification. Under this approach, separate measures of association are calculated based on the value of the confounder (Figure 9.6). Stratification can be employed when the confounder is categorical (or can be categorized via a cut point). For example, suppose that in the positive confounder example from earlier, sedentary lifestyle can be dichotomized as "yes" or "no" and the researcher found a crude relative risk of 4.0 when comparing the risk of heart attack in those who were obese versus not (top of Figure 9.6). Further suppose that in this example after stratification by sedentary lifestyle, the stratum-specific relative risk estimates were 2.0 and 2.1 of heart attack in those who were obese versus not, among those who were sedentary or not. In the bottom of Figure 9.6, C+ would indicate a sedentary lifestyle, and C− would indicate an active lifestyle. If the stratified measures of association are reasonably close between the crude and adjusted estimates, the stratified variable may not be a confounder. If, as in this example, the measures of association differ between the crude and adjusted estimates, the stratified variable may be inducing confounding. Importantly, it is the magnitude of the differences in estimates that is of primary concern, and a general rule of thumb is 10%. While confounding can also be assessed statistically, the result of the statistical test should not be *sine qua non* evidence of confounding without a theoretical basis for the effect. Indeed,

	Disease (D+)	No Disease (D-)
Exposed (E+)	a	b
Unexposed (E-)	c	d

Crude relationship

- -

Adjusted relationship

Confounder Present (C+)				Confounder Absent (C-)	
	Disease (D+)	No Disease (D-)		Disease (D+)	No Disease (D-)
Exposed (E+)	e	f		i	j
Unexposed (E-)	g	h		k	l

Figure 9.6 A stratified approach to detecting confounding and effect modification.

even without a statistically significant relationship, a large magnitude of difference should be considered first and foremost as evidence of potential confounding.

As a brief aside, if the stratified adjusted effects differ with respect not only to the crude effects, but also with respect to the strata (C+ and C− in Figure 9.6), then the variable may be an *effect modifier* as opposed to a confounder. In the obesity and heart disease example, suppose the stratum-specific estimates for C+ and C− were 2.5 and 1.5, respectively. These estimates still differ from the crude relative risk of 4.0, yet, in contrast to the confounding example, the stratum-specific estimates now differ from each other, suggesting effect modification. Whereas the researcher needs to account for the confounder as an extraneous variable, an effect modifier should not be regarded as a nuisance condition, but rather a special etiological phenomenon. In this situation, one would normally present the stratified results indicating effect modification and conclude that an active lifestyle can modify the risk factor of obesity on later occurrence of heart disease.

To minimize the chance of confounding impacting the exposure to outcome relation, the researcher must account for it, either in the study design phase or the analysis phase. Techniques in the study design phase include randomization, restriction, and matching. *Randomization* helps to ensure an equal distribution of confounders, both known and unknown, between exposure groups, thereby implicitly controlling for its effect. The net result is that the groups are *exchangeable* with respect to all covariates, other than the exposure, as in a randomized controlled trial. Exchangeability nullifies the second criteria from earlier, namely that the confounder is differentially distributed across the exposure groups. *Restriction* through the study inclusion and exclusion criteria removes a potential confounding effect from the study. For example, if sedentary lifestyle is an important confounder in our study, we may wish to restrict recruitment to only those with (or without) a sedentary lifestyle. However, restriction is only applicable when confounders are known *a priori* and further reduces the eligible pool of participants for recruitment. *Matching* is often employed in case–control studies (see Chapter 7), and, as with restriction, is effective in controlling for known confounding by improving group exchangeability.

In the analysis phase, as shown earlier, *stratification* can be used to arrive at adjusted estimates of risk. However, as stratification is typically limited to a single categorical variable with few categories, it may not be practical in complex analyses. Further, stratification techniques can be cumbersome and tedious, and are not possible when the putative confounder is a continuous measure without obvious cut points. Instead, we will focus on adjusting for confounding through multivariable *regression* techniques, which will be covered in Chapter 11.

Despite the availably of multiple techniques to account for confounding effects in both the design phase and analysis phase, complete control for confounding may never be possible. There may always be unmeasured confounders present in the study, as well as *residual* confounding, due to incomplete or inaccurate assessment of known confounders. In summary, as with bias, the researcher's job is to understand and minimize threats to internal validity, while not always eliminating them.

For clinical researchers, there are several subtypes of confounding that are germane: confounding by indication, confounding by contraindication, and protopathic bias. Although the definitions of these three concepts sound similar and are frequently used interchangeably, they are conceptually distinct and should not be conflated (Faillie, 2015). *Confounding by indication* occurs when the reason for a medical intervention is related to the patient's disease prognosis. Confounding occurs because of an imbalance that now exists between groups, with the severity and prognosis of the disease confounding the effects of the medical intervention. For example, in a study of adjuvant chemotherapy and breast cancer recurrence, the authors noted an increased risk of recurrence after receipt of adjuvant chemotherapy, despite expecting a decreased risk (Bosco et al., 2010). They hypothesized that the indication of adjuvant chemotherapy among women with a higher risk of recurrence likely confounding the treatment effect. There are several options for dealing with this type of confounding, both in the study design and analysis phases (Joseph, Mehrabadi & Lisonkova, 2014); however, in at least one study, residual confounding persisted regardless of strategy (Bosco et al., 2010).

If, on the other hand, the decision about the medical intervention is not based on clinical disease but rather the early manifestation of preclinical disease, *protopathic bias* is most likely the resultant type of confounding. Importantly, the disease itself is undiagnosed at the time of the intervention – and thus the prognosis is unknown to the investigators. For example, in a case–control study of endometrial cancer and hormone therapy, hormone therapy may be given to those with early signs of endometrial cancer but lacking an actual diagnosis (Horwitz & Feinstein, 1980). Thus, the groups are no longer exchangeable.

Lastly, *confounding by contraindication* occurs when a medical intervention is contraindicated and has an unintended effect on the study. For example, in a study of induced labor and postpartum hemorrhage, induction may be contraindicated in women with a history of or at high risk for postpartum hemorrhage (Joseph, Mehrabadi & Lisonkova, 2014). In such cases, these women may not receive induction at the obstetrician's discretion, again creating an imbalance between the groups. As opposed to confounding by indication, confounding by contraindication is generally perceived to be less of a threat to validity, and can be mitigated in the study design phase through restriction (Joseph, Mehrabadi & Lisonkova, 2014).

Reverse causality

As one may posit, reverse causality is a situation where the temporal expectation of the exposure preceding the outcome cannot be assured (Figure 9.7). This is particularly problematic for diseases with long latent periods or insidious onset, such as many types of cancers and chronic diseases. Reverse causality is also a concern in secondary analysis of EHR data, as the timing of the exposure and outcome may not be known with certainty. For example, using data derived from an obstetrical EHR, we may wish to study the effects of prenatal care on adverse pregnancy outcomes, yet women with pregnancy complications may in

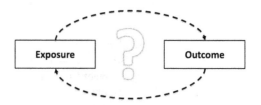

Figure 9.7 Conflation of exposure and outcome under reverse causality.

fact schedule more prenatal visits. Although at first blush the concept of reverse causality appears straightforward, there are numerous permutations depending on the health phenomena under study with resultant ambiguity (Flegal et al., 2011). Reverse causality can also be conceived as a type of residual confounding resulting from unmeasured confounding by undiagnosed preclinical disease (Robins, 2008), similar to protopathic bias. Didactically, reverse causality is treated separately in this chapter.

There are several examples in the literature of reverse causality in studies using EHR data. In a critique of an EHR-based study of neurological sequalae from SARS-CoV-2 infection, Tirozzi et al. (2022) suggested that reverse causality may explain the association in that "most of the reported disorders are themselves risk factors for COVID-19 infection, and their milder forms may go undetected." They suggest using a technique known as mendelian randomization to pseudo-randomize observational data. In a case–control study of proton pump inhibitor use as a risk factor for pancreatic cancer, Kearns, Boursi and Yang (2017) noted that proton pump inhibitors may be administered in response to preclinical diseases prior to diagnosis. Their solution involved stratifying the exposure by timing of the medication relative to the diagnosis date. In an analysis of high body mass index (BMI) as a risk factor for dementia, Kivimäki et al. (2018) described how dementia may lower someone's weight, thereby imparting an (incorrect) protective effect of high BMI due to weight loss. In this case, the remediation is to lengthen the follow-up period prior to diagnosis, which may not always be possible with historical EHR data. Lastly, in a study of systolic blood pressure (SBP) and its relationship to mortality, Ravindrarajah et al. (2017) observed that "reverse causation may apply if lower SBP values result from proximity to death." In a naïve analysis of these data, it may appear that lower SBP is a risk factor for mortality. The authors imply that observational data may be insufficient to correctly ascribe causation in studies where follow-up is limited.

Generalizability and transportability

There are two facets of external validity. *Generalizability* defines how representative the study results are in the target population. The target population need not be the one the source population was drawn from; when the results are applicable to different target population from the one studied, we say the results are *transportable*. Concerns over external validity can be framed in terms of the question: "To whom do the study results apply?" For generalizability, we may ask whether the populations captured in the study and the EHR are representative of the source population. For transportability, we may ask whether the findings from the research are applicable to other populations than the EHR used for the present analysis. These populations may differ by geography or time, for example, if the findings from a historic analysis are applicable to the present day. Unlike internal validity that has well-established methodological approaches (see quantitative bias analysis section), external validity tends toward subjectivity, although quantitative methods exist for generalizability (Cole & Stuart, 2010; Lesko et al., 2017) and transportability (Westreich et al., 2017). Rothwell (2005) provided a comprehensive list of issues that may impact external validity, which may serve as a qualitative checklist of criteria to be met. At the broadest level, this list included (1) the setting of the research study, (2) the selection of the participants, (3) the characteristics of those ultimately enrolled in the study, (4) any differences in clinical practice that may arise due to study conduct, (5) the outcome measures and follow-up, and (6) the adverse effects of the intervention (see Panel 2 in Rothwell for an enumeration of the entire list). Although this list was specific to experimental research, much of it is also applicable to observational research; see also Szklo (1998) for a similar discussion of external validity criteria for population-based cohort studies.

It is possible to have results that lack internal validity while maintaining external validity if the population is unbiased with respect to the source. Yet in practice, internal validity is often a prerequisite to external validity. The target population can differ from the source population without external validity being compromised. For example, a study drawn from the catchment area of a hospital in an urban city center may be generalizable to hospitals in other cities. In an EHR-based study, geography may be the first factor that defines differences between observational studies; additional factors may include racial or ethnic groups, age groups, socioeconomic groups, and other micro- and macro-level characteristics. Importantly, the EHR population under study can differ from other populations without affecting external validity: the issue is whether there is some unknown or unmeasured effect modifier in other areas.

To further drive home this point, suppose we are working with hypothetical EHR data to assess the relationship between an incident hospital-onset infection and a dichotomous exposure of surgery. We have access to three different EHRs representing three distinct patient cohorts and our presumed internally valid analysis found the following relative measures of association in each EHR cohort:

EHR 1. Relative risk (infection | surgery) = 1.5 (95% CI: 1.1, 1.9)
EHR 2. Relative risk (infection | surgery) = 2.0 (95% CI: 1.4, 2.8)
EHR 3. Relative risk (infection | surgery) = 2.5 (95% CI: 1.6, 4.1).

A natural question we may grapple with is whether this finding demonstrates a true difference in the hospitals or is driven by some compositional difference in the populations. Before we apply these results to other hospitals, we must be able to answer this important question, which motivates examining differences in the characteristics of each EHR population. If the differences in the source population and target population are not deemed to be important in the exposure to outcome relation, there is stronger evidence of external validity. Readers seeking a more thorough and formal treatment of external validity should consult these references (Degtiar & Rose, 2023; Lesko et al., 2017; Westreich et al., 2017).

Refining the definitions of validity

The concepts of internal and external validity have been well discussed in epidemiology (Hernán & Robins, 2020). There are theoretical (e.g., directed acyclic graphs) and mathematical representations of these two constructs, which, when ignored, may negate the value of a particular study. Internal and external validity can be confusing and ambiguous, such as the relationship between selection bias and representativeness or between generalizability and transportability. The concept of target validity has been proposed as a way of unifying this view, eschewing the need for a distinction between internal and external validity and focusing on a single measure known as target bias (Westreich et al., 2019). When target bias is zero, the study can be said to be valid. Another way to appreciate the concepts of internal and external validity is via simple, visual schematics borrowing the metaphor of inputs and outputs from computer science. The basis of these visual aids is conceptualizing internal validity as inputs to the analysis and external validity as outputs from the analysis. In other words, decisions and assumptions made about the participants or their health measures from the EHR (i.e., the inputs) impact the analysis, whereas the evidence garnered from the EHR's analysis (i.e., the outputs) impacts the inference made to various populations. Fundamental to this presentation is the study is etiologic in nature, seeking to measure a health outcome related to some putative exposure.

Figure 9.8 depicts a study that is free from bias; the inputs and outputs were both valid. When drawing the study sample or population from the EHR, there were no systematic errors in selecting participants or measuring variables, and all relevant variables were included. Sampling error was minimized, and the study

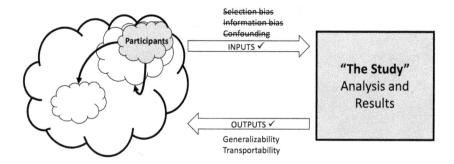

Figure 9.8 A study where the inputs and outputs are valid: internal and external validity.

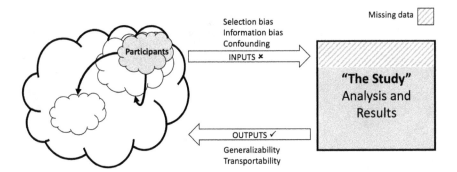

Figure 9.9 A study where the inputs are invalid, but the outputs are valid: external validity
without internal validity.

was analyzed correctly. The results are applicable to the broader population that
the study sample was drawn from as well as other, different populations. In other
words, the participants were exchangeable with other groups.

Figure 9.9 depicts a study where there was a systematic error that resulted in a lack
of internal validity, and thus one or more of the inputs were flawed. The study
population may have been preferentially selected based on the exposure and outcome (selection bias), may have mismeasured an important variable (information
bias), and/or may have failed to adequately consider an influential extraneous
variable (confounding). Internal validity has also been described as problem of
missing data (Howe, Cain & Hogan, 2015), in that data may be missing on the
non-participants (selection bias), the true value of measurements (information bias),
or the measurement of influential variables (confounding). In any or all these cases,
these "missing data" impact the results obtained during analysis. It is also important to recognize that decisions on the treatment of missing data may result in a
manifestation of any of these concepts; for example, a complete case analysis that
has excluded participants differentially on the exposure and outcome can induce
a selection bias. Despite the potential for external validity, in that the participants
may have been representative of a community targeted for inference (except in the
case of a selection bias), without internal validity we should be cautious in making
any such inference. Internal validity is a prerequisite to external validity, and to
quote another computer science adage, "garbage in, garbage out."

Figure 9.10 depicts a study that is internally valid yet lacks external validity and
thus one or more of the outputs are problematic. The participants may be non-
representative of some target population: they lack exchangeability. For example,
suppose study participants were randomly drawn from a hospital that is highly
regarded for the treatment of cancer and the desired inference was the local community. The participants in the study are likely not representative of the hospital's
catchment area, yet the study was free from any selection bias because we did not
preferentially select patients contingent on an exposure and outcome, and the
sample was randomly obtained. In this case, the study lacks generalizability to the

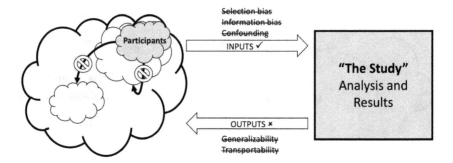

Figure 9.10 A study where the inputs are valid, but the outputs are invalid: internal validity without external validity.

local community but may be transportable to other settings with similar characteristics to the patients who have traveled to this hospital. In another example, suppose the study participants were again randomly drawn from a hospital, but this time at an urban safety net hospital that serves groups that have been historically marginalized. Again, we did not preferentially select patient's contingent on an exposure and outcome, so the results are not subject to selection bias, but in this case the participants were representative of their local community (the one served by this safety net hospital). In this case, the results may not transport from the marginalized group seen at the local hospital to a more affluent group seen at a different hospital in a different community. In other words, there is a lack of transportability to another, more affluent community, but the study maintains generalizability to the local community. A key feature of both threats to external validity shown in Figure 9.10 and presented in these two examples is the presence of an effect modifier. Some feature of the target population to which we wish to apply our inference is modifying the exposure to outcome relation. Continuing with the examples, this could be socioeconomic position as a surrogate for access to healthcare. As with the case of flawed inputs, problematic outputs are a warning for the epidemiologist to reconsider any exposure to outcome effect outside of the confines of the study participants.

Under this computer science metaphor, inputs capture the processes antecedent to analysis, while outputs represent the application of the results to various places and populations. This builds upon the concepts of internal and external validity by identifying a directionality to the mechanisms and providing a logical connection between the steps typically undertaken in an epidemiological study. Although inputs and outputs are depicted separately in the figures, they are by no means mutually exclusive. One can have problems with both the inputs and outputs concurrently (a combination of Figures 9.9 and 9.10), nor is it possible to identify a hierarchy to them (inputs are not greater than outputs, and outputs are not greater than inputs) (Westreich et al., 2019). Additionally, the notion of a study free from all biases may be an impossibility as there may always be a conceivable reason why an input or output is not perfect. Rather than striving for perfection, epidemiologists should focus on understanding the presence and impact of threats to validity, and, if necessary, perform a quantitative bias analysis, discussed in the next section.

Revisiting the inferential goals can help identify which type of validity is of greatest concern. If the target of inference is population-level, such as measures of disease prevalence or risk factors, then some error may be acceptable as these are "lower risk" situations. In this case, one might posit that external validity is of greater importance than internal validity. On the other hand, if the target of inference is individual prognosis or risk prediction, such as risk of infection in the hospital or disease prognosis due to an intervention, then more precise errors are needed as there is greater potential for harm from getting the wrong answer. In other words, internal validity may matter more than external validity, such as in a randomized controlled trial.

Bias analysis

Quantitative bias analysis (QBA) seeks to understand the sensitivity of the study results when there are threats to internal validity. Such bias analyses assess the impact of systematic errors resulting in selection bias, uncontrolled confounding, and information bias, and range from straightforward calculations to advanced probabilistic- and simulation-based approaches. A full treatment of QBA is outside the scope of this book, and, in fact, already exists as a standalone text (Fox, MacLehose & Lash, 2021). Rather, what follows is a high-level overview of QBA and its application to EHR-based epidemiology.

To conduct a bias analysis, one first needs to ascertain the *bias parameters*, which indicate the degree to which systematic error may be involved in the study. For simplicity, the bias parameters in this section all assume the simple case of a dichotomous exposure and outcome; more complex cases are covered in Fox, MacLehose, and Lash (2021). For selection bias, bias parameters include the probability of selection according to four strata: presence or absence of the exposure for those with and without the outcome. For uncontrolled confounding, bias parameters include the prevalence of the latent confounder with and without the exposure, as well as the presumed strength of the association between the latent confounder and the outcome. This can also be extended for effect modification by including bias parameters for the association between the latent confounder and the outcome, given presence or absence of the effect modifier. For information bias, bias parameters include the sensitivity and specificity of the misclassified variable. When differential misclassification is suspected, the sensitivity and specificity need to be calculated for both presence and absence of the other variable. When dependent misclassification is suspected, the amount of correlated error is also needed.

Bias parameters may come from several sources including a validation study, literature review, or even educated guesses; what is best for a particular study may be determined by availability of data or perceived importance of the parameter. Validation studies may be internal to the study at hand, and a matter of recognizing the availability of the data needed to compute the bias parameters, or external, requiring the recruitment of a new sample with the explicit goal of measuring the needed data. Consideration of all sources – validation study, literature review, educated guesses – will result in the most informative parameter selection.

Before proceeding further, let us consider several hypothetical examples of threats to internal validity applying the QBA techniques from Fox, MacLehose, and Lash (2021).[3] Chapter 8 presented the results from an EHR-based case–control study of very low birthweight neonates and staph infection while in the neonatal intensive care unit. For convenience, those data are presented in Table 9.1. A naïve analysis of these data will find that on average, very low birthweight neonates have 4.6 times the odds of also being diagnosed with a staph infection in the NICU compared to not very low birthweight neonates (95% confidence interval 2.8, 7.5).

Let us suppose that neonates who were not very low birthweight and did not have an infection were 50% less likely to participate in the study due to a systematic error that occurred during recruitment. With this bit of info and application of QBA, the selection bias adjusted odds ratio is 9.3. In other words, where this type of selection bias is present in the study, the researchers would have substantially underestimated the true effect. Now let us suppose that the outcome of staph infection was missed in 25% of cases when the infant was not very low birthweight, 10% of cases when the infant was very low birthweight, and there were no false diagnoses present. Application of QBA results in a nondependent differential misclassification adjusted odds ratio of 4.0, indicating a bias away from the null in the naïve analysis that could otherwise not have been anticipated. Finally, let us suppose that we failed to consider maternal infection as a possible confounder of this relationship. Suppose that the prevalence of maternal infection among very low birthweight infants was 20%, the prevalence of maternal infection among infants not very low birthweight was 10%, and the odds ratio of maternal infection on staph infection in the neonates was 2.5. Post-QBA, the Mantel–Haenszel adjusted odds ratio is 3.8, suggesting positive residual confounding. While these three hypothetical examples are straightforward to calculate, they lack estimates of precision, treat the bias parameters as deterministic, and only consider a single source of bias. Probabilistic- and simulation-based techniques build upon simple QBA by providing for more flexibility and rigor in the analyses (Fox, MacLehose & Lash, 2021).

A question may arise, when are QBA methods needed and appropriate? Lash et al. (2014) addressed this question in their article "Good practices for quantitative

Table 9.1 The very low birthweight and staph infection case-control contingency table

Independent variable	Dependent variable		Totals
	Case (D+)	*Control (D−)*	
Exposed (E+)	45	60	105
Unexposed (E−)	55	340	395
Totals	100	400	500

bias analysis."[4] They counsel that QBA is needed when there is causal inference from modest results or policy recommendations or action will result from the work. They then go on to describe how to identify which bias(es) to address with QBA, selection of the most appropriate QBA technique(s), operationalization of the bias parameters, and interpreting and disseminating the QBA results.

When researchers are particularly concerned over issues of unmeasured or uncontrolled confounding, the *e*-value is a newer and popular technique that is easy to calculate and interpret (VanderWeele & Ding, 2017). The *e*-value defines the minimum strength of an association that an unmeasured confounder would need to exert to fully negate the observed association. For an odds ratio (OR) for a rare outcome, the *e*-value may be calculated as OR + sqrt(OR $\star$ (OR − 1)).[5] Continuing with the earlier very low birthweight and staph infection example, the *e*-value is 8.67 for the point estimate of 4.6, and 5.04 for the lower bound of the confidence interval of 2.8. This can also be shown visually, as in Figure 9.11. The *e*-value in this figure corresponds to the inflection point in the curve at which point a confounder at or greater than this strength would fully explain the observed exposure to outcome relation. An interpretation of the *e*-value itself is one where "the observed risk ratio of 4.6 could be explained away by an unmeasured confounder that was associated with both very low birthweight and staph infection

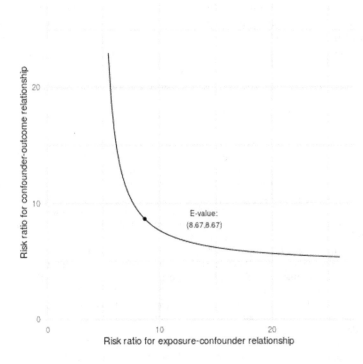

Figure 9.11 The *e*-value for an observed odds ratio of 4.6.

Image created from https://www.evalue-calculator.com and used with permission of MB Mathur.

by an odds ratio of 8.67 each, above and beyond the measured confounders, but weaker confounding could not do so" (VanderWeele & Ding, 2017). The *e*-value on its own does not demonstrate causality nor guarantee that confounding is not possible; it provides additional evidence to the plausibility of unmeasured confounding negating the observed results. It is also not a panacea to confounding, proper study design, or hypothesis testing (Ioannidis, Tan & Blum, 2019). Other techniques are available for assessing the impact of unmeasured confounding beyond those presented here (Lin, Psaty & Kronmal, 1998).

In addition to the book by Fox, MacLehose, and Lash (2021) that lays out the foundations of QBA, there are published tutorials on the topic. Newcomer et al. (2019) tackle outcome misclassification and offer a primer on using predictive values to perform a simple (deterministic) QBA. Banack, Hayes-Larson, and Mayeda (2022) detail how Monte Carlo simulations may be used to perform a QBA in the context of selection bias. Goldstein et al. (2022) demonstrate how to apply probabilistic-based techniques to account for misclassification of ICD codes. All these tutorials are applicable to EHR data. A systematic assessment of the use of QBA in epidemiological research between 2006 and 2019 noted that the majority of the 238 reviewed papers focused on misclassification, followed by uncontrolled confounding, and, least often, selection bias (Petersen et al., 2021). Readers may wish to consult this review for specific demonstrations of QBA that may be applicable to their EHR research projects. Lastly, aside from traditional QBA approaches, there are other options for researchers facing imperfect data. Shepherd and Yu (2011) describe an innovative approach to adjusting regression estimates using accuracy data obtained from an audit: this could be directly applicable to the situation where medical data have been abstracted from the EHR and a random subset is sampled for chart review and audit (see Chapter 6).

Notes

1 The article "Why representativeness should be avoided" by Rothman, Gallacher, & Hatch (2013) generated an interesting series of commentaries and letters arguing for and against representativeness. A listing of them can be found here: https://pubmed. ncbi.nlm.nih.gov/24062287/.

2 Such diagrams go by different names, depending on the field and framework. For example, directed acyclic graphs (DAGs) are common in epidemiology. They are particularly useful for revealing causal pathways in a study, drawing attention to concerns over validity (Greenland, Pearl, & Robins, 1999), but can be complicated to draw and interpret. This book uses more generic conceptual diagrams, which lack a rigid structure.

3 These examples may be reproduced based on the observed data in Table 9.1, the bias parameters that follow in text, and the spreadsheets for selection bias ("Selection Bias" tab), uncontrolled confounding ("OR" tab), and misclassification ("Outcome Misc" tab) that may be downloaded from the QBA book accompanying website: https://sites. google.com/site/biasanalysis.

4 An interesting and related article is "Bias Analysis Gone Bad" that covers three examples of suboptimal application of these techniques (Lash et al., 2021).

5 An *e*-value calculator for different epidemiologic measures is available at: https:// www.evalue-calculator.com (Mathur et al., 2018).

References

Banack HR, Hayes-Larson E, Mayeda ER. Monte Carlo simulation approaches for quantitative bias analysis: A tutorial. Epidemiol Rev. 2022;43(1):106–117.

Björk J, Nilsson A, Bonander C, Strömberg U. A novel framework for classification of selection processes in epidemiological research. BMC Med Res Methodol. 2020;20(1):155.

Bodnar LM, Siega-Riz AM, Simhan HN, Diesel JC, Abrams B. The impact of exposure misclassification on associations between prepregnancy BMI and adverse pregnancy outcomes. Obesity (Silver Spring). 2010;18(11):2184–2190.

Bosco JL, Silliman RA, Thwin SS, Geiger AM, Buist DS, Prout MN, Yood MU, Haque R, Wei F, Lash TL. A most stubborn bias: No adjustment method fully resolves confounding by indication in observational studies. J Clin Epidemiol. 2010;63(1):64–74.

Brennan AT, Getz KD, Brooks DR, Fox MP. An underappreciated misclassification mechanism: Implications of nondifferential dependent misclassification of covariate and exposure. Ann Epidemiol. 2021;58:104–123.

Brooks DR, Getz KD, Brennan AT, Pollack AZ, Fox MP. The impact of joint misclassification of exposures and outcomes on the results of epidemiologic research. Curr Epidemiol Rep. 2018;5(2):166–174.

Choi AL, Cordier S, Weihe P, Grandjean P. Negative confounding in the evaluation of toxicity: The case of methylmercury in fish and seafood. Crit Rev Toxicol. 2008;38(10):877–893.

Chubak J, Dalmat RR, Weiss NS, Doria-Rose VP, Corley DA, Kamineni A. Informative presence in electronic health record data: A challenge in implementing study exclusion criteria. Epidemiology. 2023 Jan 1;34(1):29–32.

Cole SR, Stuart EA. Generalizing evidence from randomized clinical trials to target populations: The ACTG 320 trial. Am J Epidemiol. 2010;172(1):107–115.

Degtiar R, Rose S. A review of generalizability and transportability. Annu Rev Statist Appl. 2023;10(1):501–524.

Desai RJ, Levin R, Lin KJ, Patorno E. Bias implications of outcome misclassification in observational studies evaluating association between treatments and all-cause or cardiovascular mortality using administrative claims. J Am Heart Assoc. 2020;9(17):e016906.

Edwards JK, Cole SR, Troester MA, Richardson DB. Accounting for misclassified outcomes in binary regression models using multiple imputation with internal validation data. Am J Epidemiol. 2013;177(9):904–912.

Edwards JK, Cole SR, Westreich D. All your data are always missing: Incorporating bias due to measurement error into the potential outcomes framework. Int J Epidemiol. 2015;44(4):1452–1459.

Faillie JL. Indication bias or protopathic bias? Br J Clin Pharmacol. 2015;80(4):779–780.

Feinstein AR, Horwitz RI, Spitzer WO, Battista RN. Coffee and pancreatic cancer. The problems of etiologic science and epidemiologic case-control research. JAMA. 1981;246(9):957–961.

Flegal KM, Graubard BI, Williamson DF, Cooper RS. Reverse causation and illness-related weight loss in observational studies of body weight and mortality. Am J Epidemiol. 2011;173(1):1–9.

Flegal KM, Keyl PM, Nieto FJ. Differential misclassification arising from nondifferential errors in exposure measurement. Am J Epidemiol. 1991;134(10):1233–1244.

Flood TL, Zhao YQ, Tomayko EJ, Tandias A, Carrel AL, Hanrahan LP. Electronic health records and community health surveillance of childhood obesity. Am J Prev Med. 2015;48(2):234–240.

Fox MP, MacLehose RF, Lash TL. Applying Quantitative Bias Analysis to Epidemiologic Data. 2nd edition. New York, NY: Springer, 2021.

Funk MJ, Landi SN. Misclassification in administrative claims data: Quantifying the impact on treatment effect estimates. Curr Epidemiol Rep. 2014;1(4):175–185.

Funk LM, Shan Y, Voils CI, Kloke J, Hanrahan LP. Electronic health record data versus the national health and nutrition examination survey (NHANES): A comparison of overweight and obesity rates. Med Care. 2017;55(6):598–605.

Gianfrancesco MA, Goldstein ND. A narrative review on the validity of electronic health record-based research in epidemiology. BMC Med Res Methodol. 2021;21(1):234.

Gianfrancesco MA, McCulloch CE, Trupin L, Graf J, Schmajuk G, Yazdany J. Reweighting to address nonparticipation and missing data bias in a longitudinal electronic health record study. Ann Epidemiol. 2020;50:48–51.e2.

Goldstein BA, Bhavsar NA, Phelan M, Pencina MJ. Controlling for informed presence bias due to the number of health encounters in an electronic health record. Am J Epidemiol. 2016;184(11):847–855.

Goldstein ND, Kahal D, Testa K, Burstyn I. Inverse probability weighting for selection bias in a Delaware community health center electronic medical record study of community deprivation and hepatitis c prevalence. Ann Epidemiol. 2021;60:1–7.

Goldstein ND, Kahal D, Testa K, Gracely EJ, Burstyn I. Data quality in electronic health record research: An approach for validation and quantitative bias analysis for imperfectly ascertained health outcomes via diagnostic codes. Harv Data Sci Rev. 2022 Spring;4(2). 10.1162/99608f92.cbe67e91.

Goldstein BA, Phelan M, Pagidipati NJ, Peskoe SB. How and when informative visit processes can bias inference when using electronic health records data for clinical research. J Am Med Inform Assoc. 2019;26(12):1609–1617.

Greenhouse JB, Kaizar EE, Kelleher K, Seltman H, Gardner W. Generalizing from clinical trial data: A case study. The risk of suicidality among pediatric antidepressant users. Stat Med. 2008;27(11):1801–1813.

Greenland S, Pearl J, Robins JM. Causal diagrams for epidemiologic research. Epidemiology. 1999;10(1):37–48.

Gustafson P. Measurement Error and Misclassification in Statistics and Epidemiology: Impacts and Bayesian Adjustments. Boca Raton, FL: CRC Press/Taylor & Francis, 2003.

Gustafson P, Le Nhu D. Comparing the effects of continuous and discrete covariate mismeasurement, with emphasis on the dichotomization of mismeasured predictors. Biometrics. 2002;58(4):878–887.

Haneuse S, Daniels M. A general framework for considering selection bias in EHR-based studies: What data are observed and why? EGEMS. 2016;4(1):1203.

Hernán MA, Robins JM. Causal Inference: What If. Boca Raton, FL: Chapman & Hall/CRC, 2020.

Horwitz RI, Feinstein AR. The problem of "protopathic bias" in case-control studies. Am J Med. 1980;68(2):255–258.

Howe CJ, Cain LE, Hogan JW. Are all biases missing data problems? Curr Epidemiol Rep. 2015;2(3):162–171.

Ioannidis JPA, Tan YJ, Blum MR. Limitations and misinterpretations of e-values for sensitivity analyses of observational studies. Ann Intern Med. 2019;170(2):108–111.

Joseph KS, Mehrabadi A, Lisonkova S. Confounding by indication and related concepts. Curr Epidemiol Rep. 2014;1:1–8.

Jurek AM, Maldonado G, Greenland S. Adjusting for outcome misclassification: The importance of accounting for case-control sampling and other forms of outcome-related selection. Ann Epidemiol. 2013;23(3):129–135.

Kearns MD, Boursi B, Yang YX. Proton pump inhibitors on pancreatic cancer risk and survival. Cancer Epidemiol. 2017;46:80–84.

Keogh RH, Shaw PA, Gustafson P, Carroll RJ, Deffner V, Dodd KW, Küchenhoff H, Tooze JA, Wallace MP, Kipnis V, Freedman LS. STRATOS guidance document on measurement error and misclassification of variables in observational epidemiology: Part 1-basic theory and simple methods of adjustment. Stat Med. 2020;39(16):2197–2231.

Kivimäki M, Luukkonen R, Batty GD, Ferrie JE, Pentti J, Nyberg ST, Shipley MJ, Alfredsson L, Fransson EI, Goldberg M, Knutsson A, Koskenvuo M, Kuosma E, Nordin M, Suominen SB, Theorell T, Vuoksimaa E, Westerholm P, Westerlund H, Zins M, Kivipelto M, Vahtera J, Kaprio J, Singh-Manoux A, Jokela M. Body mass index and risk of dementia: Analysis of individual-level data from 1.3 million individuals. Alzheimers Dement. 2018;14(5):601–609.

Lash TL, Ahern TP, Collin LJ, Fox MP, MacLehose RF. Bias analysis gone bad. Am J Epidemiol. 2021;190(8):1604–1612.

Lash TL, Fox MP, MacLehose RF, Maldonado G, McCandless LC, Greenland S. Good practices for quantitative bias analysis. Int J Epidemiol. 2014;43(6):1969–1985.

Lesko CR, Buchanan AL, Westreich D, Edwards JK, Hudgens MG, Cole SR. Generalizing study results: A potential outcomes perspective. Epidemiology. 2017;28(4):553–561.

Lin DY, Psaty BM, Kronmal RA. Assessing the sensitivity of regression results to unmeasured confounders in observational studies. Biometrics. 1998;54(3):948–963.

Lin KJ, Singer DE, Glynn RJ, Murphy SN, Lii J, Schneeweiss S. Identifying patients with high data completeness to improve validity of comparative effectiveness research in electronic health records data. Clin Pharmacol Ther. 2018;103(5):899–905.

MacMahon B, Yen S, Trichopoulos D, Warren K, Nardi G. Coffee and cancer of the pancreas. N Engl J Med. 1981;304(11):630–633.

Mathur MB, Ding P, Riddell CA, VanderWeele TJ. Web site and r package for computing e-values. Epidemiology. 2018;29(5):e45–e47.

McGee G, Haneuse S, Coull BA, Weisskopf MG, Rotem RS. On the nature of informative presence bias in analyses of electronic health records. Epidemiology. 2022;33(1):105–113.

Merola D, Schneeweiss S, Schrag D, Lii J, Lin KJ. An algorithm to predict data completeness in oncology electronic medical records for comparative effectiveness research. Ann Epidemiol. 2022;76:143–149.

Newcomer SR, Xu S, Kulldorff M, Daley MF, Fireman B, Glanz JM. A primer on quantitative bias analysis with positive predictive values in research using electronic health data. J Am Med Inform Assoc. 2019;26(12):1664–1674.

Petersen JM, Ranker LR, Barnard-Mayers R, MacLehose RF, Fox MP. A systematic review of quantitative bias analysis applied to epidemiological research. Int J Epidemiol. 2021;50(5):1708–1730.

Porta M. A Dictionary of Epidemiology. New York, NY: Oxford University Press, 2014.

Raphael K. Recall bias: A proposal for assessment and control. Int J Epidemiol. 1987;16(2):167–170.

Rassen JA, Murk W, Schneeweiss S. Real-world evidence of bariatric surgery and cardiovascular benefits using electronic health records data: A lesson in bias. Diabetes Obes Metab. 2021;23(7):1453–1462.

Ravindrarajah R, Hazra NC, Hamada S, Charlton J, Jackson SHD, Dregan A, Gulliford MC. Systolic blood pressure trajectory, frailty, and all-cause mortality >80 years of age: Cohort study using electronic health records. Circulation. 2017;135(24):2357–2368.

Richiardi L, Pizzi C, Pearce N. Commentary: Representativeness is usually not necessary and often should be avoided. Int J Epidemiol. 2013;42(4):1018–1022.

Robins JM. Causal models for estimating the effects of weight gain on mortality. Int J Obes. 2008;32(3):S15–S41.

Rothman KJ, Gallacher JE, Hatch EE. Why representativeness should be avoided. Int J Epidemiol. 2013;42(4):1012–1014.

Rothwell PM. External validity of randomised controlled trials: "to whom do the results of this trial apply?" Lancet. 2005;365(9453):82–93.

Royston P, Altman DG, Sauerbrei W. Dichotomizing continuous predictors in multiple regression: A bad idea. Stat Med. 2006;25(1):127–141.

Sayon-Orea C, Moreno-Iribas C, Delfrade J, Sanchez-Echenique M, Amiano P, Ardanaz E, Gorricho J, Basterra G, Nuin M, Guevara M. Inverse-probability weighting and multiple imputation for evaluating selection bias in the estimation of childhood obesity prevalence using data from electronic health records. BMC Med Inform Decis Mak. 2020;20(1):9.

Shepherd BE, Yu C. Accounting for data errors discovered from an audit in multiple linear regression. Biometrics. 2011;67(3):1083–1091.

Srugo SA, Gaudet L, Corsi D, Fakhraei R, Guo Y, Fell DB. Examining the effects of pre-pregnancy weight and gestational weight gain on allergic disease development in offspring: A protocol for a population-based study using health administrative databases in Ontario, Canada. BMJ Paediatr Open. 2021;5(1):e000893.

Szklo M. Population-based cohort studies. Epidemiol Rev. 1998;20(1):81–90.

Tirozzi A, Santonastaso F, de Gaetano G, Iacoviello L, Gialluisi A. Does COVID-19 increase the risk of neuropsychiatric sequelae? Evidence from a Mendelian randomization approach. World J Psychiatry. 2022;12(3):536–540.

Tran NK, Lash TL, Goldstein ND. Practical data considerations for the modern epidemiology student. Glob Epidemiol. 2021;3:100066.

VanderWeele TJ, Ding P. Sensitivity analysis in observational research: Introducing the e-value. Ann Intern Med. 2017;167(4):268–274.

Westreich D, Edwards JK, Lesko CR, Cole SR, Stuart EA. Target validity and the hierarchy of study designs. Am J Epidemiol. 2019;188(2):438–443.

Westreich D, Edwards JK, Lesko CR, Stuart E, Cole SR. Transportability of trial results using inverse odds of sampling weights. Am J Epidemiol. 2017;186(8):1010–1014.

Yland JJ, Wesselink AK, Lash TL, Fox MP. Misconceptions about the direction of bias from nondifferential misclassification. Am J Epidemiol. 2022;191(8):1485–1495.

10 Epidemiologic Analysis I

The focus of this chapter and the next is moving from data to results. These chapters present a refresher in biostatistics, including crude measures of association and multivariable modeling, model diagnostics, sensitivity analysis, and methods in missing data. This material is not intended to be a full introduction to analytic techniques nor an advanced study in the methodology needed to analyze observational data. Rather, this material is a concise summary of the procedures and techniques most applicable to EHR analysis. The presentation is generic although wherever possible, EHR-specific concerns are addressed. Readers with expertise in this material may elect to skim these chapters or skip to the sections of greatest relevance to their research projects.

Any epidemiological analysis, whether descriptive or analytic, generates statistics and it is up to the researcher to understand how to interpret the results from the statistics. In this chapter, we revisit some of the most common statistics encountered in analytic epidemiology organized by the statistical procedure and offer practical interpretation of the relevant output. The goal is not to instruct how to perform these tests but rather revisit their proper interpretation. Unless otherwise indicated, all hypothesis tests are interpreted as statistically significant if the p-value is less than an α of 0.05, the *de facto* standard, and for simplicity, all assumptions behind these statistical tests have been met.

The analytic procedures and output were produced using R statistical software (R Core Team, 2020) but are applicable to any statistical software; the interpretation of the statistics remains consistent regardless of the software used. The chapter begins with a review of key assumptions in statistical analysis within the framework of descriptive epidemiology, and then transitions to analytic epidemiology. To introduce analytic epidemiology, bivariate analyses where a single exposure and outcome are modeled are presented along with the fundamentals of regression techniques. Later in the chapter we turn to multivariable analysis that is presented within the context of the epidemiological study design and inferential goal.

An example analytic dataset

Many of the sample codes, graphs, and figures in this chapter and the next are derived from an example dataset of risk factors associated with low birthweight of infants, *birthwt*, available in the *MASS* package (Venables & Ripley, 2002) in

DOI: 10.4324/9781003258872-13

Table 10.1 The *birthwt* data dictionary

Variable	Type	Values	Missing	Comment
low	Categorical	0 = no 1 = yes	0 (0%)	Low birthweight defined as <2,500 grams
age	Numeric	14...45	0 (0%)	Maternal age, in years
lwt	Numeric	80...250	0 (0%)	Maternal weight at last menstrual period, in pounds
race	Categorical	1 = White 2 = Black 3 = other	0 (0%)	Maternal race
smoke	Categorical	0 = no 1 = yes	0 (0%)	Smoking status during pregnancy
ptl	Categorical	0, 1, 2, 3	0 (0%)	Number of previous preterm labor
ht	Categorical	0 = no 1 = yes	0 (0%)	History of maternal hypertension
ui	Categorical	0 = no 1 = yes	0 (0%)	Presence of uterine irritability
ftv	Categorical	0, 1, 2, 3, 4, 5, 6	0 (0%)	Number of doctor visits during first trimester
bwt	Numeric	709...4990	0 (0%)	Birthweight, in grams
gestation	Numeric	34...43	0 (0%)	Gestational age at birth

the R statistical software (R Core Team, 2020). The data in *birthwt* represent a cross-sectional study of infants at a medical center and can be conceptualized as a secondary data analysis from the EHR. While the data are cross-sectional, we will analyze them under various study designs to demonstrate the methods, however this is for didactic purposes alone and does not necessarily represent true causality. Example code to load the *birthwt* dataset from the *MASS* package and save it as a universally readable CSV file can be found in Code #3.1 in Appendix 2.

Table 10.1 is the data dictionary for *birthwt*. Notice the inclusion of a new variable not in the original dataset, "gestation." This variable was simulated to represent the gestational age of the infant at birth and will be treated as a measure of maternal follow-up time in a cohort analysis. Deliberately, gestational age was set to vary with respect to a maternal history of smoking, where a positive history was associated with an increase in preterm birth. For users of R, sample code to load the dataset and simulate the gestation variable can be found in Code #10.1 in Appendix 2.

Describing the variables and verifying assumptions

Almost every epidemiological or clinical analysis that utilizes human participants will typically include a description of the study population or sample as the first exhibit in the resultant publication: the so-called "table one." This table summarizes key participant characteristics and helps the reader assess whether any anomalies are present that may impact internal or external validity. We may also review the distribution of variables and assess whether any statistical assumptions are potentially violated. The appropriate descriptive statistics will depend upon the type of variable. For categorical variables, the statistics typically include a count of the number of observations in that category and percent. Categories with a small number of observations – generally less than five – may need to be appropriately condensed (see chapter 5). For continuous variables, the statistics include a measure of central tendency, such as the mean or median, and a measure of variability, such as the standard deviation or interquartile range, which indicates the spread of the data. The decision to use mean or median depends on the distribution of the variable: if the distribution is approximately normal (Figure 10.1a), the mean is appropriate to present, while if the distribution is heavily skewed (Figure 10.1b), a median may be more appropriate. There are many types of distributions possible including nonparametric ones that do not conform to any expected shape. Since many statistical tests assume

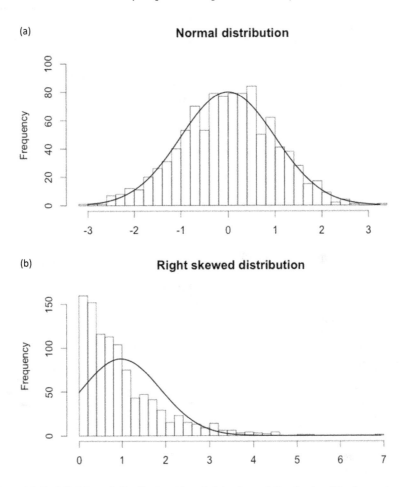

Figure 10.1(a & b) Normal distribution (a) and right skewed distribution (b) of a continuous variable.

approximate normality, checking all variable distributions is a typical first step in the analysis.

When the variable is not normally distributed, it may be transformed through a mathematical operation, such as taking the natural log of the variable, or used in a nonparametric statistical test that does not assume a given distribution. When working with EHR data, many variables will satisfy the normality assumption due to the large sample sizes, but it is nevertheless still prudent to verify this assumption.

Examining the *birthwt* data dictionary (Table 10.1), there are seven categorical variables ("low," "race," "smoke," "ptl," "ht," "ui," and "ftv") and four continuous variables ("age," "lwt," "bwt," and "gestation"). For the categorical variables, we can use a frequency table (Table 10.2) to check the distribution of categories and ensure no category has fewer than five observations, our heuristic of choice. We can see that the variables "low," "race," "smoke," "ht," and "ui" do not violate the small counts assumption, while "ptl" and "ftv" have cells with counts fewer than five. Based upon this finding, both "ptl" and "ftv" require re-parameterization. The easiest option may to collapse the small cell count categories, as follows. Previous

Table 10.2 Distribution of the categorical variables in the *birthwt* dataset

Characteristic (variable)	Count	Frequency
Low birthweight (low)		
No	130	69%
Yes	59	31%
Maternal race (race)		
White	96	51%
Black	26	14%
Other	67	35%
Smoking during pregnancy (smoke)		
No	115	61%
Yes	74	39%
Previous preterm labor (ptl)		
None	159	84%
One	24	13%
Two	5	3%
Three	1	<1%
Maternal hypertension (ht)		
No	177	94%
Yes	12	6%
Uterine irritability (ui)		
No	161	85%
Yes	28	15%
First trimester doctor visits (ftv)		
None	100	53%
One	47	25%
Two	30	16%
Three	7	4%
Four	4	2%
Five	0	0%
Six	1	<1%

preterm labor becomes a dichotomous category representing a history of preterm labor (yes or no), and three through six first trimester doctor visits become three or more doctor visits. Compare Tables 10.2 and 10.3 to see the re-parameterization of these two variables to account for the small cell counts.

Equally important to the distribution of cell counts is whether these categories conceptually capture the characteristics of interest. For example, the definition of maternal race is nonspecific as it does not consider racial groups other than White and Black, which have not been clearly defined, such as the inclusion of non-African-American Black races. Without the proper categories defined in advance, teasing out nuanced differences in the study population will be impossible.

Histograms can be used to verify the distributions of the four continuous variables (Figure 10.2). Visual inspection indicates "age" and "lwt" that are slightly right skewed, "gestation" is slightly left skewed, while "bwt" is not appreciably skewed. There may also be outliers present, which can be identified using boxplots (Figure 10.3). There are many outliers in the "lwt" variable, while the other

Table 10.3 Characteristics of the *birthwt* analytic dataset

Characteristic (variable)	Count or Mean	Frequency or Standard deviation
Low birthweight (low)		
No	130	69%
Yes	59	31%
Maternal age, years (age)	23	5
Maternal weight (lwt_170)		
<170 pounds	168	89%
≥170 pounds	21	11%
Maternal race (race)		
White	96	51%
Black	26	14%
Other	67	35%
Smoking during pregnancy (smoke)		
No	115	61%
Yes	74	39%
Previous preterm labor (ptl)		
No	159	84%
Yes	30	16%
Maternal hypertension (ht)		
No	177	94%
Yes	12	6%
Uterine irritability (ui)		
No	161	85%
Yes	28	15%
First trimester doctor visits (ftv)		
None	100	53%
One	47	25%
Two	30	16%
Three or more	12	6%
Birthweight, grams (bwt)	2945	729
Gestational age, weeks (gestation)	39	2

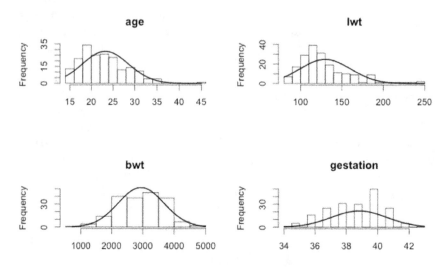

Figure 10.2 Distributions of the continuous variables in the *birthwt* dataset.

three continuous variables only have a single outlier. Based on the visual evidence, it is reasonable to suggest that "age," "bwt," and "gestation" satisfy the criteria for being approximately normal, while "lwt" can be transformed to resemble a normal distribution or re-parameterized as a categorical variable, depending on the research goals. Suppose we are particularly concerned about the effect of maternal weight on birth outcomes, and based on prior literature, a cut point of

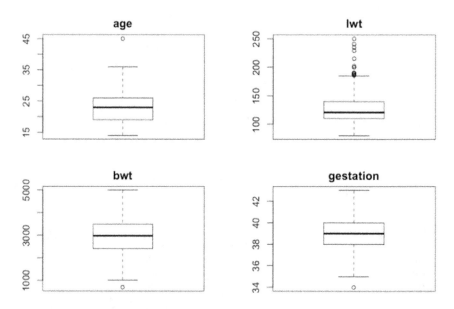

Figure 10.3 Boxplots of the continuous variables in the *birthwt* dataset.

170 pounds has been posited as an inflection point. We can dichotomize the continuous variable "lwt" into a categorical variable, "lwt_170", representing weight above (lwt_170 = 1) and below (lwt_170 = 0) this threshold.[1]

We have now preliminarily verified distributions and re-parameterized variables to accommodate potential violations of select statistical assumptions. While this is not meant to be an exhaustive or rigorous review of all theoretical assumptions, these quick checks represent an initial review of the data necessary for descriptive analysis. We can now construct a "table one" that depicts the characteristics of the *birthwt* dataset (Table 10.3). Note that in this table the continuous and categorical variables are presented together where the column labels and row indents (for levels of categorical variables) indicate the appropriate statistic to the reader. See Code #10.2 in Appendix 2 to generate Table 10.3.

Crude analysis

The term "crude analysis" is not meant in a pejorative way, but rather to state that an association is unadjusted for potential confounding effects. As demonstrated herein, crude analyses are used for bivariate comparisons between an exposure and outcome. Such associations are useful to identify differences in the distribution of characteristics across groups, such as for hypothesis formation, confounder identification, hypothesis testing, and so on. Such techniques are also applicable if confounding is not suspected, as is expected under a randomized controlled trial that achieved intervention exchangeability.

T-test

The t-test is one of the most used statistical tests and is applicable when comparing the mean of numeric characteristics across two groups that follow an approximately normal distribution. In the *birthwt* dataset, suppose we were interested in determining whether maternal age was associated with having a low birthweight baby. The researcher's hypothesis was that low birthweight babies were more frequent among mothers of younger age. The output from this analysis is shown in Figure 10.4, where group 0 is the not low birthweight infants and group 1 is the low birthweight infants.

```
> t.test(analytic_dataset$age ~ analytic_dataset$low)

        Welch Two Sample t-test

data:  analytic_dataset$age by analytic_dataset$low
t = 1.7737, df = 136.94, p-value = 0.07834
alternative hypothesis: true difference in means is not equal to 0
95 percent confidence interval:
 -0.1558349  2.8687423
sample estimates:
mean in group 0 mean in group 1
       23.66154        22.30508
```

Figure 10.4 A t-test comparing maternal age by low birthweight babies.

The mean maternal age of low birthweight infants was 22.3 years of age, while the mean maternal age of nonlow birthweight infants was 23.7 years of age. Although it may appear that on average low birthweight babies were "associated with"[2] mothers of a younger age, we do not have enough evidence to conclude this was not a chance finding (p-value = 0.08). Therefore, we may conclude there was no apparent mean age difference in mothers with low birthweight babies.

Analysis of variance (ANOVA)

When the researcher wishes to compare the mean between more than two groups, one-way ANOVA is commonly used. As with the t-test, its use is most appropriate when the numeric characteristics are represented by a continuous variable that follows an approximately normal distribution. The one-way ANOVA is a global test that will identify if at least one group is statistically different from any other group, but it will not indicate which group is different. To identify which group differs from others requires *post hoc* testing.

In the *birthwt* dataset, suppose we were interested in determining whether maternal age was associated with race, which was represented by three categories: groups 1, 2, and 3. The researcher's hypothesis was that maternal age varied with respect to race. The output from this analysis is shown in Figure 10.5a.

Based on the result of the ANOVA, there was statistical evidence to suggest that the mean maternal age varied with respect to race (p = 0.02). Note that we cannot identify which group(s) differed from this test alone, for that we must perform a *post hoc* analysis, as shown in Figure 10.5b. This *post hoc* analysis produces

(a)

```
> anova(aov(analytic_dataset$age ~ as.factor(analytic_dataset$race)))
Analysis of Variance Table

Response: analytic_dataset$age
                                  Df Sum Sq Mean Sq F valu  Pr(>F)
as.factor(analytic_dataset$race)   2  230.1 115.040   4.238  0.01585 *
Residuals                        186 5048.2  27.141
---
Signif. codes:  0 '***' 0.001 '**' 0.01 '*' 0.05 '.' 0.1 ' ' 1
```

(b)

```
> TukeyHSD(aov(analytic_dataset$age ~ as.factor(analytic_dataset$race)))
  Tukey multiple comparisons of means
    95% family-wise confidence level

Fit: aov(formula = analytic_dataset$age ~ as.factor(analytic_dataset$race))

          diff       lwr         upr       p adj
2-1 -2.7532051 -5.474434 -0.03197581 0.0466676
3-1 -1.9036070 -3.863030  0.05581649 0.0589215
3-2  0.8495982 -1.994371  3.69356754 0.7603654
```

Figure 10.5(a & b) A one-way ANOVA (a) and *post hoc* comparison (b) of maternal age by race.

pairwise comparisons: a comparison for each possible grouping of races. The three rows of the highlighted output indicate there were three comparisons performed: race 2 versus race 1, race 3 versus race 1, and race 3 versus race 2. Each comparison is interpreted independently:

- Race 2 averaged 2.7 years younger than race 1; this difference was likely not do to chance ($p < 0.05$) and was statistically significant.
- Race 3 averaged 1.9 years younger than race 1; this difference may be due to chance ($p = 0.06$) and therefore we would not conclude this was a statistically significant difference.
- Race 3 averaged 0.8 years older than race 2; this finding may be due to chance ($p = 0.76$) and therefore we would not conclude this was a statistically significant difference.

As can be inferred, the number of *post hoc* comparisons increases rapidly based on the number of groups being compared. As such, the probability of committing a type I error and having a false positive result increases based on the number of statistical tests being conducted on the data. One approach to guarding against this occurrence is by using a more conservative statistical significance threshold, for example an α 0.01 instead of 0.05, or by dividing the α based on the number of comparisons, known as a Bonferroni correction = $0.05/3 = 0.02$. Had we employed either of these strategies, none of the *post hoc* comparisons would have reached statistical significance, and we may have concluded there was no evidence to suggest that maternal age varied with respect to race.

Wilcoxon rank-sum or Mann-Whitney test

The Wilcoxon rank-sum or Mann-Whitney test is similar to the t-test in that two groups are being compared but is employed when the distribution of the characteristic does not follow a normal distribution, which violates a core assumption of the t-test. In this case, rather than test the mean difference between the groups, the distribution of the values is compared between groups to determine if the characteristics are statistically different.

In the *birthwt* dataset, suppose we were interested in determining whether maternal weight was associated with having a low birthweight baby and we had reason to believe that maternal weight was a skewed distribution. As such, the mean would be an inappropriate measure of central tendency, and we should use a test of the medians. The researcher's hypothesis was that low birthweight babies were more frequent among mothers of lower weight. The output from this analysis is shown in Figure 10.6, where group 0 is the not low birthweight infants and group 1 is the low birthweight infants.

As can be seen from the output, the median maternal weight of low birthweight babies was 120.0 pounds, while the median maternal weight of nonlow birthweight babies was 123.5 pounds. Low birthweight babies were correlated with mothers who weighed less ($p = 0.01$).

```
> wilcox.test(analytic_dataset$lwt ~ analytic_dataset$low)

    Wilcoxon rank sum test with continuity correction

data:  anal                        analytic_dataset$low
W = 4702.5,  p-value = 0.01278
alternative                        ocation shift is not equal to 0

> median(analytic_dataset$lwt[analytic_dataset$low==0])
[1] 123.5
> median(analytic_dataset$lwt[analytic_dataset$low==1])
[1] 120
```

Figure 10.6 A Wilcoxon rank-sum test comparing maternal weight by low birthweight babies.

Chi-squared test

A chi-squared test also seeks to determine if a characteristic is statistically different between groups. Unlike the preceding tests where the characteristic was numeric, a chi-squared test examines differences in categorical variables via a comparison of proportions. In the *birthwt* dataset, suppose we were interested in determining whether maternal race was associated with having a low birthweight baby. The researcher's hypothesis was that low birthweight babies are associated with mothers of a certain race, which is represented by three categories: groups 1, 2, and 3. As race was also a categorical variable, the analysis compared proportion of low birthweight babies for each race using a chi-squared test. The output from this analysis is shown in Figure 10.7, where group 0 is the not low birthweight infants and group 1 is the low birthweight infants.

Based on the p-value, we can conclude that there was likely no association of low birthweight babies with maternal race ($p = 0.08$). The cells in the output table provide some sense of proportions among the various race categories for low birthweight and nonlow birthweight babies. By using column percentages, in that the percentages in each column sum to 100%, we can easily compare the distribution of racial groups by birthweight. For example, 56% of women of race 1 did not have a low birthweight baby while 39% of women of race 1 had a low birthweight baby. Even though this may appear to be a large difference, we cannot conclude this was not due to chance alone. Nevertheless, and as will be discussed in Chapter 11, focusing on p-values alone, as opposed to the magnitude of the estimate, is problematic.

Regression analysis

The biostatistical approach most used in analytic epidemiology is regression. Regression is both a predictive and etiologic modeling method, where given the value of one or more *independent* variables (termed X_i for the *i*th variable, the exposure of interest plus covariates) the change in the *dependent* variable (termed Y, or the outcome) is estimated. When only a single independent variable is modeled ($i = 1$), the regression model corresponds to the slope of a line under the formula

```
> CrossTable(analytic_dataset$race, analytic_dataset$low, prop.r=F,
    prop.t=F, prop.chisq=F, chisq=T)

  Cell Contents
|-------------------------|
|                       N |
|            N / Col Total |
|-------------------------|


Total Observations in Table:  189
```

| | analytic_dataset$low | | |
analytic_dataset$race	0	1	Row Total
1	73 0.562	23 0.390	96
2	15 0.115	11 0.186	26
3	42 0.323	25 0.424	67
Column Total	130 0.688	59 0.312	189

```
Statistics for All Table Factors


Pearson's Chi-squared test
----------------------------------------------------
Chi^2 =  5.004813     d.f. =  2     p =  0.0818877
```

Figure 10.7 A chi-squared test comparing maternal age by race.

$Y = M \times X + B$, where M is the slope and B is the intercept. Unlike a crude bi-variable analysis that assesses the statistical relationship of only one exposure and outcome, a regression analysis allows the researcher to specify multiple covariates, thereby controlling for potential confounding. In other words, it is used to isolate the independent contributions on the outcome from each modeled variable. Doing so may provide stronger evidence of a link between the exposure and outcome since the other variables that may influence the relationship have been held constant in the analysis.

The regression results allow us to estimate measures of disease association, such as relative risks and odds ratios. As seen in Chapter 8, these measures of association are contingent upon the type of study and outcome: a cohort study that examines incident outcomes uses a relative risk of disease incidence, whereas a case-control study that examines presence of an outcome will use an odds ratio of exposure presence. Importantly, regression analyses will *only* provide associational estimates – the probability of an event occurring or having occurred – the context and philosophy brought to the analysis provide causal inference (discussed in Chapter 11). Multivariable analysis within the context of study design is presented in Chapter 11; here we review the fundamentals of regression models.

There are four core assumptions in standard regression techniques: (1) normality, (2) independence, (3) linearity, and (4) equal variance. The first assumption, normality, states that all variables follow an approximately normal distribution: multivariate normality. Instead of checking each variable individually, the *residuals*, or the difference between each predicted value and actual value, are usually assessed. The second assumption, independence, states that each observation in the dataset can be treated as a stand-alone entity that is not influenced by any other observations. When this assumption is violated, such as occurs with longitudinal data stored in long format or multilevel/hierarchical data, special techniques are needed to account for the nonindependence. These techniques are discussed in Chapter 11. The third assumption, linearity, states that a linear relationship is sufficient to explain the independent and dependent variables. A straight line – the regression line – represents a constant linear relationship between the observations over the range of the data, defined by the slope M in the earlier equation. When a linear relationship is *not* sufficient to explain the independent and dependent variables, the data must be transformed or require a nonparametric approach to modeling, such as spline or quantile regression. The final assumption, equal variance, states that the variability is constant through the predicted ranges of a variable, also known as *heteroscedasticity*. An often-used example is the relationship between income and age. At younger ages, incomes are generally lower and have a smaller range as younger workers tend to make similar starting salaries. At older ages, income becomes highly variable because some people make a lot of money while others make little money. Therefore, the variability in the data changes over age, thus violating the equal variance assumption. These four assumptions will be revisited in the model diagnostics section.

There are many types of regression techniques one can perform on epidemiological data, whether to account for potential violations in assumptions, offer improved control over confounding, more accurately represent a time-varying effect, accommodate different data types, or account for other nuances in the data. Linear regression techniques are used when the dependent, or outcome, variable is continuous. The independent variables' effects are interpreted as an average change in the outcome measure. For a continuous independent variable, the effect is based on a per-unit change of that variable. For a categorical independent variable, the effect is based on a relative comparison of the levels of the categories to some referent level.

Logistic regression is a generalized form of linear regression, and the same assumptions for linear regression hold true for logistic regression. In logistic regression, the dependent variable is binary – it either occurs or does not occur – such as being a case or control. The dichotomous outcome variable is "transformed" to a continuous value (the log-odds of the outcome) by use of the *logit* function, which is performed automatically in the logistic regression algorithm. As with linear regression, the independent variables can either be continuous or categorical, where the effect is based on a per-unit change of the continuous variable or a relative comparison of the levels of categorical variable to some referent level. Using the default *logit* link function, the estimates from a logistic regression will be odds ratios, the benefit of which should be apparent when analyzing a case-control study where the outcome is dichotomous.

Two other types of commonly used regression techniques include Poisson regression and Cox proportional hazards regression, also known as survival analysis. Poisson regression is appropriate when the dependent variable captures count data, such as the number of events that occur, and is especially useful for modeling the cumulative incidence or incidence rate when person time is available. The independent variables' effects are interpreted as a relative risks or rate ratios of the outcome. Cox regression is used when the dependent variable is binary and the primary interest is time-to-event, such as hospital discharge. The independent variables' effects are interpreted as a hazard ratio of the outcome, which is interpretable similar to a relative risk. As with the other regression techniques, for a continuous independent variable, the effect is based on a per-unit change of that variable and for a categorical independent variable, the effect is based on a relative comparison of the levels of the categories to some referent level.

Examples of linear and logistic regression from the birthwt analytic dataset

Figure 10.8 depicts the association between two continuous variables in the *birthwt* dataset: maternal weight at last menstrual period ("lwt") and infant's birthweight ("bwt"). The data were graphed via scatterplot, and a linear regression model was fit to estimate the relationship between the independent predictor of maternal weight and the dependent outcome of birthweight. There is both a qualitative and

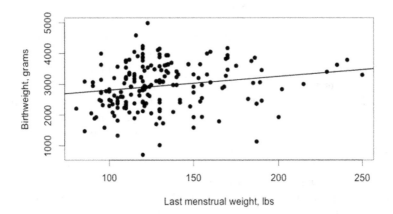

Figure 10.8 A regression model between maternal weight at last menstrual period (the independent predictor) and infant's birthweight (the dependent predictor).

```
Call:
lm(formula = bwt ~ lwt, data = analytic_dataset)

Residuals:
     Min       1Q    Median       3Q      Max
-2192.12  -497.97     -3.84   508.32  2075.60

Coefficients:
            Estimate Std. Error t value Pr(>|t|)
(Intercept) 2369.624    228.493  10.371   <2e-16 ***
lwt            4.429      1.713   2.585   0.0105 *
---
Signif. codes:  0 '***' 0.001 '**' 0.01 '*' 0.05 '.' 0.1 ' ' 1

Residual standard error: 718.4 on 187 degrees of freedom
Multiple R-squared:  0.0345,   Adjusted R-squared:  0.02933
F-statistic: 6.681 on 1 and 187 DF,  p-value: 0.0105
```

Figure 10.9 Example linear regression estimates with a continuous predictor using R.

quantitative interpretation of this figure. Qualitatively, the positive slope of the line indicates that as maternal weight increases so does infant birthweight. This is not necessarily a causal relation, but rather an associational one.

Quantitatively, we can estimate the change in birthweight by examining the coefficients from the linear regression equation (Figure 10.9). The estimate for the "lwt" variable indicates that, on average, for each one pound increase in maternal weight, the infant's birthweight increased by 4.4 grams. The last column is the p-value, corresponding to the statistical significance of the result, and indicates that this result was unlikely due to chance alone ($p = 0.01$).

When the exposure, or any independent variable, is not continuous, the variable becomes modeled as a relative comparison to some referent level (this referent state for a continuous variable is a one-unit difference in its value). For example, suppose instead of maternal weight expressed as a continuous variable, we decided to use the categorical version of it[3] that was dichotomized by a weight of 170 pounds, where a value of 0 indicates weight below 170 pounds, and a value of 1 indicates weight equal to or above 170 pounds (Figure 10.10).

The interpretation of the categorical predictor is slightly different from the interpretation of a continuous predictor. Recall that when operationalized continuously, the regression estimate was for each one pound increase in maternal weight. Under the categorical paradigm, compared to mothers who weighed less than 170 pounds at the last menstrual period, mothers who weighed more had an infant whose birthweight was 256 grams higher, on average. In the statistical software R, the referent group of mothers weighing less than 170 pounds at last menstrual period was implied by the "1" appended to the variable name seen in the output. This tells us the estimate corresponds to when the value of this variable equals 1 and is compared for reference to the birthweight change when the variable equals 0. The referent group can be deduced from the category not included in the

```
Call:
lm(formula = bwt ~ as.factor(lwt_170), data = analytic_dataset)

Residuals:
     Min        1Q    Median        3Q       Max
 -2207.17   -506.17     31.83    527.83   2073.83

Coefficients:
                     Estimate Std. Error t value Pr(>|t|)
(Intercept)           2016.17      56.06   52.01    <2e-16 ***
as.factor(lwt_170)1    255.73     168.19    1.52      0.13
---
Signif. codes:  0 '***' 0.001 '**' 0.01 '*' 0.05 '.' 0.1 ' ' 1

Residual standard error: 726.7 on 187 degrees of freedom
Multiple R-squared:  0.01221, Adjusted R-squared:  0.006929
F-statistic: 2.312 on 1 and 187 DF,  p-value: 0.1301
```

Figure 10.10 Example linear regression estimates with a categorical predictor using R.

regression output, in this case when the variable "lwt_170" = 0, or weighing less than 170 pounds. The p-value indicates that this result was equally likely due to chance ($p = 0.13$) and therefore we cannot conclude with any statistical evidence this was a meaningful association.

That the continuous implementation of the maternal weight variable detected a statistically significant association versus the categorical implementation demonstrates how categorizing a variable may mask (or uncover) an effect. In a sensitivity analysis (discussed later), the researcher can alter the parameterization of the categorical variable to see if significant results are detected, yet there should be a sound reason for doing so, as chance alone may explain this relationship if the variable is manipulated too many times. As such, a theory driven model prior to running any analytic procedures is the preferred approach in epidemiology.

Instead of modeling infant birthweight as a continuous outcome, suppose we wish to assess low birthweight according to a 2500-gram threshold: the variable "low". Running this logistic regression model yields the output shown in Figure 10.11. In contrast to linear regression, the output from logistic regression is provided in log-odds and, to interpret the coefficient corresponding to a maternal weight of less than 170 pounds at last menstrual period, we first must reverse the log transformation by exponentiating the coefficient: $\exp(-0.73) = 0.45$. This exponentiation transforms the coefficient to the odds ratio (OR) scale and can be interpreted like other ORs. Specifically, on average mothers who weighed more than 170 pounds at the last menstrual period had 0.45 times the odds of also having a low birthweight infant compared to mother's who weighed less than 170 pounds. While it may appear counterintuitive that a greater maternal weight was protective of low birthweight, there was no statistical evidence of this occurring ($p = 0.21$). Therefore, in practice, we might conclude that low birthweight infants on average had equivalent odds of being born to mothers who weighed more than 170 pounds

```
Call:
glm(formula = low ~ as.factor(lwt_170), family = binomial(link = logit),
    data = analytic_dataset)

Deviance Residuals:
    Min       1Q   Median       3Q      Max
-0.8906  -0.8906  -0.8906   1.4944   1.8211

Coefficients:
                      Estimate Std. Error z value Pr(>|z|)
(Intercept)             0.7301     0.1644   4.380 1.19e-05 ***
as.factor(lwt_170)1    -0.7269     0.5795  -1.254     0.21
---
Signif. codes:  0 '***' 0.001 '**' 0.01 '*' 0.05 '.' 0.1 ' ' 1

(Dispersion parameter for binomial family taken to be 1)

    Null deviance: 234.67  on 188  degrees of freedom
Residual deviance: 232.91  on 187  degrees of freedom
AIC: 236.91

Number of Fisher Scoring iterations: 4
```

Figure 10.11 Example logistic regression estimates with a categorical predictor using R.

and mothers who weighed less than 170 pounds. As with linear regression, the type of independent variable affects the interpretation, and modeling a continuous variable would be interpreted as a per-unit change in the OR of the outcome.

Code #10.3 in Appendix 2 can be used to reproduce the output shown in Figures 10.9–10.11. Examples of Poisson regression and Cox proportional hazards regression may be found in Chapter 11.

Model diagnostics

Broadly speaking, models should be parsimonious, in that they contain the fewest number of covariates to satisfactorily explain the exposure and outcome relation, as well as assessed for "goodness of fit" and regression assumption violations. There are many options available for assessing model fit depending on the statistical package; what follows in this section is a high-level overview of common tests used for these purposes. As appropriate, these model diagnostics may be included in the output shown in Figures 10.9–10.11.

Goodness of fit tests assess how well the model explains the data. In linear models, the R-squared or adjusted R-squared estimate is a simple representation of how much variability in the data is explained by the model. It is calculated as a percentage where a score of 100% indicates a perfect fit to the data and a score of 0% represents absolute lack of fit to the data. There really is no rule of thumb for the value of R-squared that indicates a good model (Nau, 2021), so the value can be presented without speculating as to how well the model fits the data. Its utility becomes more relevant when comparing models by including additional covariates and assessing if those variables explained more of the association between the exposure and the outcome, or conversely, introduced noise into the model. The *F*-statistic is a global goodness of fit assessment that tells whether any of the regressed variables were statistically associated with the outcome, implying the overall utility of the regression model. A p-value less than 0.05 indicates the model fit was not likely due to chance while a p-value equal to or greater than 0.05 indicates the model fit may be due to chance alone, and the regression model has limited usefulness with respect to the independent variables.

In logistic models, the likelihood function along with its derivatives of the Akaike information criterion and the Bayesian information criterion represent a relative measure of how well the model fits the data. A better model fit is indicated by a lower likelihood value although an absolute interpretation is not possible. Rather, these statistics are again more useful for model comparisons. While there is a "pseudo" *R*-squared available for logistic models, its use is generally discouraged. Analogous to the *F*-statistic global goodness of fit test in linear regression, a chi-squared statistic representing the results from a Hosmer–Lemeshow test will often be included in the regression output. It is interpreted similarly to the linear regression F-test, where a p-value less than 0.05 indicates an acceptable model fit. The exact test utilized will be based on the researcher's statistical software and options available during the regression modeling.

Occasionally, as the result of introducing many covariates in the model, some predictors may be closely related to each other, known as *multicollinearity*. For example, income and education are often tightly intertwined. One extreme manifestation of multicollinearity is failed model convergence, where the regression algorithm cannot estimate the parameters. If the model converges but multicollinearity is present, the variance inflation factor statistic is useful for detecting this phenomenon. In addition to multicollinearity, outliers in the data may result in imbalance in the model. This can be detected through measures of *leverage* and *influence*, which are assessed similarly in both linear and logistic regression models.

The *residuals*, or predictive error, from the regression model are useful for detecting departure from regression assumptions. The Q-Q plot shows departure from normality, where a deviation from a 45° straight line indicates nonnormal data. A plot of residuals versus predicted values can be used to detect departure from linearity as well as heteroscedasticity. Independence can be deduced from a thorough knowledge of the data; statistically it can also be measured with a residual time series plot, or plot of residual autocorrelations.

Sensitivity analysis

Assumptions were made while operationalizing the variables and performing the regression analyses. For example, earlier in this chapter, two variables were collapsed in the *birthwt* dataset for analysis – history of preterm labor and number of doctor visits – and maternal weight was dichotomized into a categorical variable based on the 170-pound threshold. Suppose these decisions were wrong. A sensitivity analysis allows us to test analytic decisions such as these. This should not be misconstrued as "fishing" for statistical significance. The sensitivity analysis is directed based on *a priori* suspicions about the assumptions used and not the results of the analysis. Rigorous epidemiology should include sensitivity analyses along with transparent reporting when disseminating the results.

In a traditional sensitivity analysis, variables may be re-parameterized, the regressions rerun, and the results compared, with two possible outcomes. If the results are found to be robust, they will not meaningfully differ during the sensitivity analyses. This provides further evidence about the validity of the assumptions. If the results are found to be sensitive to changes in variable operationalization or regression assumptions, the researcher has several options: (1) report the original findings and acknowledge as a limitation in the work, (2) present the findings believed to be the closest to some reality and justify, (3) revisit the original assumptions and data, and (4) consider alternatives, redoing the analysis in the process. The way forward will largely depend on the importance of the variable and assumptions.

More sophisticated sensitivity analysis techniques include mitigating bias, imputing missing data, and adjusting for unaccounted confounding. The techniques for quantifying the impact of bias were introduced in bias analysis section of Chapter 9. Missing data methods are presented next.

Missing data

Up to this point in the chapter, we have assumed that the analytic dataset was complete, and in fact, in the *birthwt* dataset, there were no missing data points. As argued in previous chapters, this does not represent reality, especially in EHR-based research (Haneuse et al., 2016). Missing data can have a profound impact on the analysis, particularly if the data are not missing at random, and may compromise internal validity as discussed in Chapter 9. At one extreme, missing data may be treated as inconvenience where any observations containing incomplete data are discarded at the point of analysis. This is known as complete case analysis and is the default analytic approach by most regression fitting algorithms implemented in statistical software. Despite this being the most convenient option, this practice should be avoided when missing data are greater than ~10%, or the data are not missing at random (Marino et al., 2021). Even if these two cases do not apply, complete case analysis needlessly results in a loss of precision. On the other hand, when data are missing extensively on key variables (greater than ~40%) the study findings have limited utility for hypothesis testing purposes (Marino et al., 2021). Some have advocated for a missing data indicator to "control" for the effects of missing data; however, when used in observational studies, this missing data indicator can induce bias in the analysis (Donders et al., 2006; Greenland & Finkle, 1995; Groenwold et al., 2012).

As an example of missing data, consider a simple research study to assess if smoking was related to preterm birth where postpartum mothers were asked if they smoked during pregnancy. The participants may either choose to answer the question (providing a "yes" or "no" response) or not answer the question without providing any response. The researcher may omit all women from the analysis who did not provide an answer but suppose these women were more likely to be smokers and have babies who were born preterm. The analysis may become biased because these data were not included in the analysis.

There are two alternatives to discarding missing data and conducting a complete case analysis: (1) imputation of missing values and (2) weighting of complete records based on a probability of completeness (Greenland & Finkle, 1995). When *imputing* missing values, we infer what the data might have been were they collected. There are a variety of approaches for imputing missing data, each with corresponding advantages and disadvantages. Beaulieu-Jones et al. (2018) evaluated 18 algorithmic approaches to impute data, including mean/median imputation, random sample imputation, K-nearest neighbors imputation, singular value decomposition, matrix imputation, and multiple imputation by chained equations. They tested these methods on four EHR-derived datasets obliterating data completely at random, at random, not at random, and by realistic patterns in the original data, this last condition attempting to recreate a real-world scenario. Unsurprisingly, they found that when the missing data mechanism was predictable, the imputation methods performed well, as opposed to vice versa.

Although Beaulieu-Jones et al. do not believe it is possible – or even wise – to choose a single best method, they provide some general guidance for researchers. Simple deterministic approaches including mean/median and K-nearest neighbors imputation tended to have the largest bias and most likely should be avoided. While coding population-based imputations may be computationally easier, it will result in inferences that are potentially flawed compared to other techniques. More sophisticated deterministic approaches such as singular value decomposition and matrix imputation performed well but were not suitable for what is known as multiple imputation, where multiple copies of the data are created, imputed, and then compared. Multiple imputation essentially simulates new datasets that are sampled from the original data while filling in the missing observations with several possible values based on the algorithm chosen. The multiple datasets are then merged during analysis for single point estimates of risk as well as corresponding estimates of precision. This stochastic approach to imputation – multiple imputation by chained equations – had lower overall bias but was conditional on specifying the correct imputation equation and the data being missing at random. Figure 10.12 is a general summary of the trade-off in imputation approaches for observational data under the missing-at-random mechanism.

Other studies that have examined imputation approaches for imperfect EHR data provide additional guidance for researchers faced with this dilemma. Li, Chen & Moore (2019) noted how incorporating genetic information, if available in the EHR, can help improve accuracy of imputation for cardiovascular-related measurements including low-density lipoprotein, heart failure, and aortic aneurysm disease. Wells et al. (2013) noted that "the probability of missing data may be linked to disease severity and healthcare utilization since unhealthier patients are more likely to have comorbidities and each interaction with the healthcare system provides an opportunity for documentation." As such, any multiple imputation method that can incorporate measures of overall health status such as the Charlson

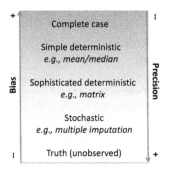

Figure 10.12 Trade-off of imputation approaches when the data are missing at random.

Comorbidity Index, healthcare utilization, or even external data sources such as census data may improve the accuracy of multiple imputation. Petersen et al. (2019) and Glance et al. (2009) corroborate that multiple imputation is a recommended approach when working with missing data in the EHR, provided that the missing-at-random assumption can be posited. Petersen et al. (2019) recommend that health indicators be included in such models, but further note that the missing-at-random assumption may not be true if "individuals with high or low levels of the health indicators are monitored" more or less frequently. Researchers should keep in mind that multiple imputation by chained equations is not a panacea to missing data and has potential drawbacks including joint distribution and covariate interaction issues (Stuart et al., 2009). Special consideration is also needed when imputing data in a meta-analysis (Koopman et al., 2008).

For longitudinal analyses of EHR data, there are more data points available for imputation, hopefully improving the algorithmic accuracy. Engels and Diehr (2003) examined 14 single imputation methods for longitudinal data. In terms of limiting the bias and variance, they found "last & next" and "next observation carried backward" imputations to be the strongest performers, and population median or mean to be the weakest, in line with the simple deterministic approaches evaluated by Beaulieu-Jones et al. (2018).

In short, there is no single best approach to imputing missing data in the EHR, aside from ignoring it altogether (Cole et al., 2023). While many have extolled the benefits of multiple imputation, it should not be seen as a magic bullet for recovering data, especially if the missing data are informative (Groenwold, 2020). In practice, the results of different approaches for dealing with missing data can be contrasted in a sensitivity analysis. If the results are robust, they provide a level of assurance to the investigator about their missing data assumptions. Ideally, one would be able to conduct a validation study to obtain a sample of the missing data, using the knowledge gained from this exercise to identify the type of missingness and provide direction as to the most appropriate remediation approach (Haneuse et al., 2016). Readers requiring a more thorough treatment of the missing data problem are referred to the references throughout this section, and researchers employing imputation should be transparent and disclose all pertinent details (Klebanoff & Cole, 2008).

Notes

1 Generally, dichotomizing continuous predictors in clinical research should be avoided: see Royston, Altman, and Sauerbrei (2006) and Heavner et al. (2010) for a detailed discussion. Herein it is done for illustrative purposes only.
2 One may want to be more explicit and say "born to," however, at this point in our work we are not inferring a causality between maternal age and low birthweight babies. We are merely noting presence (or absence) of a statistical association. This may appear to be semantics but has important implications for causal inference, discussed in chapter 11. All ensuing analyses are interpreted with this same caveat in mind.
3 Depending on the statistical software, it may be necessary to identify that this variable was categorical and not continuous. Each statistical software has its own implementation categorizing a variable, such as the "class" statement in SAS or the "factor" statement in R. Failure to correctly identify a categorical variable is a common mistake that can lead to invalid statistical inference.

References

Beaulieu-Jones BK, Lavage DR, Snyder JW, Moore JH, Pendergrass SA, Bauer CR. Characterizing and managing missing structured data in electronic health records: Data analysis. JMIR Med Inform. 2018 Feb;6(1):e11.

Cole SR, Zivich PN, Edwards JK, Ross RK, Shook-Sa BE, Price JT, Stringer JSA. Missing outcome data in epidemiologic studies. Am J Epidemiol. 2023 Jan 6;192(1):6–10.

Donders ART, van der Heijden GJ, Stijnen T, Moons KG. A gentle introduction to imputation of missing values. J Clin Epidemiol. 2006 Oct;59(10):1087–1091.

Engels JM, Diehr P. Imputation of missing longitudinal data: A comparison of methods. J Clin Epidemiol. 2003 Oct;56(10):968–976.

Glance LG, Osler TM, Mukamel DB, Meredith W, Dick AW. Impact of statistical approaches for handling missing data on trauma center quality. Ann Surg. 2009 Jan;249(1):143–148.

Greenland S, Finkle WD. A critical look at methods for handling missing covariates in epidemiologic regression analyses. Am J Epidemiol. 1995 Dec;142(12):1255–1264.

Groenwold RH. Informative missingness in electronic health record systems: The curse of knowing. Diagn Progn Res. 2020 Jul;4:8.

Groenwold RH, White IR, Donders ART, Carpenter JR, Altman DG, Moons KG. Missing covariate data in clinical research: When and when not to use the missing-indicator method for analysis. CMAJ. 2012 Aug;184(11):1265–1269.

Haneuse S, Bogart A, Jazic I, Westbrook EO, Boudreau D, Theis MK, Simon GE, Arterburn D. Learning about missing data mechanisms in electronic health records-based research: A survey-based approach. Epidemiology. 2016 Jan;27(1):82–90.

Heavner KK, Phillips CV, Burstyn I, Hare W. Dichotomization: 2 x 2 (x2 x 2 x 2...) categories: Infinite possibilities. BMC Med Res Methodol. 2010 Jun;10:59.

Klebanoff MA, Cole SR. Use of multiple imputation in the epidemiologic literature. Am J Epidemiol. 2008 Aug;168(4):355–357.

Koopman L, van der Heijden GJ, Grobbee DE, Rovers MM. Comparison of methods of handling missing data in individual patient data meta-analyses: An empirical example on antibiotics in children with acute otitis media. Am J Epidemiol. 2008 Mar;167(5):540–545.

Li R, Chen Y, Moore JH. Integration of genetic and clinical information to improve imputation of data missing from electronic health records. J Am Med Inform Assoc. 2019 Oct;26(10):1056–1063.

Marino M, Lucas J, Latour E, Heintzman JD. Missing data in primary care research: importance, implications and approaches. Fam Pract. 2021 Mar 29;38(2):200–203.

Nau R. What's a Good Value for R-Squared? Duke University Fuqua School of Business. https://people.duke.edu/~rnau/rsquared.htm (accessed December 2, 2021), 2021.

Petersen I, Welch CA, Nazareth I, Walters K, Marston L, Morris RW, Carpenter JR, Morris TP, Pham TM. Health indicator recording in UK primary care electronic health records: Key implications for handling missing data. Clin Epidemiol. 2019 Feb;11:157–67.

R Core Team. R: A Language and Environment for Statistical Computing. Vienna: R Foundation for Statistical Computing (accessed March 27, 2020), 2020. https://www.R-project.org/.

Royston P, Altman DG, Sauerbrei W. Dichotomizing continuous predictors in multiple regression: A bad idea. Stat Med. 2006 Jan;25(1):127–41.

Stuart EA, Azur M, Frangakis C, Leaf P. Multiple imputation with large data sets: A case study of the Children's Mental Health Initiative. Am J Epidemiol. 2009 May;169(9):1133–9.

Venables WN, Ripley BD. Modern Applied Statistics with S Fourth Edition. New York, NY: Springer, 2002.

Wells BJ, Chagin KM, Nowacki AS, Kattan MW. Strategies for handling missing data in electronic health record derived data. EGEMS. 2013 Dec;1(3):1035.

11   Epidemiologic Analysis II

This chapter continues the overview of epidemiologic analyses relevant to observational EHR data. In Chapter 10, we introduced simple descriptive statistics, unadjusted bivariable analyses, and regression models. This was intended not to provide a full discourse on biostatistics, but rather revisit at a high-level techniques most applicable to secondary analysis of EHR data. Toward the end of the chapter, we also discussed the importance of sensitivity analyses and approaches to dealing with missing data, which can be quite extensive in EHRs (see Chapter 6). We now turn to the problem of producing statistical and causal inference from the most common EHR-based observational study designs. We begin by discussing analytic epidemiology, the phenomena of confounding, and how proper study design and analysis can improve internal validity. Then, continuing with the *birthwt* dataset, the most relevant study designs are analyzed through hypothetical examples to demonstrate the multivariable regression techniques used to obtain adjusted estimates of association. Finally, we conclude by discussing statistical versus causal inference, and how one may approach going from estimates of association to estimates of causation.

As a reminder, the analytic procedures and output were produced using R statistical software (R Core Team, 2020) but are applicable to any statistical software; the interpretation of the statistics remains consistent regardless of the software used. Chapter 10 includes more details about the *birthwt* dataset and how to operationalize the variables used in the analyses for both chapters.

Analytic epidemiology

The crux of analytic epidemiology is hypothesis testing, where a hypothesis is a concrete, testable assertion about the data and its relationship to a risk factor of interest. The assertions one makes about the data are a corollary to the study design. For example, to assess whether smoking during the first trimester of pregnancy leads to an increased risk of low birthweight infants motivates a cohort study, to compare incidence proportions between exposure groups. We may also assert that among low birthweight infants, they are at increased odds of having a mother who smoked during the first trimester, in which a case–control study may be used to compare the risk of the exposure. Using the data from the *birthwt* dataset, we

DOI: 10.4324/9781003258872-14

can create three hypothetical study designs to motivate analytic epidemiological analysis, as follows:

1   The data represent a cross-sectional study. We wish to describe the prevalence of the outcome and compare prevalence proportions between groups of smokers and nonsmokers.
2   The data represent a cohort study. We wish to describe the incidence of the outcome, make a relative comparison between exposure groups, and an estimate the burden of low infant birthweight due to smoking in an absolute measure.
3   The data represent a case–control study. We wish to describe the odds of the exposure given in the outcome and make a relative comparison between exposure groups.

In practice, the appropriate analysis corresponds to the study design. Therefore, if we have knowledge that the original study design was cross-sectional, only this analysis will be appropriate. As a hypothetical, in this chapter, we will analyze the data as a cohort and case–control study to demonstrate the process.

Confounder selection

Multivariate regression models control for (properly measured) confounders. As such, selecting the appropriate covariates to include in these models is a starting point for analysis. There are theoretical and statistical approaches for assessing confounding, and typically each confounder is addressed as a separate entity, unless the joint effects of multiple confounders are of concern. From the *birthwt* dataset, confounder selection will model the relationship between the exposure of early pregnancy smoking (assume smoking was assessed during the first trimester) and the outcome of low birthweight (Figure 11.1).

Statistical perspective

From a statistical perspective, the potential confounder must be correlated with both the exposure and the outcome. One simple way to assess this is by creating a descriptive table stratified by the exposure (Table 11.1) and the outcome

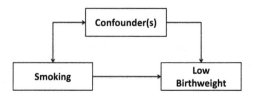

Figure 11.1 Relationship of one or more confounders to the exposure and outcome in the *birthwt* dataset.

Table 11.1 Assessing potential confounders for the smoking exposure in the *birthwt* dataset

Potential confounder	No history of smoking	History of smoking	p-Value[a]
Maternal age, years	23 (5.5)[b]	23 (5.0)	0.54
Maternal weight (pounds)			0.71
<170	103 (90%)	65 (88%)	
≥170	12 (10%)	9 (12%)	
Maternal race			<0.01
White	44 (38%)	52 (70%)	
Black	16 (14%)	10 (14%)	
Other	55 (48%)	12 (16%)	
Previous preterm labor			0.01
No	103 (90%)	56 (76%)	
Yes	12 (10%)	18 (24%)	
Maternal hypertension			0.85
No	108 (94%)	69 (93%)	
Yes	7 (6%)	5 (7%)	
Uterine irritability			0.39
No	100 (87%)	61 (82%)	
Yes	15 (13%)	13 (18%)	
First-trimester doctor visits			0.12
None	55 (48%)	45 (61%)	
One	35 (30%)	12 (16%)	
Two	19 (17%)	11 (15%)	
Three or more	6 (5%)	6 (8%)	
Gestational age, weeks	40 (1.0)	37 (1.1)	<0.01

[a] Statistical testing using Student's *t*-test for continuous variables, and the chi-squared test for categorical variables, $\alpha = 0.20$.

[b] Estimates are given as mean (standard deviation) for continuous variables, and count (frequency) for categorical variables.

(Table 11.2), with the potential confounders enumerated on the rows. Using the appropriate statistical techniques depending on whether the potential confounders are continuous or categorical, a simple hypothesis test can assess whether there is a statistical association that is unlikely due to chance alone. Often one uses a more conservative α, say 10% or 20%, when searching for potential confounders, where a p-value below this threshold for both the association with the exposure and the association with the outcome satisfies this criterion.

Based on the associations with the exposure and outcome, and a cut point of 0.20 for the p-value, there are three variables that can be considered potential confounders in the *birthwt* dataset: "maternal race" (p<0.01 for exposure; p=0.08 for outcome), "previous preterm labor" (p=0.01 for exposure; p<0.01 for outcome), and "gestational age" (p<0.01 for exposure; p=0.04 for outcome). Analytic code to reproduce these tables may be found in Appendix 2 (Code #11.1).

In addition to assessing the potential confounders by the stratified associations with the exposure and outcome, they can be assessed by a change in the exposure to outcome relation, where a change of more than 10% indicates potential confounding (Rothman, Greenland & Lash, 2012). This can also be depicted via a table structured with potential confounders enumerated on the rows along with

Table 11.2 Assessing potential confounders for the low birthweight outcome in the *birthwt* dataset

Potential confounder	Not low birthweight	Low birthweight	p-Value[a]
Maternal age, years	24 (5.6)[b]	22 (4.5)	0.08
Maternal weight (pounds)			0.20
<170	113 (87%)	55 (93%)	
≥170	17 (13%)	4 (7%)	
Maternal race			0.08
White	73 (56%)	23 (39%)	
Black	15 (12%)	11 (19%)	
Other	42 (32%)	25 (42%)	
Previous preterm labor			<0.01
No	118 (91%)	41 (70%)	
Yes	12 (9%)	18 (31%)	
Maternal hypertension			0.04
No	125 (96%)	52 (88%)	
Yes	5 (4%)	7 (12%)	
Uterine irritability			0.02
No	116 (89%)	45 (76%)	
Yes	14 (11%)	14 (24%)	
First-trimester doctor visits			0.27
None	64 (49%)	36 (61%)	
One	36 (28%)	11 (19%)	
Two	23 (18%)	7 (12%)	
Three or more	7 (5%)	5 (9%)	
Gestational age, weeks	39 (1.7)	38 (1.9)	0.04

[a] Statistical testing using Student's *t*-test for continuous variables, and the chi-squared test for categorical variables, $\alpha = 0.20$.

[b] Estimates are given as mean (standard deviation) for continuous variables, and count (frequency) for categorical variables.

three columns capturing: (1) the relationship between the exposure and outcome *without* the confounder, (2) the relationship *with* the confounder, and (3) the percent difference between them. Table 11.3 is the resulting table.

Based on this "change in effect" analysis and a cut-point of 10%, we have four candidates for potential confounding in the *birthwt* dataset: "maternal race" (59% change in effect), "previous preterm labor" (24% change), "first-trimester doctor visits" (11% change), and "gestational age" (38% change). Analytic code to reproduce this table may be found in Appendix 2 (Code #11.2).

Theoretical perspective

The results of the confounder selection process differed with respect to the two statistical techniques offered. By fitting an automated covariate-fitting algorithm (e.g., stepwise selection, forward selection, backward selection, etc.), this difference may not have been detected if only the significance of the covariate assessed by the p-value was used as the criterion for selection. In practice, such automated confounding assessments should be avoided. In addition to examining statistical

Table 11.3 Assessing potential confounders through a change in effect between the exposure and outcome in the *birthwt* dataset

Potential confounder	Exposure to outcome relation[a]		
	Without confounder	*With confounder*	*Percent change (%)*
Maternal age	0.7041	0.69185	2
Maternal weight	0.7041	0.7231	3
Maternal race	0.7041	1.1160	59
Previous preterm labor	0.7041	0.5365	24
Maternal hypertension	0.7041	0.7119	1
Uterine irritability	0.7041	0.6780	4
First-trimester doctor visits	0.7041	0.6296	11
Gestational age	0.7041	0.43421	38

[a] Estimates are the log(odds ratio) of smoking exposure with low birthweight as the outcome, with and without the potential confounder included in the equation.

evidence for confounding, the researcher should be able to justify a theoretical basis for including or excluding each covariate. For example, we may see evidence that a covariate is strongly associated with both the exposure and outcome, but suspect it is a mediator rather than a confounder. Therefore, we may not wish to control for its effects unless we are performing a decomposition analysis. Furthermore, the two statistical techniques from earlier gave us differing results. The change in effect analysis identified "first-trimester doctor visits" as a potential confounder, whereas the stratified association tables did not; specifically, the p-value was greater than 0.20 in the variable's association with the low birthweight outcome. As the analyst, we must decide which one to trust. A literature review, and possibly expert opinion, can help inform our decision.

In addition to assessing the inclusion of potential confounders, we must also guard against including irrelevant covariates. Including irrelevant covariates reduces the degrees of freedom, which may result in model fit and multicollinearity issues, as well as introduces the possibility of inducing residual confounding. In short, we need to justify from a theoretical standpoint which variables to include or exclude as confounders additional to the statistical assessment.

Multivariate procedures by study design

Cross-sectional

Data from a cross-sectional study are analyzed as prevalence rates. Prevalence rates can be compared between groups as a *prevalence rate ratio* or *prevalence odds ratio*. The word prevalence assumes that the variable is categorical, in that a health state or condition is found among those in the study. If the health state or condition is a continuous measure, it must first be made categorical, such as using a threshold value, as was done in Chapter 10 for maternal weight.

A prevalence rate ratio is calculated by dividing the prevalence rate in one group over the prevalence rate in a comparison group. This approach is a common measure of association in cross-sectional studies but also can be used to describe the baseline (enrollment) characteristics of a cohort. If the prevalence rate ratio is calculated with respect to a study endpoint, it is not necessarily equivalent to the relative risk calculated from incidence, unless certain criteria are satisfied (see Chapter 8).

Focusing on the outcome of low birthweight (the variable "low"), the overall prevalence in the *birthwt* analytic dataset is 31% (=59/189 × 100). To assess whether there is a relationship between low birthweight and early pregnancy smoking (assume smoking was assessed during the first trimester), we can compute a prevalence rate ratio by dividing the prevalence in the smoking group (41% =30/74 × 100) by the prevalence in the nonsmoking group (25%, =29/115 × 100). The prevalence rate ratio is 41/25 = 1.6, which suggests that on average women who smoked during pregnancy are 60% more likely to also have low birthweight infants, compared to women who did not smoke. Note that this analysis is unadjusted for confounding: it is a bivariate, crude relation.

To adjust for confounding, we can either stratify the above estimates by the potential confounder in a simple case or, more commonly, use logistic regression. A logistic regression model allows for the estimation of the prevalence odds ratio. We regress the outcome of low birthweight by the predictor of smoking history while also include any potential confounders as covariates. For comparison, we will first estimate the crude prevalence odds ratio for the bivariate relationship via logistic regression (Figure 11.2). Recall in logistic regression, we must

```
> summary(glm(low ~ as.factor(smoke), data=analytic_dataset,
    family=binomial(link=logit)))

Call:
glm(formula = low ~ as.factor(smoke), family = binomial(link = logit),
    data = analytic_dataset)

Deviance Residuals:
    Min       1Q    Median        3Q       Max
-1.0197   -0.7623   -0.7623    1.3438    1.6599

Coefficients:
                  Estimate Std. Error z value Pr(>|z|)
(Intercept)        -1.0871     0.2147  -5.063 4.14e-07 ***
as.factor(smoke)1   0.7041     0.3196   2.203   0.0276 *
---
Signif. codes:  0 '***' 0.001 '**' 0.01 '*' 0.05 '.' 0.1 ' ' 1

(Dispersion parameter for binomial family taken to be 1)

    Null deviance: 234.67  on 188  degrees of freedom
Residual deviance: 229.80  on 187  degrees of freedom
AIC: 233.8

Number of Fisher Scoring iterations: 4

> exp(0.7041)
[1] 2.022026
```

Figure 11.2 Prevalence odds ratio for smoking history and low birthweight.

exponentiate the coefficients to arrive at the odds ratio since the dependent variable is dichotomous.

The prevalence odds ratio of 2.0 has overestimated the manually calculated prevalence rate ratio of 1.6. This is not unexpected given the high prevalence of low birthweight infants in this sample (31%). In cases where the outcome is not rare, the prevalence rate ratio will be a less biased measure (Thompson, Myers & Kriebel, 1998). We can directly estimate the prevalence rate ratio using log-binomial regression instead of logistic regression (Figure 11.3). Log-binomial modeling of the relative risk can be more difficult to statistically fit, resulting in failed model convergence, therefore many analysts fall back on logistic models that estimate the odds ratio and interpret them with caution when the prevalence is not rare (Williamson, Eliasziw & Fick, 2013). Again, as the dependent variable is dichotomous, we must exponentiate the coefficients to arrive at the rate ratio.

The log-binomial estimate for the regression modeling agrees with the manually calculated prevalence rate ratio of 1.6. To estimate the precision of this measure, we can request a 95% confidence interval using the R code: confint(model). We can be 95% confident that the true prevalence rate ratio is captured in the interval of (1.1, 2.5). Despite the more accurate approximation of the log-binomial model to estimate the prevalence rate ratio when the outcome is common, the same caution needs to be exercised when interpreting this measure, specifically

```
> summary(glm(low ~ as.factor(smoke), data=analytic_dataset,
     family=binomial(link=log)))

Call:
glm(formula = low ~ as.factor(smoke), family = binomial(link = log),
    data = analytic_dataset)

Deviance Residuals:
    Min       1Q    Median       3Q       Max
-1.0197   -0.7623   -0.7623    1.3438    1.6599

Coefficients:
                    Estimate Std. Error z value Pr(>|z|)
(Intercept)          -1.3776     0.1606  -8.579   <2e-16 ***
as.factor(smoke)1     0.4748     0.2136   2.223   0.0262 *
---
Signif. codes:  0 '***' 0.001 '**' 0.01 '*' 0.05 '.' 0.1 ' ' 1

(Dispersion parameter for binomial family taken to be 1)

    Null deviance: 234.67  on 188  degrees of freedom
Residual deviance: 229.80  on 187  degrees of freedom
AIC: 233.8

Number of Fisher Scoring iterations: 6

> exp(0.4748)
[1] 1.607693
```

Figure 11.3 Prevalence rate ratio for smoking history and low birthweight.

with respect to inferring any causal effects. As the data have been captured in a cross-sectional study, we cannot be sure of temporality or that smoking status was ascertained without bias.

To adjust for confounding, we include the potential confounder variables in the model specification. Based on the statistical and theoretical confounder selection process, four potential confounders were identified earlier: maternal race, previous preterm labor, first-trimester doctor visits, and gestational age. The fully adjusted model and prevalence odds ratio[1] is provided in Figure 11.4.

The adjusted prevalence odds ratio can be interpreted as before, yet importantly, the prevalence of smoking is no longer statistically associated with the prevalence of low birthweight infants.[2] Instead, it appears that both maternal race and previous preterm labor are statistically associated with the prevalence of low birthweight infants. As the adjusted odds ratio has decreased from the crude odds ratio − 1.4 versus 2.0, respectively − there was positive confounding present in the crude analysis, exaggerating the smoking and low birthweight association. Of equal importance, the magnitude of effects from each covariate can also be interpreted in the context of a prevalence odds ratio. For example, the presence of previous preterm labor was associated with 4.1 times (=exp(1.4148)) the prevalence

```
> summary(glm(low ~ as.factor(smoke) + as.factor(race) + as.factor(ptl_collapsed) +
as.factor(ftv_collapsed) + gestation, data=analytic_dataset, family=binomial(link=logit)))

Call:
glm(formula = low ~ as.factor(smoke) + as.factor(race) + as.factor(ptl_collapsed) +
    as.factor(ftv_collapsed) + gestation, family = binomial(link = logit),
    data = analytic_dataset)

Deviance Residuals:
    Min       1Q   Median       3Q      Max
-1.7248  -0.8425  -0.6108   1.0447   2.1754

Coefficients:
                          Estimate Std. Error z value Pr(>|z|)
(Intercept)                 4.3008     6.5480   0.657  0.51130
as.factor(smoke)1           0.3667     0.6162   0.595  0.55173
as.factor(race)2            1.1103     0.5101   2.176  0.02952 *
as.factor(race)3            0.9095     0.4253   2.138  0.03250 *
as.factor(ptl_collapsed)1   1.4148     0.4522   3.128  0.00176 **
as.factor(ftv_collapsed)1  -0.4916     0.4610  -1.066  0.28626
as.factor(ftv_collapsed)2  -0.3531     0.5083  -0.695  0.48722
as.factor(ftv_collapsed)3   0.2311     0.6591   0.351  0.72588
gestation                  -0.1516     0.1645  -0.922  0.35677
---
Signif. codes:  0 '***' 0.001 '**' 0.01 '*' 0.05 '.' 0.1 ' ' 1

(Dispersion parameter for binomial family taken to be 1)

    Null deviance: 234.67  on 188  degrees of freedom
Residual deviance: 208.06  on 180  degrees of freedom
AIC: 226.06

Number of Fisher Scoring iterations: 4

> exp(0.3667)
[1] 1.442965
```

Figure 11.4 Prevalence odds ratio for smoking history and low birthweight adjusted for potential confounding by maternal race, previous preterm labor, first-trimester doctor visits, and gestational age.

of low birthweight infants (95% confidence interval: 1.7, 10.3) compared to no history of preterm labor, adjusted for smoking history, maternal race, and first-trimester doctor visits. Using a multivariate regression model has isolated the independent contributions from all characteristics specified in the model.

Cohort

If we assume the *birthwt* dataset represents the population of all births captured in an EHR for some period, the data can be analyzed as a retrospective cohort study. Again, our interest is the relationship of early pregnancy smoking (assuming smoking was assessed during the first trimester) to low birthweight infants. As the data were collected at each obstetrical office visit, we have strengthened the temporality assumption between the exposure and outcome.[3] Through a cohort study, we can estimate the incidence of low birthweight for this population.

There are several types of regression measures of association for incidence, including the cumulative incidence relative risk and the incidence rate ratio. As before, we assume a dichotomous outcome, indicating the event has either occurred or not. If follow-up time is available, modeling the incidence rate ratio will provide a more accurate representation of incidence. Without follow-up time, a cumulative incidence relative risk may be the best option. In the *birthwt* dataset, we can compare both methods by assuming gestational age represents follow-up time provided the cohort was recruited periconception and followed through birth.

We can compute a crude cumulative incidence relative risk and a crude incidence rate ratio by first calculating incidence in the exposed smoking group and dividing it by incidence in the unexposed nonsmoking group. Users of R can refer to the *epitools* package (Aragon, 2020), which includes functions to calculate these measures with corresponding confidence intervals and hypothesis testing. As shown in Figure 11.5, the cumulative incidence relative risk indicates that on average women who smoked during the first trimester of pregnancy had 1.6 times the incidence (95% confidence interval: 1.1, 2.4) of low birthweight infants, compared to women who were nonsmokers during the first trimester. As shown in Figure 11.6, the incidence rate ratio, which accounts for follow-up time and time-to-event, is slightly larger (1.7 times the incidence, 95% confidence interval: 1.0, 2.9) and is perhaps a more accurate measure of the true incidence. Yet considering the substantial overlap in the confidence intervals, the cumulative incidence was not necessarily an unbiased measure.

To control for the potential confounders enumerated earlier, namely maternal race, previous preterm labor, and first-trimester doctor visits, requires multivariate regression techniques. There are several regression model options to estimate an incidence ratio: logistic regression, log-binomial regression, Poisson regression, and Cox proportional hazards regression. For incidence rate ratios, gestational age is treated as follow-up time, rather than a nuisance parameter adjusted for potential confounding. For cumulative incidence relative risk, the availability of gestational age is ignored since we are assuming we do not have follow-up time.

```
> no_outcome_unexposed = sum(!analytic_dataset$low[analytic_dataset$smoke==0])
> outcome_unexposed = sum(analytic_dataset$low[analytic_dataset$smoke==0])
> no_outcome_exposed = sum(!analytic_dataset$low[analytic_dataset$smoke==1])
> outcome_exposed = sum(analytic_dataset$low[analytic_dataset$smoke==1])
> riskratio(c(no_outcome_unexposed,outcome_unexposed,no_outcome_exposed,outcome_exposed))
$data
          Outcome
Predictor Disease1 Disease2 Total
  Exposed1       86       29   115
  Exposed2       44       30    74
  Total         130       59   189

$measure
          risk ratio with 95% C.I.
Predictor estimate    lower    upper
  Exposed1 1.000000       NA       NA
  Exposed2 1.607642 1.057812 2.443262

$p.value
              two-sided
Predictor midp.exact fisher.exact chi.square
  Exposed1        NA           NA         NA
  Exposed2 0.02914865    0.0361765 0.02649064

$correction
[1] FALSE

attr(,"method")
[1] "Unconditional MLE & normal approximation (Wald) CI"
```

Figure 11.5 Cumulative incidence relative risk for the relationship between maternal smoking during the first trimester and low birthweight infants.

```
> outcome_unexposed = sum(analytic_dataset$low[analytic_dataset$smoke==0])
> outcome_exposed = sum(analytic_dataset$low[analytic_dataset$smoke==1])
> persontime_unexposed = sum(analytic_dataset$gestation[analytic_dataset$smoke==0])
> persontime_exposed = sum(analytic_dataset$gestation[analytic_dataset$smoke==1])
> rateratio(c(outcome_unexposed,outcome_exposed,persontime_unexposed,persontime_exposed))
$data
          Outcome
Predictor Cases Person-time
  Exposed1    29        4594
  Exposed2    30        2742
  Total       59        7336

$measure
          rate ratio with 95% C.I.
Predictor estimate    lower    upper
  Exposed1 1.000000       NA       NA
  Exposed2 1.732858 1.035777 2.903155

$p.value
              two-sided
Predictor midp.exact       wald
  Exposed1        NA         NA
  Exposed2 0.0363954 0.03246861

attr(,"method")
[1] "Median unbiased estimate & mid-p exact CI"
```

Figure 11.6 Incidence rate ratio for the relationship between maternal smoking during the first trimester and low birthweight infants.

Logistic regression is appropriate to model the cumulative incidence if there is complete follow-up for all study participants with no withdrawals, and time-to-event is unimportant. As before, the regression estimates are odds ratios and therefore need to be interpreted with the same caution when approximating the relative risk. In certain cases, such as a rare disease with less than 10% prevalence, little loss to follow-up, and time-independent outcomes, the estimates from the logistic regression will be robust for the true relative risk. However, logistic regression is often used as an estimator of relative risk despite assumption violations due to its ease of use and interpretability of results. If using this approach, the researcher needs to justify why this is appropriate. Figure 11.7 is the fully adjusted model for cumulative incidence. The odds ratio of 2.2 suggests that smoking during the first trimester resulted in two times the odds of incident low birthweight (95% confidence interval: 1.0, 4.9), compared to nonsmoking, adjusted for maternal race, previous preterm labor, and first-trimester doctor visits.

Similar to prevalence rate regression, a cumulative incidence relative risk can be estimated using log-binomial regression instead of logistic regression. This may improve estimates of the true relative risk rather than relying on the odds

```
> summary(glm(low ~ as.factor(smoke) + as.factor(race) + as.factor(ptl_collapsed) +
as.factor(ftv_collapsed), data=analytic_dataset, family=binomial(link=logit)))

Call:
glm(formula = low ~ as.factor(smoke) + as.factor(race) + as.factor(ptl_collapsed) +
    as.factor(ftv_collapsed), family = binomial(link = logit),
    data = analytic_dataset)

Deviance Residuals:
    Min       1Q    Median       3Q      Max
-1.7871   -0.8563   -0.5717   0.9906   2.0876

Coefficients:
                             Estimate Std. Error z value Pr(>|z|)
(Intercept)                   -1.7286     0.4233   -4.083 4.44e-05 ***
as.factor(smoke)1              0.8031     0.3966    2.025  0.04290 *
as.factor(race)2               1.0370     0.5022    2.065  0.03894 *
as.factor(race)3               0.9140     0.4245    2.153  0.03133 *
as.factor(ptl_collapsed)1      1.3821     0.4489    3.079  0.00208 **
as.factor(ftv_collapsed)1     -0.5393     0.4560   -1.183  0.23696
as.factor(ftv_collapsed)2     -0.3304     0.5066   -0.652  0.51431
as.factor(ftv_collapsed)3      0.2456     0.6601    0.372  0.70987
---
Signif. codes:  0 '***' 0.001 '**' 0.01 '*' 0.05 '.' 0.1 ' ' 1

(Dispersion parameter for binomial family taken to be 1)

    Null deviance: 234.67  on 188  degrees of freedom
Residual deviance: 208.91  on 181  degrees of freedom
AIC: 224.91

Number of Fisher Scoring iterations: 4

> exp(0.8031)
[1] 2.232451
```

Figure 11.7 Adjusted cumulative incidence relative risk estimated via logistic regression for the relationship between maternal smoking during the first trimester and low birthweight infants.

```
> poissonmod = glm(low ~ as.factor(smoke) + as.factor(race) + as.factor(ptl_collapsed) +
as.factor(ftv_collapsed), data=analytic_dataset, family=poisson())
>
> library(sandwich) #robust standard errors
> poissonmod.cov.matrix = vcovHC(poissonmod, type="HC0")
> poissonmod.std.err = sqrt(diag(poissonmod.cov.matrix))
> poissonmod.r.est = cbind(Estimate= coef(poissonmod), "Robust SE" = poissonmod.std.err,
"Pr(>|z|)" = 2 * pnorm(abs(coef(poissonmod)/poissonmod.std.err), lower.tail=FALSE), LL =
coef(poissonmod) - 1.96 * poissonmod.std.err, UL = coef(poissonmod) + 1.96 *
poissonmod.std.err)
>
> exp(poissonmod.r.est[, c(1,4,5)])
                              Estimate        LL         UL
(Intercept)                  0.1684278 0.1003517 0.2826848
as.factor(smoke)1            1.6135619 1.0217064 2.5482681
as.factor(race)2             1.9017448 1.1001043 3.2875366
as.factor(race)3             1.7586008 1.0963883 2.8207858
as.factor(ptl_collapsed)1    2.0821380 1.3763560 3.1498382
as.factor(ftv_collapsed)1    0.7189413 0.4039205 1.2796494
as.factor(ftv_collapsed)2    0.8085030 0.3904517 1.6741560
as.factor(ftv_collapsed)3    1.1786302 0.5854615 2.3727763
```

Figure 11.8 Adjusted cumulative incidence relative risk estimated via modified Poisson regression for the relationship between maternal smoking during the first trimester and low birthweight infants.

ratio to approximate it. Thus, its use is more appropriate when the odds ratio is believed to be a biased measure compared to the relative risk (Wacholder, 1986). Unfortunately, fitting a log-binomial regression model may prove challenging (Williamson, Eliasziw & Fick, 2013). Instead, a Poisson regression with robust error variance via sandwich estimation is a more appropriate model for estimating the relative risk from cohort data with a binary outcome (Zou, 2004). Figure 11.8 is the fully adjusted model for cumulative incidence using the modified Poisson approach.[4] As the dependent variable is dichotomous, we must exponentiate the coefficients to arrive at the relative risk. The relative risk of 1.6 suggests that smoking during the first trimester was associated with a 60% increased risk of incident low birthweight (95% confidence interval: 1.0, 2.5), compared to non-smoking, adjusted for maternal race, previous preterm labor, and first-trimester doctor visits. Compared to the logistic regression model, the odds ratio was an overestimate given the high prevalence of the outcome, and the relative risk is a less biased estimator.

A final option to model the cumulative incidence relative risk that incorporates time-to-event and follow-up time is Cox proportional hazards regression. This technique is particularly appropriate when the exposure is assumed to immediately increase risk of the outcome, as we might hypothesize with smoking. Unlike the previous approaches, Cox proportional hazards analysis considers the time of occurrence of an event as well as time of censoring when the outcome did not occur. The estimates correspond to a hazard ratio and can be interpreted as the cumulative incidence relative risk. Figure 11.9 is the fully adjusted model for the Cox cumulative incidence relative risk. As the dependent variable is dichotomous, we must exponentiate the coefficients to arrive at the hazard rate. The hazard rate of 12.9 suggests that smoking during the first trimester resulted in a nearly

```
> summary(coxph(Surv(gestation, low)~as.factor(smoke) + as.factor(race) +
as.factor(ptl_collapsed) + as.factor(ftv_collapsed), data=analytic_dataset))
Call:
coxph(formula = Surv(gestation, low) ~ as.factor(smoke) + as.factor(race) +
    as.factor(ptl_collapsed) + as.factor(ftv_collapsed), data = analytic_dataset)

  n= 189, number of events= 59

                               coef exp(coef) se(coef)       z Pr(>|z|)
as.factor(smoke)1           2.55781  12.90756  0.39852   6.418 1.38e-10 ***
as.factor(race)2            0.52115   1.68396  0.37766   1.380   0.1676
as.factor(race)3            0.73973   2.09537  0.33204   2.228   0.0259 *
as.factor(ptl_collapsed)1   0.73585   2.08726  0.29874   2.463   0.0138 *
as.factor(ftv_collapsed)1  -0.39525   0.67351  0.36445  -1.084   0.2781
as.factor(ftv_collapsed)2  -0.02919   0.97123  0.42573  -0.069   0.9453
as.factor(ftv_collapsed)3   0.33754   1.40150  0.48587   0.695   0.4872
---
Signif. codes:  0 '***' 0.001 '**' 0.01 '*' 0.05 '.' 0.1 ' ' 1

                           exp(coef) exp(-coef) lower .95 upper .95
as.factor(smoke)1            12.9076    0.07747    5.9105    28.188
as.factor(race)2             1.6840     0.59384    0.8033     3.530
as.factor(race)3             2.0954     0.47724    1.0930     4.017
as.factor(ptl_collapsed)1    2.0873     0.47910    1.1622     3.749
as.factor(ftv_collapsed)1    0.6735     1.48475    0.3297     1.376
as.factor(ftv_collapsed)2    0.9712     1.02962    0.4216     2.237
as.factor(ftv_collapsed)3    1.4015     0.71352    0.5408     3.632

Concordance= 0.82  (se = 0.044 )
Rsquare= 0.3    (max possible= 0.941 )
Likelihood ratio test= 67.5   on 7 df,    p=4.717e-12
Wald test            = 64.16  on 7 df,    p=2.22e-11
Score (logrank) test = 82.74  on 7 df,    p=3.775e-15
```

Figure 11.9 Adjusted cumulative incidence relative risk estimated via Cox proportional hazards regression for the relationship between maternal smoking during the first trimester and low birthweight infants.

13 times increased risk in incident low birthweight (95% confidence interval: 5.9, 28.2), compared to nonsmoking, adjusted for maternal race, previous preterm labor, and first-trimester doctor visits.

In terms of estimating an incidence rate ratio, Poisson rate regression models a true rate incorporating a time element. The outcome now becomes a count of the number of low birthweight infants in the cohort and follow-up time becomes part of the intercept term specified as an offset in the form of a log-transformed variable. Figure 11.10 is the fully adjusted model for the Poisson incidence rate ratio. As the dependent variable is dichotomous, we must exponentiate the coefficients to arrive at the rate ratio. The rate ratio of 1.7 suggests that smoking during the first trimester resulted in a 70% increase in incident low birthweight (95% confidence interval: 1.0, 3.0), compared to nonsmoking, adjusted for maternal race, previous preterm labor, and first-trimester doctor visits.

In addition to the usual regression diagnostics, users of Poisson regression and Cox proportional hazards regression need to guard against additional assumption violations. In Poisson modeling, users need to guard against overdispersion, which can be spotted if the residual deviance is much greater than the degrees of

```
> summary(glm(low ~ as.factor(smoke) + as.factor(race) + as.factor(ptl_collapsed) +
as.factor(ftv_collapsed), offset=log(gestation), data=analytic_dataset, family=poisson()))

Call:
glm(formula = low ~ as.factor(smoke) + as.factor(race) + as.factor(ptl_collapsed) +
    as.factor(ftv_collapsed), family = poisson(), data = analytic_dataset,
    offset = log(gestation))

Deviance Residuals:
    Min      1Q   Median      3Q     Max
-1.4286  -0.7621  -0.5887  0.5229  1.5138

Coefficients:
                            Estimate Std. Error z value Pr(>|z|)
(Intercept)                  -5.4663     0.3376 -16.192  <2e-16 ***
as.factor(smoke)1             0.5540     0.3019   1.835  0.0665 .
as.factor(race)2              0.6330     0.3709   1.707  0.0879 .
as.factor(race)3              0.5662     0.3217   1.760  0.0784 .
as.factor(ptl_collapsed)1     0.7287     0.2993   2.434  0.0149 *
as.factor(ftv_collapsed)1    -0.3370     0.3614  -0.933  0.3510
as.factor(ftv_collapsed)2    -0.2093     0.4208  -0.497  0.6190
as.factor(ftv_collapsed)3     0.1657     0.4778   0.347  0.7288
---
Signif. codes:  0 '***' 0.001 '**' 0.01 '*' 0.05 '.' 0.1 ' ' 1

(Dispersion parameter for poisson family taken to be 1)

    Null deviance: 138.76  on 188  degrees of freedom
Residual deviance: 121.65  on 181  degrees of freedom
AIC: 255.65

Number of Fisher Scoring iterations: 6

> exp(0.5540)
[1] 1.7402
```

Figure 11.10 Adjusted incidence rate ratio estimated via Poisson regression for the relationship between maternal smoking during the first trimester and low birthweight infants.

freedom. In Cox modeling, users need to assess the independence of censoring and survival as well as the proportional hazards assumption. The proportional hazards assumption states that the exposure multiplies the risk by a constant factor compared to the unexposed. It can be checked with both statistical methods and visual inspection of the survival plot.

Based on the earlier example, the survival plot is a graphic representation of the risk for low birthweight as gestation increases by the smoking groups (Figure 11.11). As our example had two exposure groups representing smokers and nonsmokers, there are two curves on the plot. Note that it is common for the *y*-axis to represent survival (lack of the outcome), which is equivalent to 1 minus the risk, and when interpreting a survival plot, the curve closer to the bottom represents a greater risk of the outcome, or in this case, greater risk of low birthweight. Based on this plot, we can see that the trajectories of low infant birthweight differed by maternal smoking and gestational age. Low birthweight happened at an earlier gestational age for the smoking group, and it appears that smokers are at an elevated and earlier risk of this outcome. The exact relative risk comparing the two survival curves corresponds to the hazard ratio from the Cox regression model.

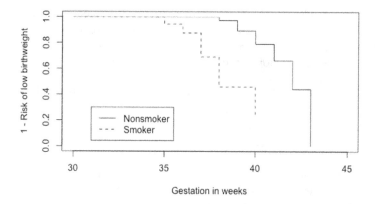

Figure 11.11 Survival curves depicting the unadjusted relationship of low birthweight and gestational age by maternal smoking status.

Cohort with correlated observations

The analytic procedures described for the preceding cohort study assumed that each observation was independent of the others. For longitudinal cohorts with repeated outcome measures, or cohorts with clustering such as multiple gestations or multiple pregnancies, the traditional regression models will be biased. In this case, we need a hierarchical model that can deal with this nonindependence of observations: longitudinal analysis or multilevel analysis.

Although longitudinal and multilevel studies generate data via different mechanisms depending on the type of study, the analysis is similar because the data form a hierarchy; therefore, these concepts are presented together. In a longitudinal or repeated outcomes measures study, an individual contributes multiple observations to the data as they have an outcome that is measured on two or more occasions. The hierarchy is at the person level. Hence any exposure to outcome relationship within that individual needs to be accounted for separately from the exposure to outcome relationship between individuals, as each individual may respond to an exposure differently. In a multilevel study, a contextual or clustering unit contributes multiple observations to the data, as two or more individuals are located within these units. The hierarchy could be at the person level, for example, if we are examining multiple gestations or multiple pregnancies, or the hierarchy could be at a contextual level, for example if patients are nested within some aspect of the care process such as clinic, bed, or ward.

The goal of analyzing cohorts with correlated, nonindependent observations is to estimate incidence from some exposure while controlling for potential confounding and accounting for the structure of the data. This exposure to outcome relationship can be described in terms of global effects, in that the effects are equivalent across everyone in the study, and is termed the fixed or marginal effects. Or, it can be described in terms of varying effects, in that the effects differ by the individual in the repeated measures study or the clustering unit in the multilevel study, and is termed the random effects. Fixed effects are akin to the standard coefficient estimates in single-level, typical regression analysis, and therefore are more intuitive to interpret. Random effects are frequently used to describe sources of variation in the data, and therefore are presented as group variances as opposed to coefficient estimates.

Assuming we would like to describe both fixed and random effects, we could fit a mixed-effects regression model. If the interest is to describe fixed effects alone, we could use a generalized estimating equations regression model, which treats the clustering as a nuisance-factor. A full comparison of the two approaches may be found in Hubbard et al. (2010); specifically, refer to their Table for a comparison of the two approaches. Model building with longitudinal or multilevel models should be treated as an iterative process that starts out with the simplest model and then sequentially adds complexity to identify the sources of variation in the data. Model convergence may be challenging in mixed-effects regression. Continuous covariates may need to be mean centered or scaled (such as through a log transformation), and there may be collinearity introduced by multiple group predictors.

If the modeled outcome is continuous, we could use linear mixed-effects regression and if the outcome is binary, we could use generalized linear mixed-effects regression. This is analogous to the linear versus logistic models introduced in Chapter 10. Linear mixed-effects regression is appropriate when the outcome is continuous and can be represented by a linear relationship. Generalized linear mixed-effects regression is appropriate when the outcome is binary and can be represented by a generalized linear relationship using a logit link function. Regardless of the type of regression model, the first step is to test for correlation among the observations using an empty model composed of the outcome and clustering unit, fit as a random intercept. If significant correlation is detected, an appropriate covariance structure can be chosen (e.g., unstructured, symmetric, autoregressive, etc.) using restricted maximum likelihood estimation. Next, the exposure can be introduced to check for a crude relationship with the outcome. Depending on the goals of the research, the exposure can be entered into the model as a fixed effect to describe the population level effect, a random effect to describe the group-specific effect, or as both a fixed and random effect. Potential confounders can also be introduced at this point with final estimates made using maximum likelihood estimation.

Typically, in a longitudinal analysis, we are interested in testing whether the exposure interacts with time to assess differences over time between groups. To do this, two nested models are built: one with an interaction term and one without. If the result of a type 3 test for interaction is significant, then the interaction term is appropriate, and one can conclude there likely are differences over time between groups by the exposure. There are additional complications in a longitudinal analysis of EHR data as the visits likely occur at irregular intervals: in statistical terms, the data are unbalanced. See Pullenayegum and Lim (2016) and Lokku et al. (2020) for analytic strategies resulting from irregular visits.

In a multilevel analysis, we may be interested in examining the change in group-level variance as we add predictors to the model, to identify where variability in the data arises from. This would again suggest a series of nested models. A full treatment of analyzing hierarchical cohort data with correlated observations is outside the scope of this text; readers are referred to other texts in these areas.

Case-control

In a case-control study, the odds of exposure are assessed given the binary occurrence of being a case or control. The odds of exposure are equivalent to the odds of disease and therefore inference can be made about risk factors and their relationship to disease. A crude relationship between the exposure and the outcome can be calculated by dividing the odds of low infant birthweight among women who smoked during their first trimester by the odds of low infant birthweight among women who did not smoke. As shown in Figure 11.12, the odds ratio is 2.0 and can be interpreted as roughly two times the odds of smoking among women who had a low birthweight infant (95% confidence interval: 1.1, 3.8), compared to women who did not have a low birthweight infant.

A fully adjusted case–control study can be modeled through logistic regression with a slight modification depending on whether matching was employed in the study design. For an unmatched or frequency-matched study, unconditional logistic regression estimates the adjusted odds ratio of the exposure compared to

```
> control_unexposed = sum(!analytic_dataset$low[analytic_dataset$smoke==0])
> case_unexposed = sum(analytic_dataset$low[analytic_dataset$smoke==0])
> control_exposed =  sum(!analytic_dataset$low[analytic_dataset$smoke==1])
> case_exposed = sum(analytic_dataset$low[analytic_dataset$smoke==1])
> oddsratio(c(control_unexposed,case_unexposed,control_exposed,case_exposed))
$data
             Outcome
Predictor  Disease1 Disease2 Total
   Exposed1       86       29   115
   Exposed2       44       30    74
   Total         130       59   189

$measure
           odds ratio with 95% C.I.
Predictor  estimate     lower     upper
   Exposed1  1.00000        NA        NA
   Exposed2  2.01268  1.073703  3.794579

$p.value
             two-sided
Predictor  midp.exact  fisher.exact  chi.square
   Exposed1         NA            NA          NA
   Exposed2  0.02914865     0.0361765  0.02649064

$correction
[1] FALSE

attr(,"method")
[1] "median-unbiased estimate & mid-p exact CI"
```

Figure 11.12 Crude odds ratio of the relationship between maternal smoking during the first trimester and low birthweight infants.

the unexposed. For an individually matched study, conditional logistic regression will similarly estimate the adjusted odds ratio, but will consider the conditional dependence of the matched data.

If we assume the *birthwt* dataset was recruited at delivery to include a sample of low birthweight infants and a random selection of controls, the data represent an unmatched case–control study. To produce a fully adjusted model, the logistic regression procedure is specified with the potential confounders as covariates shown in Figure 11.13. The odds ratio of 1.44 for the exposure of smoking is interpreted as women who smoked during the first trimester had a 44% increase in odds for low birthweight infants (95% confidence interval: 0.4, 4.9), compared to women who did not smoke, adjusted for maternal race, previous preterm labor, first-trimester doctor visits, and gestational age. As the confidence interval crossed 1.0, the smoking exposure was not a significant association. Instead, the primary drivers of the relationship appeared to be racial group and previous preterm labor.

Suppose the original study design that recruited the sample of low birthweight infants individually matched each case to a control on a potentially confounding variable, such as maternal age (see Appendix 2, Code #11.3 to create this condition). To analyze the data in a conditional logistic regression approach, the "matched" variable is conditioned upon in the procedure. Although we matched upon maternal

```
> summary(glm(low ~ as.factor(smoke) + as.factor(race) + as.factor(ptl_collapsed) +
as.factor(ftv_collapsed) + gestation, data=analytic_dataset, family=binomial(link=logit)))

Call:
glm(formula = low ~ as.factor(smoke) + as.factor(race) + as.factor(ptl_collapsed) +
    as.factor(ftv_collapsed) + gestation, family = binomial(link = logit),
    data = analytic_dataset)

Deviance Residuals:
    Min       1Q   Median       3Q      Max
-1.7248  -0.8425  -0.6108   1.0447   2.1754

Coefficients:
                          Estimate Std. Error z value Pr(>|z|)
(Intercept)                 4.3008     6.5480   0.657  0.51130
as.factor(smoke)1           0.3667     0.6162   0.595  0.55173
as.factor(race)2            1.1103     0.5101   2.176  0.02952 *
as.factor(race)3            0.9095     0.4253   2.138  0.03250 *
as.factor(ptl_collapsed)1   1.4148     0.4522   3.128  0.00176 **
as.factor(ftv_collapsed)1  -0.4916     0.4610  -1.066  0.28626
as.factor(ftv_collapsed)2  -0.3531     0.5083  -0.695  0.48722
as.factor(ftv_collapsed)3   0.2311     0.6591   0.351  0.72588
gestation                  -0.1516     0.1645  -0.922  0.35677
---
Signif. codes:  0 '***' 0.001 '**' 0.01 '*' 0.05 '.' 0.1 ' ' 1

(Dispersion parameter for binomial family taken to be 1)

    Null deviance: 234.67  on 188  degrees of freedom
Residual deviance: 208.06  on 180  degrees of freedom
AIC: 226.06

Number of Fisher Scoring iterations: 4

> exp(0.3667)
[1] 1.442965
```

Figure 11.13 Adjusted unconditional odds ratio of the relationship between maternal smoking during the first trimester and low birthweight infants.

age in the study design, we can also include it as a covariate in the regression model to control for potential residual confounding introduced in the matching process. If the matching achieved exchangeability on this covariate, the estimated coefficient of the matching variable should be approximately 1.0 and not statistically significant. Figure 11.14 is the output from the conditional logistic regression analysis.

The conditional odds ratio for the smoking exposure is interpreted the same as the unconditional odds ratio: women who smoked during the first trimester had 3.8 times the odds for low birthweight infants (95% confidence interval: 0.7, 22.7), compared to women who did not smoke, adjusted for maternal race, previous preterm labor, first-trimester doctor visits, and gestational age. As the confidence interval crossed 1.0, the smoking exposure was not a significant association. Again, the primary drivers of the relationship appeared to be racial group and previous preterm labor. Reassuringly, the maternal age covariate ("age") was not statistically significant and had an odds ratio of approximately 1.0. The larger standard errors in the conditional versus unconditional model result from the stratification by age.

Code #11.4 in Appendix 2 can be used to reproduce the output shown in Figures 11.2–11.14.

```
> summary(clogit(low ~ as.factor(smoke) + as.factor(race) + as.factor(ptl_collapsed) +
as.factor(ftv_collapsed) + gestation + age + strata(matched), data=matched_dataset))
Call:
coxph(formula = Surv(rep(1, 118L), low) ~ as.factor(smoke) +
    as.factor(race) + as.factor(ptl_collapsed) + as.factor(ftv_collapsed) +
    gestation + age + strata(matched), data = matched_dataset,
    method = "exact")

  n= 118, number of events= 59

                             coef exp(coef) se(coef)      z Pr(>|z|)
as.factor(smoke)1         1.34762   3.84825  0.90625  1.487  0.13701
as.factor(race)2          0.97729   2.65726  0.73589  1.328  0.18416
as.factor(race)3          1.37382   3.95040  0.69095  1.988  0.04678 *
as.factor(ptl_collapsed)1 2.96105  19.31821  1.13867  2.600  0.00931 **
as.factor(ftv_collapsed)1 -0.48811  0.61379  0.66803 -0.731  0.46498
as.factor(ftv_collapsed)2 0.89060   2.43659  0.81814  1.089  0.27634
as.factor(ftv_collapsed)3 1.15753   3.18206  1.09642  1.056  0.29109
gestation                 0.10170   1.10705  0.24699  0.412  0.68051
age                       0.02947   1.02991  0.24404  0.121  0.90387
---
Signif. codes:  0 '***' 0.001 '**' 0.01 '*' 0.05 '.' 0.1 ' ' 1

                          exp(coef) exp(-coef) lower .95 upper .95
as.factor(smoke)1            3.8482    0.25986    0.6514    22.734
as.factor(race)2            2.6573    0.37633    0.6281    11.241
as.factor(race)3            3.9504    0.25314    1.0198    15.303
as.factor(ptl_collapsed)1   19.3182   0.05176    2.0736    179.971
as.factor(ftv_collapsed)1   0.6138    1.62923    0.1657     2.273
as.factor(ftv_collapsed)2   2.4366    0.41041    0.4902    12.111
as.factor(ftv_collapsed)3   3.1821    0.31426    0.3710    27.289
gestation                   1.1071    0.90330    0.6822     1.796
age                         1.0299    0.97096    0.6384     1.662

Concordance= 0.729  (se = 0.082 )
Likelihood ratio test= 27.48  on 9 df,    p=0.001
Wald test            = 12.53  on 9 df,    p=0.2
Score (logrank) test = 21.28  on 9 df,    p=0.01
```

Figure 11.14 Adjusted conditional odds ratio of the relationship between maternal smoking during the first trimester and low birthweight infants.

Statistical inference

Under the frequentist paradigm of probability (Chapter 12 introduces the Bayesian paradigm), it is not enough to interpret the statistics without regard to the hypothesis under test. Although one may find a difference in statistical estimates, these may be due to chance, rather than an actual difference in the population or study sample. Statistical inference is concerned with the outcomes of hypothesis testing. One aspect of statistical inference is the p-value, where a "significant" p-value indicates that the findings are unlikely due to chance alone compared to some threshold, denoted by the Greek letter α. If the p-value is less than α, the null hypothesis is rejected, and we may conclude that the alternative hypothesis is the more plausible explanation. On the other hand, if the p-value is greater than or equal to α, the alternative hypothesis is rejected, and we may conclude that the null hypothesis is the more plausible explanation. A common way to view the p-value in health sciences research is the probability of producing a sample where an exposure to outcome relationship exists in the data but does not exist in the underlying population. Hence a tiny p-value suggests a small probability for the study to produce an association not found in the population.

Convention has established an α of 5% as a *de facto* standard, corresponding to a 1 in 20 chance of reaching a false positive conclusion. But this begs the question of why should a p-value of 0.051 be interpreted as radically different from one of 0.049? Indeed, there is more to arriving at a conclusion than simply examining a p-value. In epidemiology, there is a consensus that the p-value is overly relied upon, and language concerning statistical significance should be minimized in deference to the language of statistical precision and magnitude of effects. In fact, several leading epidemiology journals discourage reporting p-values under certain circumstances, such as inferring causality. Therefore, this issue is probably more relevant to many clinical journals, where EHR research is frequently published. Recognizing this, some have advocated abandoning its use altogether, concluding "testing null hypotheses at arbitrary *p* values of 0.05 has no basis in medicine and should be discouraged" (Grimes & Schulz, 2002). Berner and Amrhein (2022) debunked four misconceptions about the p-value: (1) the p-values themselves are subject to variation, (2) the lack of statistical significance is not evidence of a lack of effect, (3) statistically significant effect sizes are overestimates, and (4) our underlying hypotheses are flawed.

Using the p-value in this discouraged fashion is not consistent with some overall scientific truth underlying the study. As an alternative, the researcher can simply present the estimates with corresponding measures of precision, thereby letting the readers form their own conclusions, or use a Bayesian paradigm of research. For example, consider these two statements of findings:

1 We observed an odds ratio of 1.5 (p = 0.05), although it did not meet statistical significance at an α of 5% and was a marginal effect.
2 We observed an odds ratio of 1.5 (95% CI: 1.0, 2.1).

The second statement is shorter, clearer, and does not make a case for or against concluding the effect is meaningful. Returning to the topic of confounder selection presented at the start of this chapter, a case was made for both a statistical and theoretical basis, as a pure statistical approach may only include a confounder that is associated with the exposure or outcome at a specific, yet arbitrary, α. If the researcher has a strong theoretical basis for including a variable, it should be in the model. In some instances, such as global goodness-of-fit tests in regression diagnostics, only a p-value will result from the hypothesis test, so its acceptance is widely understood.

As another example, suppose a study resulted in a p-value of 0.30 for the association between smoking and lung cancer; in other words, the finding was not statistically significant. In such instances, we may be hesitant to conclude that there was no effect given the preponderance of existing evidence. Instead, it would be more prudent to focus on the "why" of this occurrence. Perhaps the sample size was too small or there were unknown or unmeasured threats to validity. The precision of the point estimate provides an important piece of evidence: a wide confidence interval may indicate an insufficient sample or large variability due to inconsistency in measurement. Now suppose in another study of this same topic, the p-value was 0.0001, indicating that the statistics were extremely unlikely due to chance alone. Even though in this case the findings corroborate our intuition, the results deserve as much scrutiny as a null effect finding before we make arrive at any conclusions from the study. After all, a more precisely measured biased effect is still a biased effect.

When the statistical analysis generates a confidence interval as the measure of uncertainty, more information can be gleaned than from the p-value alone. Consider these three examples of reported relative risks:

1   Relative risk = 3.5, 95% confidence interval: 2.7, 4.1.
2   Relative risk = 3.5, 95% confidence interval: 1.1, 7.2.
3   Relative risk = 3.5, p = 0.02.

All report the same relative risk of 3.5, interpreted as more than three times the increase in "risk," presumably associated with some harmful exposure. All are statistically significant in that the results are unlikely due to chance alone at an α of 5%. The added information from the confidence interval may be interpreted as follows. The first relative risk offers a more precise estimate due to the tighter confidence interval, while the second relative risk is less precise with potential "risk" extending all the way from almost no effect of a relative risk ˜1 to a bit over seven times the risk. In general, more precise estimates are preferable, which usually means less variability through larger sample sizes. But both relative risk estimates with corresponding confidence intervals are superior to the third estimate, where we lack information about the precision to infer whether significance was due to a true association or a huge sample size.

In addition to presenting the precision as a confidence interval, the researcher can also calculate the width and ratio of the interval, providing another indicator of the precision around the point estimate (Poole, 2001). For the two relative risk estimates with confidence intervals presented above, the width and ratios are calculated as follows:

1 Relative risk = 3.5, 95% confidence interval: 2.7, 4.1
2 Width = 4.1–2.7 = 1.4
3 Ratio = 4.1/2.7 = 1.5
4 Relative risk = 3.5, 95% confidence interval: 1.1, 7.2
5 Width = 7.2–1.1 = 6.1
6 Ratio = 7.2/1.1 = 6.5

Presenting the confidence interval along with its width or ratio provides an intuitive grasp of the precision of the estimate, useful for multiple comparisons. As can be seen, the first confidence interval is smaller than the second confidence interval: the point estimate is more than four times as precise.

Statistically versus clinically meaningful

A hypothesis test reveals statistical differences in groups unlikely due to chance alone. Consider the following hypothetical: suppose a retrospective outpatient EHR study examined the link between multivitamin use and mean differences in blood pressure after one year of supplementation. Among those in the unexposed group who did not have a multivitamin, the mean systolic blood pressure after one year was 122 millimeters of mercury (95% confidence interval: 120, 124, width: 4) and among those in the exposed group who had a multivitamin, the mean systolic blood pressure after one year was 124 millimeters of mercury (95% confidence interval: 122, 126, width: 4). As we can see from this contrived example, the mean blood pressure was very precisely measured, suggesting quite a large cohort size, common among EHR studies at large institutions. The corresponding hypothesis test provided strong evidence that the blood pressure difference was unlikely due to chance alone ($p < 0.001$). Does this statistical evidence translate to clinical importance? A two-millimeter difference in systolic blood pressure has little clinical utility, and the finding is a by-product of a study that was overpowered from a huge cohort population, indicated by the small width of the confidence intervals.

Now consider another example of a study to assess differences in systolic blood pressure among two groups. The first group, whose blood pressure was measured in a clinical environment, had a mean systolic blood pressure of 135 (95% confidence interval: 125, 155, width: 30). The second group, whose blood pressure was self-measured in the home environment, had a mean of 115 (95% confidence interval: 90, 155, width: 65). Further suppose that a test of statistical significance had a p-value of 0.04, suggesting that these differences were unlikely due to chance alone. While we may be tempted to conclude there is a clear difference, there are two observations about these statistics that may temper our enthusiasm. First, there was greater variability in the in-home testing group, with more than a doubling in the confidence interval width. Upon further investigation, we may find that there were problems using the automated sphygmomanometer. Second, the elevated blood pressure at in the clinical environment may not be due to the second group being unhealthier but rather a manifestation of so-called "white coat hypertension." These critical details may not be known from a researcher applying only statistical inference – we must also consider causal inference of the study findings.

Causal inference

In etiologic research, there is an oft-quoted expression: "Correlation does not equal causation." How do we know that the exposure led to the outcome, rather than being an artifact of poor study design, uncontrolled confounding, or random chance? In Chapter 9, we discussed how statistical associations between independent and dependent variables under study – the exposures and the outcomes – can be caused by one or more combinations of five mechanisms: (1) true causation between the exposure and the outcome, (2) *bias*, or an artificial association due to systematic errors in measurement or selection, (3) *confounding*, or a real association caused by an extraneous variable, (4) *reverse causation* where the outcome caused the exposure unbeknownst to the researcher, and (5) *random error*. Our goal as researchers is to appreciate and thereby minimize mechanisms #2–#5, so the strongest explanation for an association between the exposure and the outcome is a causal one.

Causal inference not only provides a framework for evaluating the exposure to outcome relation, but also for establishing the limits of epidemiology as a science. There are two lenses to examine causality: a philosophical lens and a technical lens. The philosophical lens is a "set of convictions about how epidemiologists should think about causality," whereas the technical sense "concerns a collection of mathematical tools and methods" (Vandenbroucke, Broadbent & Pearce, 2016). The EHR research methods in this book are not married to any causal camp; although they may arise out of a specific philosophical approach, they can be viewed as a distinct entity. In fact, this is how epidemiological training often proceeds. Trainees typically take a course on causal inference that is weighted toward the philosophical aspects of the concept, while the tools and techniques to achieve causal inference are taught in advanced epidemiological or biostatistical methods courses. In addition, causal inference should not be conflated with statistical inference as these are distinct concepts. Statistical software always and only gives associational estimates from the model: our subjective context and philosophy provide causal inference. Thus, we can summarize by stating that the theory of causation is firmly grounded in philosophy, while the tools for causal inference arise from modeling causation (Figure 11.15).

There are many different schools of thought with respect to causal thinking (Beebee, Hitchcock & Menzies, 2009). Philosophical causality invokes theories of regularity, probabilism, causal processes, interventionism, and counterfactualism, to name but a few. Counterfactualism has become the *de facto* school of thought for epidemiology and posits that had an exposure not been present, the outcome would not have manifested (Maldonado & Greenland, 2002). It is implied that

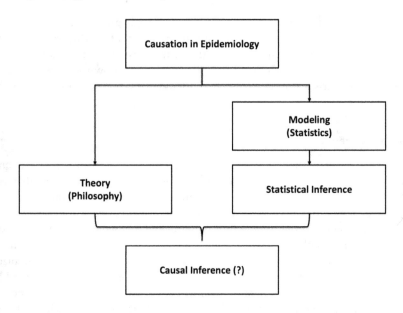

Figure 11.15 Philosophical versus technical lenses of causality.

the event and nonevent are observed in the same person: an impossibility. Thus, we rely on study designs that attempt to recreate the counterfactual condition between exposure groups. In the idealized setting, nothing will differ between individuals except the exposure, and, if causally related, the eventual outcome. One way of achieving this is through comparable, exchangeable treatment groups. In methodological language, this is known as the potential outcome approach: what is the potential outcome by varying treatment assignment? Some purists draw a distinction between the potential outcome approach and philosophical counterfactualism, and argue that potential outcomes are in fact an intervention-ist approach to causal thinking (Vandenbroucke, Broadbent & Pearce, 2016). The interventionist approach to epidemiology suggests that for a clinical question to be addressable through causal methods, we must be able to intervene in the exposure. Whether this distinction is important for the EHR researcher is up to the reader to decide. An intervention is the essence of the randomized controlled trial and randomization is used to achieve exchangeability. However, EHR research is more likely to fall under observational epidemiology.[5]

In observational epidemiology, the paradigm has become how to best mimic the randomized trial through study design and analysis, essentially replicating the unbiased exposure assignment inherent in the trial (Hernan & Robbins, 2016). Some have argued this view is too limited (Vandenbroucke, Broadbent & Pearce, 2016). For example, interventions are rarely well-specified, may be inconsequential to specify, and can change over time because what is not intervenable today may very well be tomorrow. Furthermore, some interventions are impossible: one cannot intervene upon age, sex, or other immutable characteristics which are linked to health-related outcomes. Regardless of the philosophical lens we bring to our science, the methods used in epidemiology are frequently described in terms of potential outcomes framework largely due to the work of Donald Rubin and the Rubin Causal Model (Rubin, 1978).

To compare the potential outcomes, epidemiologists strive to create the counterfactual condition. We cannot estimate the causal effect for an individual because the counterfactual does not exist nor are we necessarily interested in the individual effect, so we estimate average causal effects. The unobserved outcome can be thought of as a missing data problem. The counterfactual condition can be achieved through exchangeability of the exposure groups through true randomization when possible, Mendelian randomization and instrumental variables (see Sheehan et al., 2008), difference-in-differences (see Lechner, 2011), and other approaches. For the observational epidemiologist, the exchangeability criteria are paramount: how do we ensure that when the exposure groups are not randomized in the true sense of the word, we have selected, measured, and analyzed a study population as if they were? And this assumes that we have, in fact, a study population available to us. What if the treatment was hypothetical or planned? Observed data may not even exist. Our methods then become one of speculation. Suppose a person had received treatment, what would have happened? The potential outcomes are the outcomes that could be observed for each unit under the different exposure conditions.

Let us turn our attention to methods for causal inference used in epidemiology to answer the etiologic question, does X cause Y? In the most simplistic case, let us assume there is no confounding or missing data, X and Y are perfectly measured, there is a consistent linear relationship between the two variables, and Y does not cause X (no reverse causality). If this were the case – along with other assumptions omitted here – then we could fit a simple linear regression model and, if we see a statistical association, infer a causal one. Yet these assertions cannot be guaranteed in EHR research, or for that matter, even experimental research. Therefore, we need to turn to more sophisticated methods that can deal with a host of such methodological challenges. The survey of methods below is not meant to be exhaustive, nor mutually exclusive, as one may employ multiple methods, but rather a starting point for considering the causal approach to take.

- **Observed data methodology**: observational data already exist or can be collected. Secondary analysis of EHR data falls under this category.

  - *Traditional regression* with covariates informed from causal diagrams such as directed acyclic graphs. This is probably the most frequent analysis undertaken because of its simplicity, yet it also carries the greatest number of assumptions that are not likely to be met in practice. Methods include the regression approaches discussed in this chapter in line with the various study designs.
  - Methods for improved control of confounding, covariate balancing, and reduced model dependency.

    - *G-computation.* Estimating parameters had the observational study been a perfectly randomized experimental study (see Robins, 1986).

- *Propensity (exposure) scoring* and *doubly robust estimation* through propensity score matching and multivariable regression. The propensity score estimates the probability of exposure to mitigate the dimensionality of multiple potential confounders (see Rosenbaum & Rubin 1983).
- Time-varying effects of exposures or confounders. The exposure (or covariates) may be influenced by covariates (or exposure) or the outcome over time. An overview of these methods is provided by Daniel et al. (2013).

  - Structural nested models fit via *G-estimation* (see Robins et al., 1992).
  - Marginal structural models fit via *inverse probability weighting* (see Robins, Hernan & Brumback, 2000).

- Decomposing exposure to outcome effects in the context of endogenous variables.[6] An overview of these methods is provided by VanderWeele (2016).

  - *Structural equation modeling* and traditional mediation analysis, such as Baron and Kenny effect decomposition or Sobel product of coefficients, with a variety of extensions (see Baron & Kenney, 1986).
  - *Counterfactual approach*. Simulation-based approach to mediation analysis, similar to G-computation (see Imai, Keele & Tingley, 2010).

- Negative controls. Negative controls are an example of a design strategy that eschews exchangeability between groups to have a comparison group that differs in an important way to detect possible biases (see Lipsitch, Tchetgen & Cohen, 2010).

- **Unobserved and synthetic data methodology**: observational data do not exist nor can be collected at the present time. This may be useful for proposed clinical interventions that cannot be evaluated in practice (as an example, see Goldstein et al., 2018).

  - Observed data methodology can be applied over a synthetic data set or existing data set but with missing outcomes, for example, G-computation to predict outcomes scaling up an existing intervention.
  - Systems modeling approaches. See Galea, Riddle & Kaplan (2010) for a discussion of these approaches in causal inference.

    - *Agent-based models*. This class of models simulate an exposure among individual agents to estimate the outcome effect. Sometimes called complex systems (dynamic) approaches.
    - *Dynamic transmission models*. This class of models also simulates an exposure, yet operates at group levels, thus has fewer assumptions than agent-based models. Sometimes called system dynamic models.

Many of these methods have various extensions, such as dealing with case–control and survival (time-to-event) data, missing data, semi- and nonparametric approaches, as well as have a variety of assumptions that must be met. Sensitivity analyses are recommended to check for the robustness of assumptions and are a final step to guard against bias before inferring causality.

Causal inference in epidemiology is a complex matter, and can fill an entire book (see, for example, Hernan & Robins, 2020). Aside from the frameworks discussed thus far, there are other, simpler frameworks that help to assess the question of causality. One of the first formalized frameworks for establishing causality in epidemiology resulted from Doll and Hill's investigations of lung cancer mortality as related to tobacco smoking (Doll & Hill, 1950; Doll & Hill, 1954). As the ideas from this work coalesced, Hill articulated nine criteria for ascribing causality (Hill, 1965). This framework has been extensively quoted, used, and to some extent, modified, and is an accepted way of vetting an association between an antecedent exposure and subsequent outcome before inferring causality. Paraphrased, these criteria are:

1 *Strength*. A greater magnitude of association provides stronger evidence of causality compared to a weaker measure of association.
2 *Consistency*. Results from a study should be repeatable, especially among studies of inherently dissimilar designs.
3 *Specificity*. A well-articulated exposure needs to be associated with a well-articulated outcome. This minimizes the chance for misspecification, misinterpretation, and measurement error.
4 *Temporarily*. The exposure must temporally precede the outcome to have a causal effect.
5 *Biological gradient*. A dose-response relationship should be demonstrable, where greater exposure confers more (or worse) outcomes.
6 *Plausibility*. As far as current science allows, the relationship between the exposure and outcome must be biologically possible.
7 *Coherence*. Data generated from a given study should not seriously conflict with what is known about the natural history and biology of the disease process.
8 *Experiment*. The association should be demonstrable in a controlled manner.
9 *Analogy*. A claim could be made with similar exposure and outcomes, and this finding should not contradict similar relationships.

Fully satisfying these criteria is rarely, if ever possible, nor should this be viewed as a checklist. However, the more evidence provided, the greater the likelihood of the association between causal. Arguably, the most important criterion is temporality.

Causal pies are a conceptual framework for delineating between sufficient and necessary causes of an outcome (Rothman, 1995). A *sufficient* cause is one that inevitably produces the outcome. It does not need to be a single cause, but can represent a constellation of causes, which are individually termed *component* causes. A *necessary* cause is a component that is required in every sufficient cause. A necessary cause on its own may not produce the outcome but is needed with other factors to produce the outcome. The concept of sufficient and necessary causes can

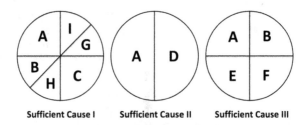

Figure 11.16 Three causal pies.

be modeled through "causal pies." Figure 11.16 depicts three causal mechanisms, where *A* is a necessary cause in each sufficient cause I, II, and III.

Good epidemiology is built on study design, variable measurement, and causal inference. Careful consideration of study design, implementation, and interpretation of the findings can hopefully minimize the mistake of inferring causation when only correlation is present. However, as has been discussed in numerous places in this book, secondary analysis of the EHR means that study design and variable measurement may be suboptimal. Thus, we must bring causal inference to the forefront. Inferring causality is less about concrete work and more about abstract thought. As a researcher – and reader of other research – there should be an underlying causal model driving the scientific inquiry. For some research questions, establishing true causality may not be a prerequisite if interventions or guidelines operate on risk factors instead of the actual causal agents.

Notes

1 Logistic regression was used as the log-binomial model failed to converge.
2 This is a hypothetical analysis and should not be assumed to be due to lack of a true causal effect.
3 From a causal inference perspective, we may question whether the timing is appropriate, or perhaps exposure to smoking periconception is more critical for the fetus than smoking during the first trimester.
4 Users of R may find implementation details here: https://stats.oarc.ucla.edu/r/dae/poisson-regression/.
5 The notion of a pragmatic clinical trial using EHR data has gained popularity in recent years. In contrast to a traditional randomized clinical trial that may lack external validity, a pragmatic trial is built around existing patient populations to compare effectiveness of real-world interventions thereby maximizing external validity, similar to an observational study. Causal inference techniques are still required beyond mere bivariable analyses to account for imbalance that may result in treatment groups, for example, due to non-adherence. Pragmatic trials is discussed further in Chapter 12.
6 Mediation analyses examine how endogenous variables (the mediators) fully or partially explain the relationship between an exposure and outcome. Such analysis may be useful in understanding the how and why of an exposure effect. If the mediator fully explains this relationship, after including it in the analysis, the exposure would no longer be independently predictive of the outcome. In reality, partial mediation, or a fraction of the total exposure to outcome effect, is expected. Assumed in this relationship is that the exposure has preceded the mediator, and the mediator preceded the outcome.

References

Aragon TJ. epitools: Epidemiology Tools. R package version 0.5-10.1, 2020. https://CRAN. R-project.org/package=epitools

Baron RM, Kenny DA. The moderator–mediator variable distinction in social psychological research: Conceptual, strategic, and statistical considerations. J Pers Soc Psychol. 1986;51(6):1173–1182.

Beebee H, Hithcock C, Menzies P (eds.). The Oxford Handbook of Causation. Oxford University Press. 2009.

Berner D, Amrhein V. Why and how we should join the shift from significance testing to estimation. J Evol Biol. 2022;35(6):777–787.

Daniel RM, Cousens SN, De Stavola BL, Kenward MG, Sterne JA. Methods for dealing with time-dependent confounding. Stat Med. 2013;32(9):1584–1618.

Doll R, Hill AB. Smoking and carcinoma of the lung: Preliminary report. Br Med J. 1950;2(4682):739–748.

Doll R, Hill AB. The mortality of doctors in relation to their smoking habits: A preliminary report. Br Med J. 1954;1(4877):1451–1455.

Galea S, Riddle M, Kaplan GA. Causal thinking and complex system approaches in epidemiology. Int J Epidemiol. 2010;39(1):97–106.

Goldstein ND, Jenness SM, Tuttle D, Power M, Paul DA, Eppes SC. Evaluating a neonatal intensive care unit MRSA surveillance programme using agent-based network modelling. J Hosp Infect. 2018;100(3):337–343.

Grimes DA, Schulz KF. An overview of clinical research: The lay of the land. Lancet. 2002;359(9300):57–61.

Hernán MA, Robins JM. Causal Inference: What If. Boca Raton, FL: Chapman & Hall/CRC, 2020.

Hernán MA, Robins JM. Using big data to emulate a target trial when a randomized trial is not available. Am J Epidemiol. 2016;183(8):758–764.

Hill AB. The environment and disease: Association or causation? Proc R Soc Med. 1965;58:295–300.

Hubbard AE, Ahern J, Fleischer NL, Van der Laan M, Lippman SA, Jewell N, Bruckner T, Satariano WA. To GEE or not to GEE: Comparing population average and mixed models for estimating the associations between neighborhood risk factors and health. Epidemiology. 2010;21(4):467–474.

Imai K, Keele L, Tingley D. A general approach to causal mediation analysis. Psychol Methods. 2010;15(4):309–334.

Lechner M. The Estimation of Causal Effects by Difference-in-Difference Methods. St. Gallen: Department of Economics, University of St. Gallen: 2011.

Lipsitch M, Tchetgen Tchetgen E, Cohen T. Negative controls: A tool for detecting confounding and bias in observational studies. Epidemiology. 2010;21(3):383–388. Erratum in: Epidemiology. 2010 Jul;21(4):589.

Lokku A, Lim LS, Birken CS, Pullenayegum EM, TARGet Kids! Collaboration. Summarizing the extent of visit irregularity in longitudinal data. BMC Med Res Methodol. 2020 May 29;20(1):135.

Maldonado G, Greenland S. Estimating causal effects. Int J Epidemiol. 2002;31(2):422–429.

Poole C. Low p-values or narrow confidence intervals: Which are more durable? Epidemiology. 2001;12(3):291–294.

Pullenayegum EM, Lim LS. Longitudinal data subject to irregular observation: A review of methods with a focus on visit processes, assumptions, and study design. Stat Methods Med Res. 2016;25(6):2992–3014.

R Core Team. R: A Language and Environment for Statistical Computing. Vienna: R Foundation for Statistical Computing, 2020. https://www.R-project.org/.

Robins J. A new approach to causal inference in mortality studies with a sustained exposure period—Application to control of the healthy worker survivor effect. Math Model. 1986;7(9–12):1393–1512.

Robins JM, Blevins D, Ritter G, Wulfsohn M. G-estimation of the effect of prophylaxis therapy for pneumocystis carinii pneumonia on the survival of AIDS patients. Epidemiology. 1992;3(4):319–336.

Robins JM, Hernán MA, Brumback B. Marginal structural models and causal inference in epidemiology. Epidemiology. 2000;11(5):550–560.

Rosenbaum PR, Rubin DB. The central role of the propensity score in observational studies for causal effects. Biometrika. 1983;70(1):41–55.

Rothman KJ. Causes 1976. Am J Epidemiol. 1995;141(2):90–95; discussion 89.

Rothman KJ, Greenland S, Lash TL.Modern Epidemiology. Philadelphia, PA: Lippincott Williams & Wilkins, 2012.

Rubin DB. Bayesian inference for causal effects: The role of randomization. Ann Statist. 1978;6(1):34–58.

Sheehan NA, Didelez V, Burton PR, Tobin MD. Mendelian randomisation and causal inference in observational epidemiology. PLoS Med. 2008;5(8):e177.

Thompson ML, Myers JE, Kriebel D. Prevalence odds ratio or prevalence ratio in the analysis of cross sectional data: What is to be done? Occup Environ Med. 1998;55(4):272–277.

Vandenbroucke JP, Broadbent A, Pearce N. Causality and causal inference in epidemiology: The need for a pluralistic approach. Int J Epidemiol. 2016;45(6):1776–1786.

VanderWeele TJ. Mediation analysis: A practitioner's guide. Annu Rev Public Health. 2016;37:17–32.

Wacholder S. Binomial regression in GLIM: Estimating risk ratios and risk differences. Am J Epidemiol. 1986;123(1):174–184.

Williamson T, Eliasziw M, Fick GH. Log-binomial models: Exploring failed convergence. Emerg Themes Epidemiol. 2013;10(1):14.

Zou G. A modified Poisson regression approach to prospective studies with binary data. Am J Epidemiol. 2004;159(7):702–706.

12 Advanced and Emerging Methods and Applications

This chapter is a high-level survey of advanced methodologies as well as emerging and newer innovations in epidemiological research relevant to the EHR. In some sense, it is a clearinghouse for the various methods and techniques that do not fit conveniently into other chapters in the book. It is also an opportunity to cover techniques that are not widely used in traditional observational epidemiology. To describe some of these approaches as cutting-edge would only serve to date the material, given how quickly computational fields such as data science evolve. Data science, for example, did not become formalized as a discipline until the mid-twentieth century. Electronic health records are even newer, becoming commonplace in the late twentieth century. As such, these are disciplines that are still defining themselves and adopting and adapting methods that have been used in other areas, including statistics, computer science, linguistics, geography, and, of course, epidemiology. This chapter is not meant for readers to become proficient in these methodologies. Far from it. Rather, it serves as an overview of techniques that may prove useful for certain EHR research studies. Numerous references are included with prototypical examples.

Data science, machine learning, and artificial intelligence

Data science is built upon many core competencies including computer science, statistics, ethics, information technology, visualization, and communication, among others (Meng,, 2019). As argued in Chapter 1, EHR research benefits from a multi-perspective collaborative, and data science can contribute in numerous ways, from predictive models that use machine learning (ML) and artificial intelligence (AI) to methods for improved data collection and capture, innovative data visualizations, simulation and complex systems modeling, data security and privacy, and linguistic processing of free text. Data scientists are often well versed in working with high dimensional data and can assist with optimizing statistical models to ensure EHR data can be used in near-real time, such as for clinical prediction and decision support. Although the field is often conflated with a sole focus on ML/AI, it is indeed much richer. Nevertheless, data scientists frequently develop and employ ML/AI techniques, and it is this area that we will explore further in this chapter. ML can be viewed as a collection of

DOI: 10.4324/9781003258872-15

tools that help us identify patterns in high dimensional data, such as the EHR; AI automates decisions based on those patterns. For example, we might develop an ML approach to predict sepsis among hospitalized inpatients using EHR data and an AI approach to provide clinical decision support in the EHR based on the ML model. Although these two concepts are frequently discussed together, for our purposes, we will only focus on ML. For those new to ML, there are review articles that provide a summary of ML for epidemiological applications (Wiemken & Kelley, 2020) and include applied examples, such as triaging emergency medicine patients, diagnosing septic shock, treating community-acquired pneumonia, and identifying COVID-19 cases at risk for clinical deterioration (Hamilton et al., 2021).

ML and AI have received an extraordinary amount of attention in epidemiology but before discussing the benefits and applications of ML to EHR research, we first need to recognize that it is not a remedy to all healthcare problems. Several high-profile examples demonstrate how harm may come from the deployment of AI systems, and unfortunately, the systems are not tested or vetted in a peer-reviewed manner, commonplace in medicine and epidemiology (Szabo, 2019). Inappropriate ML can perpetuate biases in the EHR, including missing data and measurement error, and may exacerbate existing healthcare disparities (Andaur Navarro et al., 2021; Gianfrancesco et al., 2018; Obermeyer et al., 2019). ML provides a means to complete a task, such as the construction of a statistical model, but the model is not the end goal of epidemiology. Generally, ML should be avoided when the goal of the research is to identify clinical intervention points, when there are too few data points, or when there is a need for a mechanistic or causal understanding of the clinical pathway. Further, the added value of ML is limited in traditional epidemiologic investigations of binary data points. In a secondary analysis of EHR data comparing ML to traditional regression models predicting outcomes of heart failure, ML offered a limited improvement over traditional methods (Desai et al., 2020). It is not until there is a clear clinical application and research question with accompanying high dimensional data[1] that the value of ML begins to emerge.

Despite these caveats, there are at least four areas that ML can contribute to EHR research: (1) exploratory analysis of large datasets through unsupervised learning, (2) development of predictive models, and to a limited extent, etiologic models through supervised learning, (3) handling missing data, deidentifying data, and creating synthetic data through semi-supervised learning, and (4) knowledge discovery and data mining. There are a plethora of ML algorithms and selecting the appropriate one depends on the research question, data type, hypothesized effects, interpretability, and flexibility. This chapter does not cover specific algorithms; readers are referred to this text for implementation details (James et al., 2021). In addition, collaboration with an epidemiologist or training in epidemiology should be viewed as a prerequisite to taking a data science view of EHR research because of epidemiology's rigorous focus on study design, variable measurement, and causal inference (Goldstein, LeVasseur & McClure, 2020).

Exploratory analysis

One of the most straightforward uses of ML is to identify patterns in data for reducing dimensionality. In an EHR-derived dataset, there may be hundreds or thousands of variables available for a given patient, especially if omics or laboratory measures are available. Most likely, there are many dependencies and correlations across these variables, and therefore the researcher must either choose a subset of variables that are minimally collinear or perform dimension reduction. In a traditional epidemiologic analysis, we might undertake a factor analysis or principal component analysis when the dimension reduction problem occurs independent of the health outcome (i.e., dependent variable). Alternatively, we can employ ML approaches that do not depend on the outcome being present in the data, known as *unsupervised learning* algorithms.[2]

An unsupervised learning approach seeks to learn about patterns and correlations in the independent variables regardless of the dependent variable. This is especially useful where we have broad clinical states that are heterogeneous in their presentation, and we wish to create latent homogenous groups. In other words, the goal is to identify distinct clinical phenotypes (Wang et al., 2020). Unsupervised learning has been used in EHR data to identify phenotypes of Alzheimer's disease (Alexander et al., 2021) and other aging-related diseases (Kuan et al., 2021), COVID-19 (Cui, Robins & Finkelstein, 2020), pediatric critical care (Williams, Ghosh & Wetzel, 2018), and mental health (Kung et al., 2021), among others. It also has been applied to aspects of care delivery, such as types of EHR users (Fong et al., 2022), management of sepsis (Fohner et al., 2019), and neonatal care (Chen et al., 2021).

Modeling

Regression modeling is the backbone of biostatistical techniques used in epidemiology. Regression can be used for predictive modeling to identify protective or risk factors for disease, or etiologic modeling in the hunt for causal agents for the purposes of intervening. In a traditional regression analysis, a dependent variable is regressed on one or more independent variables. Using *supervised learning* ML algorithms,[3] we may also predict the outcome based on a high dimensional input. This contrasts with unsupervised learning where the outcome is removed from the data. Supervised learning techniques are used for regression (mostly predictive, but there are emerging causal approaches), classification problems, and estimation.

Unlike traditional regression approaches where the researcher is required to specify the model, ML does not make assumptions about the data-generating process, such as the presence of interactions. Thus, predictive ML approaches can detect previously unknown associations. However, any time we fit a model, whether a regression model or ML, we are making a claim about how the dependent and independent variables are related, requiring us to bring our substantive expertise to evaluate the model. For example, tree-based algorithms may be useful for detecting unknown interactions, but ML cannot distinguish if the independent variables are mediators instead of confounders.

Data scientists speak of a *pipeline* to move from data to an ML model (Figure 12.1). This pipeline begins with typical observational epidemiology considerations of applying inclusion and exclusion criteria to arrive at the analytic sample and variable list. Once the ML algorithm is selected, the data are stratified into training and testing datasets, where the training dataset is the initial application of the algorithm to propose a model. In an iterative process, hyperparameters that control the ML algorithm are tuned, the model is tested in the testing dataset, and the output is evaluated to select a final model. Alternative ML algorithms may also be considered as part of this process. Once a model is selected, the predictive performance is evaluated through measures of sensitivity, specificity, and predictive values, which are presented in what is known as a *confusion matrix*.

ML–based prediction models have been employed heavily in EHR research. For example, researchers have built models to predict atrial fibrillation (Tiwari et al., 2020), heart failure (Wu, Roy & Stewart, 2010), infection (Bhavani et al., 2020), kidney injury (Kate et al., 2020), postoperative complications (Bronsert et al.,

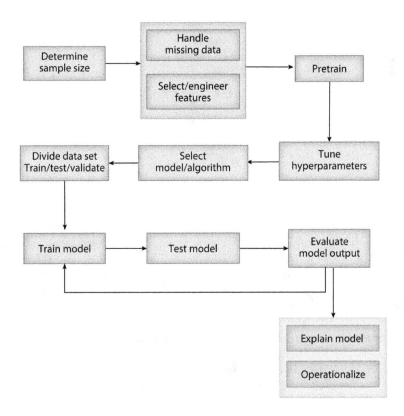

Figure 12.1 Machine learning predictive model pipeline.

2020), childhood obesity (Pang et al., 2021), diabetes (Dinh et al., 2019), and cardiovascular disease (Dinh et al., 2019); the list goes on extensively. To expound on one study further, Pang et al. developed a "comprehensive machine learning workflow [...] that includes data quality control, data processing, missing data imputation, and machine learning model development for early childhood obesity prediction" using data from a large pediatric EHR. Their ML workflow mirrors the pipeline in Figure 12.1. After applying inclusion and exclusion criteria, approximately 27,000 patients with over 100 variables were available for model development., and were divided into training (80%) and testing datasets (20%). Seven ML algorithms, including the XGBoost ensemble algorithm, were developed to predict obesity incidence in the cohort. The authors found the ensemble model performed the best (see Tables 1 and 2 in Pang et al.); unfortunately, a traditional theory-driven logistic regression model was not available for comparison. Nevertheless, the authors demonstrated a rigorous process to develop a predictive ML model using EHR data.

Aside from pure prediction, there are emerging approaches to causal modeling using ML. Supervised learning has been used to predict the counterfactual state and fit propensity score models for inverse probability weighting. Through simulation studies, Naimi, Mishler and Kennedy (2021) contrasted parametric and nonparametric (i.e., ML) based approaches, including inverse probability weighting, g-computation, augmented inverse probability weighting, and targeted minimum loss-based estimation for estimating causal effects. They noted that singly robust ML estimation of the average treatment effect was biased, but performance improved when using doubly robust estimation, where an exposure model and outcome model are combined into a single estimator. The authors offered four suggestions for researchers using ML to quantify the average treatment effect: use (1) doubly robust methods, (2) sample splitting, (3) multiple ML algorithms through an ensemble approach, and (4) interactions and transformations on selected variables.

Under *semi-supervised learning*, some of the outcome data have been removed. This approach can be used to impute missing outcome data under a variety of missing data mechanisms. Algorithms such as k-nearest neighbors, tree-based methods, and deep learning have the embedded capacity to handle missing data as part of the prediction pipeline (Figure 12.1), potentially enabling its use. In experimental settings, random forest consistently performs well for imputation compared to other more resource-intensive algorithms (Jäger, Allhorn & Bießmann, 2021). Researchers have also assessed how ML imputation methods perform for specific data structures, such as survival data (Guo, Yang & Chen, 2021). Despite this integrated capacity, among clinical prediction model studies in the literature, missing data have infrequently been handled through ML (Nijman et al., 2022).

Knowledge discovery and data mining

A third area of ML applications to EHR research is knowledge discovery. In knowledge discovery – also known as data mining – ML provides a method to automatically delve into the EHR and retrieve meaning from the data. A full treatment of knowledge discovery and data mining may be found elsewhere (Freitas, 2002); rather what follows here are applications specific to EHR research.

Knowledge discovery proceeds in a sequential fashion, beginning with data identification, followed by data preprocessing, then data mining, and concluding with evaluation. Preprocessing constitutes most of the process (Zhang, Zhang & Yang, 2003). As such, researchers have proposed pipelines for data preprocessing prior to the application of ML techniques: in Figure 12.1, this is an expansion of the second step following sample size determination. One such pipeline is known as FIDDLE (Flexible Data-Driven Pipeline), which "systematically transforms structured EHR data into representations that can be used as inputs to ML algorithm" (Tang et al., 2020). Examples of how this preprocessing pipeline works include identification of time-varying data; filtering and collapsing rare, duplicate, or uninformative data; identification of frequent versus infrequent measures; missing data imputation; and automatically reconciling heterogenous data types. The goal of a pipeline such as FIDDLE is to enable researchers to obtain EHR data beyond what is easy or convenient.

One immediate application of ML to knowledge discovery is improving EHR data abstraction beyond what has already been discussed in Chapter 4. Whereas manual chart review is cumbersome, prone to errors, and time-consuming, ML has been deployed to automate the process for both structured and unstructured data. Hu et al. (2017) explored the use of six automated approaches for identifying postoperative complications among surgical patients using structured EHR data, including diagnostic codes, microbiology tests, antibiotic administration, and other labs. The performance of each of these approaches was compared against manual chart review, which was treated as the gold standard, and all approaches performed better than chance alone (area under the curve exceeding 0.8 for all complications). In Park et al. (2020), the authors contrasted three ML algorithms for identifying hospital-acquired catheter-associated urinary tract infections from EHR data. Similar to Hu, they used structured data from the EHR, supplemented with ancillary data from nursing, and constructed a gold standard via manual chart review. Also similar to Hu, the authors observed that the algorithms performed better than chance (area under the curve exceeding 0.75 for all algorithms) and noted the feasibility of ML for data mining hospital-acquired catheter-associated urinary tract infections.

Data need not be limited to the healthcare enterprise for this application. Researchers have linked publicly available data on the built environment, neighborhood characteristics, and housing attributes to the EHR to explore in-home environmental exposures to asthma (Bozigar et al., 2022). Using an ensemble approach, four allergen prediction models were constructed to discover the presence of cockroaches, rodents, mold, and carpets. The gold standard in this analysis was an asthma flowsheet in the EHR that was only occasionally completed by the healthcare workers. The algorithms performed modestly (area under the curve between 0.55 and 0.65) but demonstrated the possibility of supplementing existing clinical data with public data to identify harmful exposures not otherwise captured in the EHR.

Data also need not be structured to automatically derive meaning. This book has emphasized the importance of free text contained in the EHR to bring context and nuance to clinical findings (see Chapter 4, for example). However, free text is more challenging to operationalize compared to discrete data. The subfield of natural language processing is concerned with extracting meaning from free text and is covered in a separate section in this chapter.

Processing free text

Chapter 5 briefly introduced strategies to capture free text in the research database. Extracting meaning from free text is a challenging yet common problem in EHR research. In fact, a whole subfield of computer science is concerned with methods for addressing this problem, which range from string parsers and regular expressions to probabilistic techniques including natural language processing (NLP). The goal of parsing narrative text in the EHR is to extract relevant information for epidemiologic analysis that may not be captured in discrete or coded fields. Textual data captures information such as patient-reported outcomes, symptoms, illness trajectory and progress notes, differential diagnoses, social and behavioral history, and so on. It is mostly nonredundant to other information in the EHR, and as such it has tremendous value for public health and epidemiologic measures not normally found in the EHR, such as the social determinants of health (see Chapter 3). However, there are numerous challenges to processing free text. These challenges include the breadth of medical terminology and abbreviations; misspellings, unconventional sentence structure, and phrases; documentation patterns specific to clinician, specialty, location, and EHR; and complexity and ability to validate more sophisticated approaches including NLP.

String parsing

To begin, we will consider the more straightforward approaches to manipulating text. These approaches assume that the free text has been extracted from the EHR and exist as a string-type variable in the research database or spreadsheet. There are a variety of functions that exist in statistical software to manipulate and parse strings, including retrieving the length of a string, subsetting or splitting a string, concatenating multiple strings together, locating the position or matching one or more characters within a string, truncating or removing a portion of the string, replacing a sequence of characters in a string with another, and standardizing the case or removing special characters. There are many other string manipulation functions and their availability depends on the statistical software in use.

Let us consider an example of a hepatitis C test result received from an outside laboratory and stored as free text in the EHR: "HCV antibody POSITIVE; HCV RNA POSITIVE 900,000 IU/L; Interpretation: chronic infection with hepatitis C." There are several approaches we may take to extracting meaning from this string. On the one hand, we may be interested in a qualitative interpretation: the patient has a chronic hepatitis C infection. On the other hand, we may be interested in a quantitative interpretation: the patient's viral load is high at 900,000 copies. For this hypothetical, we are interested in operationalizing two variables: hepatitis C antibody presence and, if positive, hepatitis C viral load. Permutations of these variables can be used to infer no infection, prior infection, or current infection, and thus these two variables are sufficient for the presumed analytic goals.

The text string includes delimiters – characters that separate data points, a semicolon in this case – and splitting the string by this delimiter will result in three new strings: "HCV antibody POSITIVE," "HCV RNA POSITIVE 900,000 IU/L," and "Interpretation: chronic infection with hepatitis C." To focus on the viral load, we now need to extract the actual value. One approach for this would be to use a string search function that identifies numbers in text (i.e., regular expression, covered later); a second option may be to take the "word" immediately preceding the unit of measure "IU/L"; and a third option may be to further parse by a space delimiter and extract the penultimate string. The validity of these approaches depends on the consistency of the lab reporting format. Following extraction of "900,000" we may need to use a character replacement function to remove the comma, otherwise, the value may not be castable as a numeric data type. This can be further complicated by patients who do not have detectable virus in their blood where the lab report may say "HCV RNA NEGATIVE Undetectable." A frequency table can be used to identify all the possible permutations and code can be written to handle the special cases. As can be seen from this simple example, string parsing is as much an art as it is a science, and what is easy for humans to accomplish through manual chart review can be quite challenging for a computer to automate. Fortunately, there are tools available to aid in the process.

For smaller research databases, Microsoft Excel (Microsoft Corp., Redmond, WA) offers many of the string manipulation functions previously discussed but in a graphical user interface obviating the need for complicated programming. Chapter 5 introduced several tools that can be used to extract meaning from free text. For example, the **Text to Columns** function can accomplish the delimiter-based parsing needed to separate antibody and viral load from the other attributes in the test result. A visual inspection of the data will allow the researcher to align the parsed fields into the appropriate columns (variables) and search for inconsistencies. Then, using the **Filter** operation on the column, outlier or nonconforming values can be isolated and addressed. While Excel makes this process intuitive, it adds additional time to the data preprocessing and will be counterproductive on large datasets.

When the use of Excel is not an option, regular expressions are a powerful alternative for retrieving patterns in text; however, constructing regular expressions requires experience with their syntax.[4] If a recurring pattern exists in the free text, regular expression searches can parse the required data. Returning to the earlier example, "HCV antibody POSITIVE; HCV RNA POSITIVE 900,000 IU/L; Interpretation: chronic infection with hepatitis C," the regular expression in Figure 12.2 will automatically parse (1) the results of the antibody test as positive or negative, (2) the RNA test as positive or negative, and (3) the viral load whether

```
. * [ANTIBODY|Antibody|antibody]\s(POSITIVE|NEGATIVE|pos
itive|negative) . * [RNA|Rna|rna]\s(POSITIVE|NEGATIVE|pos
itive|negative)\s(\d+(,\d{3})*|UNDETECTABLE|Undetectab
le|undetectable)
```

Figure 12.2 An example of a regular expression.

a number or undetectable. This regular expression allows variation in capitalization as well as the use of commas in the number and can be further enhanced to consider a multitude of reporting differences. Regular expression search engines are available in many statistical software packages.

Natural language processing

The hepatitis C lab result example in the previous section was simplistic and not representative of the reality of free text responses. Suppose we needed to operationalize a variable for male patients that captures whether they have sex with other men. Assuming sexual orientation or behavior is not captured in the EHR as a discrete variable, this information is most likely found as a free text note in the patients' social histories. Examples of such language may include: "Pt reports hx of sex with men," "Pt is MSM," "Pt identifies as homosexual," "Pt has same-gender partner." In these cases, a standard text parser would be difficult to implement. We may develop a list of key words to search for in the free text note, such as "MSM," "gay," or "homosexual," and while this may work for positive documentation, or documentation that occurs in the presence of a finding, this would fail to detect the subtleties of negative documentation, or documentation that occurs in the absence of a finding: "Pt denies same-sex behavior." Furthermore, this information may be buried in other notes taken during the patient history requiring more sophisticated processing techniques such as NLP.

There are multiple types and subfields of NLP, including classification and extraction. Herein we focus on high-level applications applied to the clinical narrative. NLP can also range from more simplistic rule-based approaches to ML algorithms, with hybrid adaptions of both. Several NLP solutions have been developed explicitly for the EHR. These EHR-specific solutions include homegrown and open-source solutions such as the clinical text analysis knowledge extraction system (cTAKES) and the clinical event recognizer (CLEVER), as well as commercial options such as Linguamatics (IQVIA, Durham, NC) and Spark NLP for Healthcare (John Snow Labs, Lewes, DE). There are additionally a variety of open-source NLP libraries available for proficient programmers. For a historical review of NLP solutions in healthcare, refer to Savova et al. (2010). Use of NLP tools depends on the free text being available and electronically extractable from the EHR; in the case of older paper-based records that may or may not have been scanned into the EHR, optical character recognition will need to be applied first to digitize their contents prior to NLP.

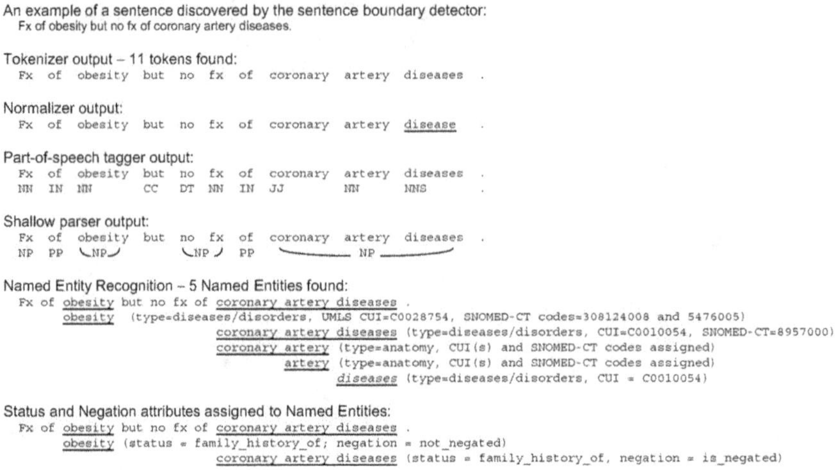

An example of a sentence discovered by the sentence boundary detector:
Fx of obesity but no fx of coronary artery diseases.

Tokenizer output – 11 tokens found:
```
Fx  of  obesity  but  no  fx  of  coronary  artery  diseases  .
```

Normalizer output:
```
Fx  of  obesity  but  no  fx  of  coronary  artery  disease  .
```

Part-of-speech tagger output:
```
Fx  of  obesity  but  no  fx  of  coronary  artery  diseases  .
NN  IN  NN       CC   DT  NN  IN  JJ        NN      NNS       .
```

Shallow parser output:
```
Fx  of  obesity  but  no  fx  of  coronary  artery  diseases  .
NP  PP  ⌣NP⌣          ⌣NP⌣  PP            ⌣_____ NP _____⌣
```

Named Entity Recognition – 5 Named Entities found:
Fx of obesity but no fx of coronary artery diseases.
    obesity (type=diseases/disorders, UMLS CUI=C0028754, SNOMED-CT codes=308124008 and 5476005)
        coronary artery diseases (type=diseases/disorders, CUI=C0010054, SNOMED-CT=8957000)
        coronary artery (type=anatomy, CUI(s) and SNOMED-CT codes assigned)
                artery (type=anatomy, CUI(s) and SNOMED-CT codes assigned)
                diseases (type=diseases/disorders, CUI = C0010054)

Status and Negation attributes assigned to Named Entities:
Fx of obesity but no fx of coronary artery diseases.
    obesity (status = family_history_of; negation = not_negated)
        coronary artery diseases (status = family_history_of, negation = is_negated)

Figure 12.3 An example sentence processed through the clinical text analysis knowledge extraction system (cTAKES).

cTAKES is a hybrid rule-based and ML NLP approach for processing clinical narratives (Savova et al., 2010). It processes text in a sequential and cumulative fashion (Figure 12.3). At a high level, the narrative is parsed into sentences; words, numbers, and dates are identified and normalized to standardize tense, spelling, and so on; terminology is mapped into the National Library of Medicine's Unified Medical Language System (UMLS, see Chapter 2); and annotations are applied to understand context, such as the negative or positive occurrence of a condition. In several validation studies, compared to an expert-abstracted gold standard measure, cTAKES achieved agreement better than 90% for ascertaining cardiovascular risk factors for a case–control study of peripheral arterial disease and treatment classification for a pharmacogenomics breast cancer treatment study (Savova et al., 2010). The cTAKES software is now part of an open-source consortium (Apache Software Foundation, Wilmington, DE) and is regularly updated.[5]

CLEVER is a tool that aids in the annotation of EHR narratives for clinical concepts (Tamang et al., 2017). The first step in the CLEVER pipeline (Figure 12.4) is to create the dictionary of terms applicable to the extraction based on expert opinion. For example, for researchers studying lupus in the EHR, this dictionary would include terms indicative of the condition. As with cTAKES, this seed dictionary is referenced against the UMLS to build a list of synonymous terms. The clinical narrative should first be cleaned for punctuation and normalized, and then the CLEVER tool can be applied to generate the annotations. Annotations will flag positive mentions of disease, for example, "patient has lupus," or negative

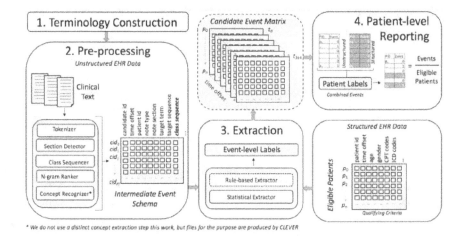

* We do not use a distinct concept extraction step this work, but files for the purpose are produced by CLEVER

Figure 12.4 The clinical event recognizer (CLEVER) pipeline.

mentions of disease, for example, "rule out lupus." Although CLEVER is still being used for NLP due to its efficiency and simplicity, it is not being actively maintained as of writing.[6] Other NLP annotation engines have been deployed into EHRs, such as the UMLS MetaMap (Aronson, 2001). Researchers have compared the accuracy in the extraction of clinical notes of these open-source NLP engines (Reátegui & Ratté, 2018).

There are abundant examples in the literature of NLP applied to free text in the EHR, many of which have been summarized in systematic reviews (Ford et al., 2016; Koleck et al., 2019; Kreimeyer et al., 2017; Shivade et al., 2014; Wang et al., 2018; Sheikhalishahi et al., 2019; Spasic & Nenadic, 2020). While there are domain-specific reviews of NLP (Abbe et al., 2016; Juhn & Liu, 2020; Pons et al., 2016; Spasić et al., 2014), herein we focus on more general applications of NLP for clinical narratives in the English language. Koleck et al. (2019) reviewed the use of NLP to extract symptoms captured in free text, such as "pain, fatigue, disturbed sleep, depressed mood, anxiety, nausea, dyspnea, and pruritus." Given their subjective nature that differs by provider and clinical specialty, symptoms could be documented in varied ways, thus hampering more straightforward data mining techniques. Among the 27 reviewed relevant articles that met the inclusion criteria, the authors observed a wide variety of NLP approaches used by the researchers including commercial software, open-source algorithms, and, in approximately 50% of the studies, homegrown solutions. Manual chart review served as the gold standard for comparison in most studies and the authors noted that most of the reviewed studies' objectives were to identify symptomology in the EHR, which in their view, suggested that NLP was a nascent field concerned with methodology over application.

Sheikhalishahi et al. (2019) conducted a review on the application of NLP to identify chronic disease because in their experience, unstructured data was far more common than structured data for documentation of diseases such as heart disease, stroke, cancer, diabetes, and lung disease. Among 106 reviewed articles covering 43 diseases in 10 disease categories, the authors found that metabolic diseases tended to have the greatest amount of structured data while diseases of the circulatory system had the greatest amount of unstructured data. As with Kolek et al., Sheikhalishahi et al. observed a diversity of NLP algorithms, with an increasing trend toward ML – in particular, support vector machines and naïve Bayes – or hybrid approaches in more recent years. Nevertheless, rule-based approaches were still quite common likely due to their relative simplicity despite the improved accuracy of what are known as deep classifiers or general deep learning methods for NLP. The authors also noted that the use of NLP for identifying co-morbidities or combining structured and unstructured data for prediction and longitudinal modeling was underutilized. In addition to calling for improvement in temporal extraction, they also called for focusing NLP to describe relationships between conditions and diagnoses beyond phenotype identification, and more public unstructured data for algorithmic development.

Spasic and Nenadic (2020) conducted a review of 110 articles focused on ML NLP in clinical narratives. Despite rich datasets being available in the reviewed studies, supervised ML was often used on subsets of the available data, owing to the burden of creating a validation dataset via manual chart review. This was identified as a major bottleneck to further development of ML for NLP. In general, the data requirements for supervised learning were more likely to be met for in-hospital death, discharge, readmission, and emergency department visits. An additional finding was the common use of single-institution EHRs, which may limit the transferability of the ML approach given how clinical narratives, among other factors, vary by institution (Sohn et al., 2018). Figure 4 in Spasic and Nenadic summarizes the clinical applications of NLP in the reviewed studies: the most common applications were enabling other tasks (i.e., NLP serving as a stepping stone, often to diagnosis), prognosis, clinical phenotyping, and care improvement. These applications most commonly mined EHR data in clinical notes, admission notes, discharge summaries, progress reports, radiology reports, allergy entries, and free-text medication orders.

To conclude this section, we will focus on two studies that have mined EHR data for social determinants that are otherwise infrequently captured via diagnostic or billing codes: homelessness (Bejan et al., 2018) and social isolation (Zhu et al., 2019). In the study by Bejan et al. (2018), the authors sought to identify homelessness from over 100 million clinical notes for 2.6 million patients in the Vanderbilt University Medical Center EHR, while comparing two data-driven NLP methodologies: lexical associations, a measure of connection between words and phrases, and word2vec, an open-source ML NLP toolkit. Seed terms were initially provided by the researchers, and the NLP engines expanded the query to form the search lexicon. The clinical notes were then compared against the vocabulary, results weighted and filtered to remove negative documentation, and subsequently assessed for relevance. Expert opinion was used to refine terms and manual review compared NLP annotations with manual annotation, resulting in the final search lexicon: homeless, homelessness, shelter, unemployed, jobless, and incarceration. Performance of the ML NLP approach surpassed the lexical association approach, with area under the curves exceeding 0.90. Based on their success, the authors further explored identifying childhood adverse experiences from the EHR and suggested that other social determinants can be operationalized from unstructured EHR data using NLP.

Indeed, this was the case with Zhu et al. (2019) who sought to identify another social determinant – social isolation – in the clinical notes of patients with prostate cancer at the Medical University of South Carolina. As opposed to Bejan et al. (2018), where the authors used homegrown or open-source NLP, Zhu et al. relied on the commercial NLP software Linguamatics (IQVIA, Durham, NC). Their approach followed the standard NLP pipeline: social isolation seed terms were provided based on content area expertise and then expanded in the NLP software, with subsequent expert review. Once a final lexicon was developed, the algorithm was deployed on a training set and performance tested against a testing data set, both of which included the gold standard manual chart review annotations. Continual refinement occurred to maximize the accuracy of the algorithm. In total, 200,000 clinical notes for 4,000 patients were mined for social isolation. These notes came from multiple places in the EHR: progress notes, telephone encounters, plan of care documents, consults, history and physical notes, discharge summaries, and emergency department notes. The sensitivity of their algorithm was 97% and the positive predictive value was 90%, leading the authors to conclude that when social isolation information is documented in the EHR, NLP is a viable option for extraction.

Despite the success of these two studies, researchers should keep in mind that (1) these are single-center studies that (2) take resources to create the gold standard and expertise to implement NLP, and (3) the context or reasons for the social determinants will not be automatically parsed from the free text. Further, (4) the tuning of these algorithms must balance potential false positives and false negatives on a case-by-case basis, and (5) NLP applications are still largely in the exploratory and algorithmic development stages.

Quasi-experimental studies

Health services research using EHR data is a growing field (Myers & Stevens, 2016). When evaluating a policy, decision, or guideline in healthcare, it is quite common to conduct what are known as before-and-after or pre-and-post studies. In these types of studies an intervention or policy is introduced and the impact is quantified over time. For example, the intervention may be a new guideline for ordering diagnostic tests, a care improvement bundle delivered to patients, or changes in environmental cleaning products. These interventions are not deployed in a randomized fashion, due to practical or ethical reasons, but rather are delivered in what is known as a quasi-experimental manner. The goal is to demonstrate causality between an intervention and an outcome, similar to etiologic research, but without the randomization. There are a variety of quasi-experimental study designs and analytic strategies that fill their own textbooks. Here, we will focus on three common quasi-experimental analytic approaches applicable to EHR research: difference-in-difference, interrupted time series, and process control charts. Although presented separately, they can be used in tandem for robust analysis (see, for example, Gandrup et al., 2020).

Before proceeding to a presentation of relevant methods, let us first address the major weakness of nonrandomization in quasi-experimental studies. This weakness threatens internal validity. Researchers have described nine categories of concern for quasi-experimental studies based on the principles of observational epidemiology (Harris et al., 2006).

1 **Temporality**. It is not always clear whether the intervention was antecedent to the outcomes being measured.
2 **Selection**. The selection into the study may be related to the factors under study.
3 **History**. Confounding events that occur concurrently with the intervention may be responsible for any observed changes.
4 **Maturation**. Secular or temporal changes over time may lead to the effect.
5 **Regression**. When units are selected based on their extreme values, these values may have been due to chance and subsequent measurements may regress toward the mean.
6 **Attrition**. Loss to follow-up may be differential by the intervention and outcome under study.
7 **Testing**. Awareness of testing may lead to the change rather than the intervention.
8 **Instrumentation**. Measurement error may explain the observed effect.
9 **Interaction**. Another variable may be interacting with the intervention and resulting in the observed changes.

As these threats were previously discussed in Chapter 9 of this book, readers are referred there to review the concepts and approaches toward remediation.

As a motivational hypothetical study, suppose we are interested in measuring the occurrence of hospital-acquired infection and the impact of a policy in the intensive care unit of universal nonsterile gloving and gowning. The intervention was nonrandom, and we have longitudinal data from the EHR on infection rates for six months before-and-after the policy went into place. For simplicity, we will assume compliance was immediate and complete.

Interrupted time series

As the name implies, an interrupted time series (ITS) is comprised of two features. The first feature is the time-series nature of the data: that is, some outcome has been measured at multiple time points. The measurements are generally, but not always, taken at even, regular intervals and can take various forms such as counts, continuous data, or dichotomous data. The number of measurements drives the power of the study but there are no fixed limits regarding the number of data points. The second feature is that of an interruption, or intervention, that has occurred at a distinct point or period during the time series. The intervention should be one that can produce an effect quickly or within a well-defined lag period. In the hypothetical example, the time series is the one-year study of infection rates in the intensive care unit, and the interruption is the universal nonsterile gloving and gowning policy that went into effect at the mid-point during the time series. Conceptually, an ITS creates a hypothetical counterfactual control, whereby the control time series is extrapolated beyond the intervention. The deviation from this counterfactual serves as the measure of effect while accounting for the temporal trends. This analysis uses the methods of conventional regression techniques and is a preferred option for testing an intervention when no control exists (Bernal, Cummins & Gasparrini, 2019).

To conduct an ITS analysis, we *a priori* specify an impact model where we posit how and when the intervention will impact the outcome. This impact model may specify a change in the slope of the time-series curve, a change in the level or amount of the outcome post-intervention, or a combination of changes in the slope and level (Figure 12.5a–c, respectively). Descriptive analysis of the data follow. This analysis can include plots and visualizations of the time series, or summary statistics of the outcome for the overall time series as well as before-and-after the intervention.

Regression modeling follows descriptive analysis. At a minimum, an ITS model will include the dependent variable of the outcome and the independent variables corresponding to time, the intervention period (pre or post), and the interaction between time and the intervention period. The coefficient for the intervention period term indicates the change in level of the outcome post-intervention while the coefficient for the interaction term indicates the change in slope of the outcome post-intervention. More complicated models incorporating lag periods, nonlinear responses, control groups, autocorrelation, or time-varying confounding are possible (Bernal, Cummins & Gasparrini, 2017; Bernal, Cummins & Gasparrini, 2018).

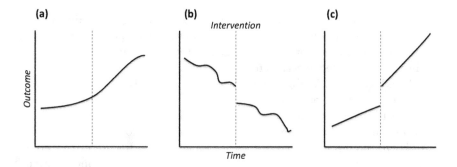

Figure 12.5(a–c). Impact models in an interrupted time series depicting a change in slope (a), a change in level (b), or a change in slope and level (c). Dashed line denotes intervention.

Autocorrelation and time-varying confounders deserve further comment. Since standard regression models assume the observations are independent of one another, this may be violated in time-series data as observations closer in time are more likely similar than observations further in time. Autocorrelation may be tested statistically via the Durbin–Watson test (Savin & White, 1977), and accounted for using autoregressive models or robust standard errors. In general, ITS models are robust to time-varying confounders when their impact is exerted on a temporal scale different than the observed time series. The net effect is that they will be balanced before-and-after the analysis but should still be included in the model. On the other hand, if time-varying confounders are posited to change rapidly, are unmeasured, or are unknown, a range of design adaptations can be used to control for these possible concurrent events (Bernal, Cummins & Gasparrini, 2017).

Suppose in our hypothetical that only the intensive care unit had enacted the universal nonsterile gloving and gowning, and another unit in the hospital, say the oncology service, had not. Now, instead of the time prior to intervention serving as the control comparison condition, we can use an entirely separate population for the pre- and post-intervention for the condition. In a controlled or comparative ITS, a control group, such as the oncology service, is selected, and the absence of an effect in the control group provides stronger evidence of the intervention. The selection of the control requires scrutiny, and there are many options, including selection based on location (as in our hypothetical), characteristics, behavior, history, or even simulation (synthetical controls). See Table 1 in Bernal, Cummins, and Gasparrini (2018) for a review of the strengths and weaknesses of these options.

ITS is frequently applied for EHR research. Gandrup et al. (2020) evaluated three rheumatoid arthritis interventions that were EHR-based. Each of these interventions had nonoverlapping starting points allowing the creation of three distinct biweekly time series. The researchers performed three statistical analyses of these data. First, they visualized the data using process control P charts (discussed later). Second, they conducted an ITS using linear regression model accounting for the autocorrelation present in the data. Third, they examined predictors of rheumatoid arthritis documentation in the EHR to identify independent characteristics associated with intervention success. The use of both control charts and ITS corroborated their findings while allowing for a quantitative investigation of the interventions' impacts. However, there was no control group in this study, and the authors acknowledge that temporal changes in documentation may have occurred unrelated to the intervention.

In Parikh et al. (2022), the authors used a commercial EHR-derived database to examine the impact of the COVID-19 pandemic on time to treatment initiation for patients newly diagnosed with a metastatic solid cancer. In contrast to Gandrup et al., Parikh et al. employed a controlled ITS approach using a historical control. The intervention time series measured changes in time to treatment initiation from early 2020 to mid-2020 with the pandemic being the "intervention," whereas the control time series was used to examine changes in time to treatment initiation from early 2019 to mid-2020. Aligning the months and days but changing the year had the intention of controlling for seasonal or secular trends that may impact the outcome aside from the pandemic. The primary ITS analysis was an interaction between year and the intervention period with an additional interaction with cancer type to explore possible effect modification. Given that the timing and impact of the pandemic on the outcome may be varying, the authors conducted a sensitivity analysis with an alternate intervention definition.

Difference-in-difference

Difference-in-difference (DID) is another quasi-experimental design for the evaluation of an intervention when a control group is available. We will continue with the hypothetical introduced in the robust ITS analysis where the intensive care unit received the intervention and the oncology service had not. An attractive feature of DID analyses is the less strict exchangeability criteria: we do not need to account for all known confounders, rather we assume that on average, the unobserved differences are the same over time. To make this more concrete, in our example, it is quite unlikely the intensive care unit and oncology unit have exchangeable patient populations and environmental characteristics, but if these unit-to-unit differences stay equivalent over the study period, the results will remain unbiased.

The data requirements for a DID analysis are fewer than an ITS. Whereas an ITS typically requires many data points measured before-and-after the intervention, a classic DID analysis requires only two measures: one before the intervention and one after the intervention. These measures may occur at different times for each observation (i.e., patient) in the intervention and control groups. The change in the pre- and post-periods are computed for the intervention group and the control group, then the difference between these differences is calculated based on the counterfactual in the control group (Figure 12.6). DID can be modeled via linear or logistic regression for continuous or binary outcomes,

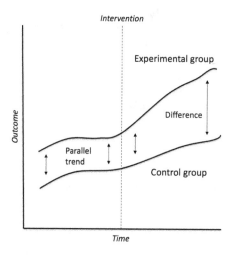

Figure 12.6 Difference-in-difference analysis.

respectively. At a minimum, independent predictors will include the study period (i.e., pre- or post-intervention), the study group (i.e., control or intervention), and an interaction term between intervention and group, which forms the DID effect estimate of inference.

The most important aspect when selecting the DID control group is known as the parallel trend assumption. This assumption states that had the intervention not occurred, the trends for both the intervention and control groups would mirror each other. While this is difficult – if not impossible – to confirm in practice, having more than just a single preintervention measure in each group can assure that this assumption is minimally satisfied. Other assumptions include exchangeability or covariate balance between groups, positivity in that everyone was theoretically eligible for the intervention, and stable group composition without interference between the groups.

There are examples in the literature of DID analyses using EHR data, although it appears to be used less frequently than ITS. Watson et al. (2021) conducted a secondary analysis of EHR data to examine the effect of an emergency department-based opioid use disorder intervention. In their analysis, the DID control group was not place-based but rather time-based, in that the intervention was compared against a time in the emergency department when someone from the intervention team was not on duty. The parallel trends assumption was tested visually and empirically by comparing four of the study outcomes between the intervention and control groups prior to the intervention date, with no systematic differences being observed. This study demonstrates not only a process to conduct DID using EHR data, but also the different types of control groups possible.

ITS versus DID

ITS and DID are similar analytical options for naturally occurring or nonrandomized experiments to evaluate the impact of an intervention when a control or comparison group is available. Generally, DID requires fewer data points than ITS in that only one before and one after measure are required. On the other hand, ITS requires time-series data with multiple measures before and after. Some have argued that given the choice between the two methods, ITS is the preferred methodology based on its ability to mitigate confounding (Bernal, Cummins & Gasparrini, 2019), although there are various extensions to DID to address its shortcomings such as the strict parallel trend assumption (Abadie, 2005; Lechner, 2011). As with many statistical choices, it may not be a question of whether one method is superior to another, but rather investigator familiarity with the alternatives. Users of SAS statistical software (SAS Institute, Cary, NC) can consult this reference for detailed examples of both techniques (Warton, 2020).

Process control charts

We may alternatively view the hypothetical study as one of a continual process improvement program to reduce hospital-acquired infections. Viewed under this paradigm, the research question deals with whether the observed variation in

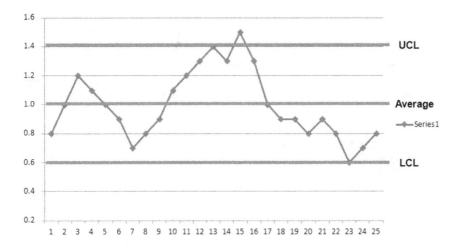

Figure 12.7 A process control chart. UCL, upper confidence limit; LCL, lower confidence limit.

infections is random or due to the intervention. Quality improvement methods fall under two general categories: visualization of the data and analysis of the data. The first step is to visualize the data for a qualitative examination of trends and changes in variability over time. One of the easiest visualizations to create is the simple run chart (Figure 12.7). In this type of chart, the *x*-axis corresponds to time, and the *y*-axis represents the outcome under study. The data need to be organized as time-series data, that is, measures of the outcome per unit time. The data will dictate the unit of time. The unit of time can be manipulated to examine trends by week, month, quarter, or year, and while this can make trends easier to visualize, it also results in a loss of data.

Process control charts, of which there are many types,[7] allow the researcher to differentiate random variability from nonrandom variability. This is also known as the signal or the result of the intervention. There are several techniques to detect nonrandom variability and establish whether an intervention impacted the outcome. These techniques are often based on an individual or series of time points occurring outside of a certain threshold, such as the 3-sigma limit, akin to exceeding the confidence interval bounds. Visualizing a run chart of the data will allow an overall sense of the trends. The run chart includes the median of the data and can be partitioned by pre and post-intervention periods. Using the so-called "Western Electric" rules, a run of 8 points above or below the median indicates an intervention effect. In Figure 12.7, at time point 15 we see a value outside the upper confidence limit, known as special cause variation. Also in this figure, from time points 18–25 we see a "run of 8" below the average. If the intervention happened prior to this, we may infer the intervention resulted in this reduction. If a trend is observed in the run chart, then the analyst can employ specific control charts based on assumptions about the data including its distribution and mean.

For those interested in *p*-values to supplement the analysis, there are a few different ways to generate these. A *p*-value for the overall intervention effect can be calculated through a nonparametric test, such as the rank-sum test, comparing the distribution of values before-and-after the intervention. A p-value for the overall trend of the data can be calculated as a test for trend, using a linear regression predicting count by time. This can further be stratified by the intervention. Depending on the data, the researcher needs to guard against violating assumptions that are not inherent in process control charts, such as nonindependence of observations. Readers interested in a more thorough treatment of quality and process improvement methodology may wish to consult Carey and Lloyd (2001) or Brownson, Colditz, and Proctor (2017).

As an example of a quality improvement program evaluated using EHR data, Paul et al. (2019) studied the effect of a bundled care intervention to reduce the risk of sudden unexpected postnatal collapse following hospital-based deliveries. The researchers mined the EHR for records of live births and sudden unexpected postnatal collapse between January 2014 and July 2017 (n = 23,107 births). The intervention was fully deployed on June 1, 2015 (n = 9,143 preintervention and 13,964 post-intervention). They created a process control G chart to evaluate the number of live births between events and noted special cause variation was reached post-intervention. There was no comparison or control series as this was a hospital-wide initiative. Thus, provided there were no temporal or cyclical forces at play outside of the intervention, the authors viewed the intervention as the most likely cause for the reduction.

Clinical trials and the EHR

Traditionally falling under the purview of clinical trials, EHRs can contribute to our understanding of disease risk factors, etiology, treatments, and interventions. The overlap between clinical trials and the EHR may occur in several ways: pragmatic clinical trials, the EHR as a data source in clinical trials, and emulating clinical trials from the EHR. Each of these are reviewed in turn.

Pragmatic clinical trials

Clinical trials may be embedded within the healthcare setting, indeed within the EHR, to study disease etiology, treatments, and interventions, minimizing the need for a complex clinical trial infrastructure with multifaceted (and unrepresentative) inclusion and exclusion criteria. This framework is known as the *pragmatic clinical trial* (Weinfurt, 2021). With the overarching goal of improving health and healthcare in the clinical setting, it is important to draw a distinction between the traditional randomized clinical trial, the pragmatic clinical trial that may also be randomized, and a quasi-experimental study of an intervention, such as a quality improvement project (quasi-experimental study designs are discussed elsewhere in this chapter). In some sense, the pragmatic trial is a hybrid of the two in that it seeks to not only create generalizable knowledge but also to improve care at a given institution and inform care and policy decisions (Weinfurt, 2021). As contrasted to a traditional randomized clinical trial that operates under ideal and often unrealistic conditions, the pragmatic trial operates within the existing healthcare setting. As such, the results are more likely to have external validity. Another distinguishing characteristic is the nature of the intervention itself. In a traditional randomized clinical trial, an intervention is compared to a placebo or other nonintervention control condition. In a pragmatic trial, the comparative effectiveness of real-world alternatives is studied, and adherence is not as rigorously enforced. Nevertheless, adherence is important to consider in the analysis, and emerging methods are becoming available to deal with issues of nonadherence or partial adherence in pragmatic trials (Ehsan et al., 2021). With this overview of pragmatic clinical trials, let us turn to the use of EHR data in these trials, followed by a real-world example.

In contrast to a traditional randomized clinical trial, where data are collected *de novo* and for the explicit purpose of the trial, a pragmatic trial utilizes existing data sources, namely, the EHR. As such the limitations of EHR data and observational inference, as identified in Chapters 6 and 9, still apply. Further, the pragmatic clinical trial research question needs to be answerable using the EHR, as discussed in Chapter 3. Richesson et al. (2021) identified how the EHR supports four major activities in pragmatic trials. First, the EHR can be used to identify the study population for the trial, estimate numerators and denominators, and target recruitment efforts. Second, the EHR serves as the baseline measure of phenotypes and prognostic characteristics – both objective and subjective – for the trial cohort. Third, the EHR may be used to implement and monitor the studied intervention, such as enhancing decision support or modifications to order entry flowsheets. Fourth, the EHR serves as the study endpoint measure of outcomes for longitudinal cohorts. This is especially important for longitudinal outcomes not captured in the present EHR but required through data linkage.

Gianfrancesco et al. (2019) studied whether an EHR intervention could guard against hydroxychloroquine toxicity. To ensure that patients did not receive higher than the recommended dosages, the authors conducted a pragmatic trial to assess the utility of modifying the hydroxychloroquine prescribing user interface to automatically calculate weight-based dosing. If a weight was not previously recorded, a value was forced to be entered. As described, this trial supports the third pragmatic trial activity enumerated by Richesson et al. (2021): enhancing decision support or modifications to order entry flowsheets. The trial was embedded within the healthcare system's EHR using the standard of care as the comparator condition, and 24 rheumatology providers were randomized evenly to receive the intervention or not receive the intervention. No difference in the proportion of prescribed dosages exceeding an *a priori* threshold was detected between the groups during an approximate two-year follow-up, suggesting that the prescribing interface may need further refinement to reduce the patient dosage. This in fact is one of the features of the pragmatic trial: to iteratively refine processes and test for resulting differences.

EHRs as a supplemental data source

The preceding section implied the use of EHR data in pragmatic clinical trials; the EHR can serve as a supplemental data source for any type of clinical trial or prospective study. In addition to pragmatic trials, there are other applications of EHR data for prospective clinical research (Cowie et al., 2017). The first is assessing the practicality of conducting a clinical trial in a specific health system, to ensure there are sufficient trial participants or relevant health conditions. If feasibility is established, EHRs can be used as a source of patient-participant identification and recruitment. A second application is the use of EHR data to supplement data collection in the clinical trial itself. As opposed to instruments developed specifically for data collection in the clinical trial, existing data in the EHR – demographics, morbidities, medications – can be mined or linked (known as tokenization[8]) for re-use in the clinical trial. This has the added feature of being objectively collected by a clinician in a manner unlikely to be biased by the trial itself. This brings into bearing the accuracy and completeness of data in the EHR (see Chapter 6), thus having a second data stream through a prospective study can also serve as the validation of data in the EHR. Relatedly, researchers can create *ambidirectional cohorts* that use retrospective data from EHRs but then prospectively recruit. Another application is the use of EHR data to monitor side effects, adverse events, and endpoints in an interventional trial. Again, this depends on the completeness of the data given the catchment of an EHR as well as the idea of informed presence bias, where a symptom or health state may be documented more often for individuals who more frequently engage in healthcare. Also, when data are needed in near-real time to monitor adverse events, there may be time delays in accessing EHR data, from delays in data entry to delays in data abstraction.

Specific to patient selection and recruitment, the EHR can serve as a high-volume screening tool for evaluating trial eligibility, especially to oversample patients who are historically not included in clinical trials. Using the EHR data in this manner raises several issues that need to be addressed at the outset. First, as was discussed in Chapter 6, entry into an EHR is not random, and this catchment process may limit the external validity of the trial results. Second, the privacy and confidentiality of patients must be protected, with ample security safeguards in place (Cowie et al., 2017). Third, the completeness of data for evaluating patient eligibility may be suboptimal. Köpcke et al. (2013) evaluated eligibility criteria from three clinical trials compared to EHR documentation from five hospitals. They found on average 55% of the eligibility criteria had discrete elements in the EHR, but only 35% of all records had sufficient data captured to be of use for patient recruitment. Across seven categories of trial eligibility criteria, the completeness of the data was: health status, 46%; diagnostic or lab tests, 20%; treatment or care, 25%; ethical considerations, 6%; demographics, 77%; lifestyle, 67%. These percentages suggest that exclusively relying on discrete EHR data is problematic, and further, there may be systematic differences between those who have more complete data and those who do not. Unfortunately, these differences may relate to loss to follow-up or treatment adherence. Rather than relying on often incomplete discrete elements, patient selection and recruitment may be improved using unstructured EHR data. Kirshner et al. (2021) employed machine learning to identify metastatic disease among cancer patients. In their real-world testing dataset, the positive predictive value of having the metastatic disease when the algorithm flagged a patient was 92% (95% confidence interval: 78%, 98%), and the negative predictive value was 99% (95% confidence interval: 97%, 100%).

Emulating clinical trials

One of the hallmarks of a randomized controlled trial is the ability to balance participant characteristics across treatment groups through randomization. This is known as exchangeability and helps to guard against possible confounding induced by an unequal distribution of covariates that may occur if participants selected into the treatment groups naturally. As discussed in Chapter 9, this lack of exchangeability is a key limiting factor in ascribing causality in observational studies. As such, it would be ideal if an observational study from the EHR could be analyzed as a clinical trial. This has come to be known as the *target trial* approach for analyzing observational studies for nonexperimental interventions or exposures. By framing the study design and analysis of observational data as if it were a randomized controlled trial – that is, the target trial – the observational analysis should yield the same effect estimates had the target trial been conducted (Hernán & Robins, 2016). This can be done for replicating existing clinical trials using observational data (for example, to improve external validity), or for observational studies of an intervention that is unable to be conducted experimentally but will be analyzed as such. Incremental errors can accrue based on researcher decisions made when undertaking an observational EHR study, inducing selection bias, information bias, and residual confounding, that otherwise are potentially avoidable in a randomized controlled trial setting (Rassen, Murk & Schneeweiss, 2021).

To explicate, Hernán and Robins (2016) presented seven features of a clinical trial protocol and demonstrated how they can be represented in an observational study.

- **Eligibility criteria**. The observational study should be enrolled using the same (actual or hypothetical) eligibility criteria used in the target trial. These restrictions are imposed with only the knowledge of the baseline or historical characteristics of the participants, as occurs in the prospective recruitment of a trial. See Köpcke et al. (2013) for a demonstration of evaluating eligibility criteria in an EHR.
- **Treatment strategies**. Under a traditional randomized clinical trial, the intervention is carefully monitored and scrutinized per the original protocol. An observational study equivalent is the pragmatic trial, discussed earlier, in which the standard of care or usual conditions serve as the comparison group. Patients who have met the eligibility criteria will be "assigned" to their treatment strategies based on the available data indicating whether they had the treatment or not.
- **Assignment procedures**. Under a traditional randomized clinical trial, the intervention would be randomized to achieve the exchangeability of the

treatment groups. In observational data, we do not expect this to be the case, therefore we handle confounding either in the study design or analysis phase. The target trial may use matching or restriction to account for confounding in the design stage, or stratification, adjustment, or other advanced techniques in the analysis stage. This implies that all confounders must be available in the EHR, whether discrete and measured, or abstractable via NLP. Inclusion of a negative control, or a condition hypothesized to be unaffected by the treatment, may help detect unmeasured confounding.

- **Follow-up period**. Follow-up time should begin commensurate with the treatment assignment or within a grace period afforded in the protocol, but not after. In observational studies, this likely is when an individual initiates treatment or has no treatment, but this is not straightforward to determine. If eligibility criteria are met at a single point in time, this can serve as the start of follow-up time, but if eligibility criteria are repeatedly met, then a series of nested trials may be necessary for analysis (Hernán et al., 2008).
- **Outcome**. The outcome must be clearly defined and available in the EHR. In the target trial framework, assessment of the outcome is likely not blinded to the treatment. Thus, either the target trial must not use a blinded design, or the outcome itself will need to be independently validated.
- **Causal contrasts**. The most common analytic strategies in the randomized clinical trial are the intent-to-treat analysis, which analyzes participants by their assigned treatments, and the per-protocol and as-treated analyses, which analyzes the participants by their received treatments (Smith, Coffman & Hudgens, 2021). All three are possible in the target trial framework depending on whether the comparison groups are formed at baseline (or the first measure of treatment) or incorporating treatment adherence throughout the entire study period.
- **Analysis plan**. The intent-to-treat analysis is severely hampered in the target trial approach unless complete control of confounding is possible at baseline, while also assuming no selection or information bias. Rather, the per-protocol analysis is typically employed using the so-called g-methods.

Regardless of whether the target trial approach is used, for EHR researchers evaluating an intervention or exposure a worthwhile exercise is to ruminate on the analogous clinical trial protocol. This mental exercise can help identify concerns with meeting these seven criteria in practice.

As an example of the target trial approach in EHR research, Katsoulis et al. (2021) evaluated how weight change, which could not be randomized in practice, affected the occurrence of cardiovascular diseases. Following the approach of Hernán and Robins (2016), the authors specified the hypothetical target trial using the seven features enumerated earlier and how this could be emulated from the EHR (provided in Table 1 in Katsoulis et al. 2021). Their analysis was per-protocol, using inverse probability weighting to account for time-fixed and time-dependent confounders that were related to adherence, and used positive and negative controls to detect possible residual confounding. Another example of target trials in EHR research may be found in Danaei et al. (2013), where the authors estimated the effect of statin therapy on the risk of coronary heart disease. As is standard practice in the target trial framework, the authors first specified what the hypothetical randomized clinical trial would entail, then specified how the EHR data may be used to emulate this trial. Danaei et al. (2013) used the sequence of nested trials approach and contrasted an intention-to-treat analysis, a per-protocol analysis, and an as-treated analysis. Inverse probability weighting was used for time-varying selection bias due to nonadherence censoring in the per-protocol analysis and time-varying confounding of adherence in the as-treated analysis.

Spatial analysis

Spatial analysis of EHR data seeks to examine how place – whether inside or outside of the healthcare setting – explains, influences, or modifies an observed health phenomenon. For example, one may ask whether community characteristics, such as poverty, or whether hospital characteristics, such as patients' rooms, influence the diagnosis of a disease. These types of analyses typically incorporate both intrinsic and extrinsic factors. By intrinsic, we mean characteristics of the patients themselves, and by extrinsic, we mean factors outside of the patient. Framing in this manner not only motivates spatial analysis as an extrinsic factor, but also the use of multilevel models, network analysis models, and ecological models. One common approach to extrinsic analysis is linking patients' addresses with community data to assess how location impacts health (Goldstein et al., 2021). The idea of geocoding and linking to census data was covered in Chapter 5 and the limitations of EHR address data were covered in Chapter 6. Herein we are concerned with the mechanics of spatial analysis.

Several applied examples can help motivate spatial analysis of EHR data and distinguish between analyses within the walls of the hospital versus analysis of where patients live. Goldstein et al. (2018) examined how infectious outcomes may correlate with features of a neonatal intensive care unit using inpatient EHR data. They found that outcomes were not distributed randomly but aligned with the NICU design, which may be useful for infection prevention and environmental sanitation. Goldstein et al. (2021) linked outpatient EHR data to census data at the ZIP code level to demonstrate that community risk factors drive the diagnosis of hepatitis C. Furthermore, they demonstrated how selection bias might arise in studies that use EHR data when inferring results to the local community. Murray et al. (2017) used inpatient EHR data to cluster patients by hospital ward, procedural, and diagnostic areas in the hospital to evaluate how space and transfer patterns over time influenced the risk for *Clostridioides difficile* infection. This study resulted in the implementation of improved cleaning practices. Hirsch et al. (2017) demonstrated how unconventional EHR data – in this case audit data – can be used to map patient locations and time spent with providers during outpatient encounters.

The big picture question that one grapples with in spatial epidemiology is whether the observed distribution of an outcome, in our case a health state in the EHR, is random over space – geography in a traditional spatial analysis – or if there is an underlying spatial process that explains the patterning. The null hypothesis is that the health state is unrelated to geography and is random, and the alternative hypothesis, is that the health state depends upon geography and is not random. This nonrandomness is termed spatial dependence or spatial autocorrelation; these terms are used interchangeably. If spatial autocorrelation is positive, an outcome in one area, say high rates of an infectious disease, will result in higher rates in neighboring areas (see, for example, Goldstein et al., 2018). If the autocorrelation is negative, high rates of infection in one area will result in lower rates of infection in neighboring areas: visualize a chessboard, where white squares may mean high rates and black squares may mean low rates. If spatial dependence is present and we are conducting an etiologic analysis, we next need to understand how the exposure to outcome relationship is influenced by the spatial effects.

To prepare spatial data for analysis, we first need a geographic representation of the area of interest in a computer-readable format, most commonly a *shapefile*. Shapefiles define the boundaries of geographical units. Geopolitical and administrative boundaries, such as congressional districts, census tracts, ZIP codes, or counties, are downloadable through the U.S. Census Bureau.[9] Geographical boundaries in arbitrary areas, such as the inside of a hospital or ward, may need to be created *de novo*.[10] EHR data may be merged with the geographic data to create a geographic health dataset: this can be on the basis of the patients' addresses, patients' rooms in the hospital,[11] or other spatially defining features. Next, we need two additional objects for spatial modeling purposes. The first is a mapping that defines "neighbors," which could be based on contiguity, where a given polygon shares a border with another, based on distance, for polygons within a given distance, or based on a user-supplied definition, for example, if we were mapping an intensive care unit and wanted to define patient to patient transmission of infectious disease as a result of healthcare workers who may have arbitrary patient assignments (Figure 12.8). The second object needed is a weighting scheme based on the neighbor definitions, which defines how much influence a given neighbor should have in the analysis. As with the algorithm that defines neighbors, the algorithm that defines weight has several approaches. For example, row standardization stipulates that each neighbor is weighted by the number of total neighbors. The choice of weighting approach to use is dictated by theory and the research question. One may also take a pragmatic approach and choose an approach that describes the data the best through, for example, the lowest measure of an information criterion.

Following the preparation of the spatial dataset, we can now assess spatial dependence to test the hypothesis of spatial randomness of the health outcome. Exploratory analysis, using a choropleth or gradient map, can provide a qualitative assessment of patterning (Figure 12.9). Quantitative assessment can mathematically quantify the autocorrelation and test the hypothesis of spatial dependence.

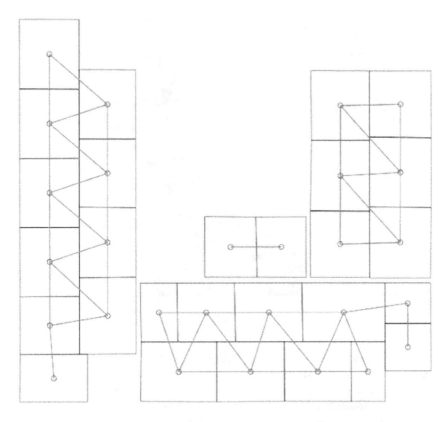

Figure 12.8 A definition of neighboring beds within a hypothetical intensive care unit based on nursing assignments.

There are several techniques for diagnosing spatial autocorrelation depending on the data type (areas versus points), cluster type (global or local), or other considerations. By far the most common approach is using *Moran's I* statistic. Under its original incarnation, Moran's I is a global test of area autocorrelation, but has also been adapted to local measures of autocorrelation. The difference between global and local measures of autocorrelation is whether the clusters are identifiable. In a global test, we assess whether any spatial dependence exists in the data, but we are unable to pinpoint, at least through the test, where the spatial dependency exists. To pinpoint the location(s) of spatial dependence, a local statistic, such as *Moran's local I*, can identify and map the exact areas where spatial autocorrelation is found. Interestingly, is possible to have local spatial autocorrelation without global spatial autocorrelation, so both statistics may be used in complement. A Moran's I value greater than zero suggests positive spatial autocorrelation, a value less than zero suggests negative spatial autocorrelation, and a value equal to zero suggests no spatial autocorrelation. One can compute or bootstrap confidence intervals around Moran's I to see if the statistic meaningfully differs from zero; depending on the statistical

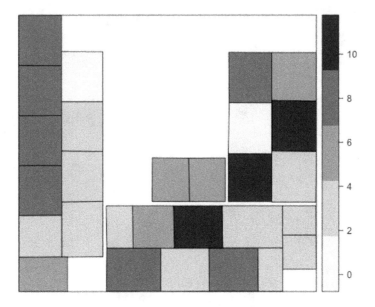

Figure 12.9 Choropleth map of a health outcome in a hypothetical intensive care unit.

software, a p-value may also be provided during the Moran's I test. Another popular test for autocorrelation is the spatial scan statistic, which is flexible to global and local tests for areas or point data and can incorporate time dependence as well (i.e., spatiotemporal autocorrelation). The freely available SaTScan software (https://www. satscan.org) can compute this measure in an intuitive, easy-to-use interface.

Modeling considerations

If there is spatial dependence in the data, a typical ordinary least squares regression model may be biased since the observations and error terms are not independent. As a starting point, we can fit this typical regression model to demonstrate whether failure to account for spatial dependence has led to biased inference by using one of the tests for spatial dependence on the residuals of the regression model. If spatial dependence is present, then a spatial regression model may be warranted, or otherwise inclusion of the variables leading to the spatial autocorrelation if those data are available. Below we will consider the more common and straightforward approaches to considering spatial dependence in the epidemiological analysis of observational data.

The simplest and most frequently used spatial regression models fall into a category called *simultaneous autoregression models*. These models are considered global in nature as the estimates apply to any location. These can also be thought of as marginal models in that the effect estimates are global, averaged across all geographies in the analysis. Starting with a typical regression model, every component of this original model may be subject to spatial autocorrelation: the independent variable(s) (denoted X), the dependent variable (denoted Y), and the error term. The spatial regression model approaches below account for the autocorrelation that may be present in various combinations across these terms.

In a *spatial error model* the error term contains the spatial effect: Y is dependent on X and an uncaptured effect (error) of the neighbors. The spatial component is measured through a parameter dubbed *lambda*: it can be viewed as nuisance parameter capturing error. The spatial error model is the most straightforward model and can be interpreted as a typical regression model.

In a *spatial lag model* or *spatially lagged Y model*, Y is dependent on X and neighboring Y. That is, there is a spillover effect present. If, for example, our Y variable corresponds to an infectious disease, a spillover suggests that higher rates of an infection in each area may be partially the result of higher rates of infection in neighboring areas. This should make intuitive sense as often geographical areas are created based on arbitrary definitions. The spatial component is captured in the parameter *rho*: the average clustering effect. Rho is not directly interpretable, but its significance will suggest whether a spatial lag effect is statistically meaningful.

Another type of spatial lag model is the *spatially lagged X model*. This model is similar to the spatially lagged Y model, the difference being Y is dependent on X and neighboring X instead of the neighboring Y. As an example of this, suppose X was vaccination. Vaccination rates will be similar in surrounding areas due to homophily, thus a spatially lagged X model may be warranted. The spatial component in the spatially lagged X model is dubbed *theta*: the average clustering effect. As with rho, theta is not directly interpretable, but its significance will suggest whether a spatial lag effect is statistically meaningful.

Finally, one may consider a model with both X and Y lags: where Y is dependent on our X, and neighboring X and Y. This is known as a *spatial Durbin model* or *lagged-mixed model*. The parameters of spatial autocorrelation are as defined in the spatial lag models for X and Y. To continue the previous example, suppose X was vaccination and Y was cases of infectious disease. One can reasonably posit that both X and Y will have spatial dependency: vaccination rates due to homophily and infection due to contagion. In this case, a Durbin model is an appropriate option. There are many permutations of spatial regression models to consider in special circumstances.[12] To help guide the decision in model choice among the many spatial models, *Lagrange multiplier tests* may be used.

Complicating inference from models with spatial lags, the parameter estimates cannot be directly interpreted. Rather effects need to be decomposed into total, direct, and indirect effects. The direct effect describes how Y is impacted in the local area, the indirect effect describes how Y is impacted from a neighboring area, and the total effect is the sum of the two. A spillover is present when outcome or covariate levels for a given geography affect the outcome for a neighboring geography, and the effects in the local and neighboring geography (direct and indirect effects) are in the same direction.

Simultaneous autoregression models are dubbed global models because they produce estimates that assume homogeneity throughout the data. That is, the estimates are marginal and apply the same to all areas under study. This is an overly restrictive assumption, and we can expect that the exposure to outcome relationship will differ by geography. Therefore, a technique known as *geographically weighted regression* (GWR) has been developed to attempt to understand the local phenomenon, or how a place may modify the relationship under study. In essence, GWR analysis creates a separate regression analysis for each geographical area in the data. As such, the output includes regression estimates and measures of precision for each geography. However, this complicates interpretation and is also sensitive to modeling assumptions. Thus, GWR should be viewed as an exploratory tool rather than confirming or disproving hypotheses and employed alongside other spatial regression approaches.

Conducting a GWR analysis is relatively straightforward. The most important part of the GWR analysis is the *kernel*. Heuristically, the kernel is the subset of data defined by neighbors and is a function of bandwidth (neighbors) and a weighting function (influence of the neighbors). It can be constant across the data – a fixed kernel – or can change over space – an adaptive kernel. First, one calibrates to determine the bandwidth size based on a typical regression model and weighting function. Second, the GWR model is estimated. As mentioned, the output from this estimation is per geography, analogous to a regression model for each geographical unit in the data. This indicates how the exposure to outcome relationship varies by geography. Third and finally, the results are mapped. There are a variety of options for mapping including plotting the slopes of each predictor and how they vary over space, or plotting the statistical significance of slopes (e.g., local t values). Diagnostic plots are also useful to assess spatial dependency post-modeling, for example, by plotting residuals on map. An informative discussion of mapping options is presented in Mennis (2006). Tabb et al. (2018) present an applied example comparing methods and inference for spatial analyses of public health data.

Bayesian analysis

Thus far, this book has presented statistics from the *frequentist* perspective. Under this paradigm, the data are collected from a given EHR and analyzed in isolation, often with some sort of a null hypothesis significance test, such as a *t*-test or regression. Inferences are made from these data, and these data alone. A *Bayesian* approach to statistical analysis would incorporate prior knowledge from other EHRs, studies, or expert opinions, to yield richer and more informative inferences. If data sharing and linkage were a nonissue, the ideal EHR study would be one that incorporates data from all EHRs, or at least a random sample from all EHRs, thereby incorporating different populations, places, and times. While this is not possible in real-world studies, it is possible conceptually and statistically using the Bayesian framework. An analogy for this would be a frequentist analysis represents a single EHR whereas a Bayesian analysis represents many and different EHRs, indeed the sum of all EHRs. Such an analytic perspective is more likely to capture and account for the substantial heterogeneities present in any single EHR while also incorporating the accumulation of knowledge gained from previous EHR research.

The crux of Bayesian analysis is the reallocation of probability. Consider a hypothetical retrospective EHR study assessing the incidence of *Clostridoides difficile* infection among inpatients. Based on the literature, other studies, or expert opinion we may expect the incidence to be 7% among hospitalized patients. Suppose we perform a study in our hospital and find a 3% infection rate. How do we reconcile this difference? A Bayesian might re-allocate the probability to 5% after considering prior evidence alongside our current study. This is known as the *posterior* probability or credibility, using Bayesian terminology. In this example, these statistics are being treated as known and measured with certainty, but in the Bayesian world, there are probabilities associated with these probabilities, specified in the form of statistical distributions. These distributions allow us to control the level of certainty represented by the probabilities. A Bayesian analysis starts with a prior distribution, incorporates the current data, and arrives as a posterior distribution. As new evidence and data accumulate, the Bayesian process is cyclical with continually refined posterior distributions.

A real-world clinical example of this is the positive (and negative) predictive values of diagnostic tests. When a patient receives a positive test result, what is the probability that the patient has the condition based on the test, and likewise when a patient receives a negative test result, what is the probability that the patient does not have the condition? This is a function of the accuracy of the test itself as well as the prevalence of the condition in the tested population; the predictive value is the reallocation of the prevalence given the data (i.e., test result). Bayesian analysis is a complex topic and readers are referred to these texts for further details (Kruschke, 2014; Moyé, 2016).

Bayesian analysis in healthcare research is rare compared to the near-ubiquitous frequentist paradigm, although given its capacity to address the multitude of biases inherent in EHR data (see Chapter 6), it is an appealing option (Fox, MacLehose & Lash, 2021). As an applied example of Bayesian analysis, we will adapt the work of Ashby, Hutton and McGee (1993) to an EHR-based study. Suppose we are interested in studying incident leukemia following treatment of Hodgkin's lymphoma, where chemotherapy versus radiotherapy is the risk factor of interest. Our source population for this study is a community hospital's oncology EHR. These data can be used to form a case–control study among patients treated for Hodgkin's lymphoma where cases are diagnosed with leukemias and controls are other incident cancers. The outcome – case versus control – as well as the type of therapy are available and abstracted from the EHR (Table 1 in Ashby, Hutton, and McGee, 1993). A frequentist paradigm would simply calculate the odds of chemotherapy among cases and the odds of chemotherapy among controls, and then compare the two via the odds ratio. Doing so using Table 1 from Ashby, Hutton, and McGee yields an odds ratio of 9.0 (95% confidence interval: 4.2, 19.2). Importantly, this analysis does not incorporate any evidence from earlier work.

Now suppose a colleague notifies us that there was another EHR study examining the same research question. A Bayesian analysis allows us to incorporate this prior work into our current study. To do so we first need to encapsulate the prior knowledge – the odds ratio from the other study – into a statistical distribution.

If there were truly no prior knowledge available, our prior distribution would not favor any particular odds ratio. If, on the other hand, we have some *a priori* knowledge, we can operationalize this knowledge into the prior distribution. The cohort study in Ashby, Hutton, and McGee can serve as this starting point. Depending on how similar the cohort study is to our study, in terms of research question, variable measurement, and patient population, we can vary the influence of this prior knowledge on the current analysis. Once the prior is defined, the probability is re-allocated using data from the present case–control analysis, and we might find a posterior distribution with a median odds ratio of 8.5 and 95% credible interval[13] of 4.9, 15.0 (Table 3 from Ashby, Hutton, and McGee 1993). Compared to the frequentists analysis from earlier, two things are notable: first, the point estimate is somewhat attenuated, and second, there is less uncertainty denoted by the smaller interval, demonstrating Bayesian learning. This process can be continued *ad infinitum* incorporating other EHR studies along the way.

Qualitative analysis

The focus of the EHR research in this book has been quantitative. As researchers, we sought to describe, measure, quantify, and analyze discrete (or discretized) data in the EHR. However, given the abundance of nondiscrete free text in medical records (discussed in Chapters 2 and 4), we may wish to employ methods that can abstract meaning from these data, aside from creating discrete measures through free text processing. Qualitative analysis of EHR data is uncommon in the biomedical literature; more common is its use to understand the process and procedures of implementing or using an EHR. In practice, qualitative analysis of secondary EHR data is akin to qualitative analysis of *any* secondary data, which has received attention in the literature (Ruggiano & Perry, 2019). Instead of traditional transcripts of interviews or focus groups, the transcript becomes the narrative recorded in the EHR's clinical notes. A typical qualitative analysis of these data would proceed from raw notes to codes to themes as follows. One would review the clinical note several times, bracketing text of importance. Each bracketed text is assigned a short label known as its *code*. Codes are expected to be re-used from note to note. *Themes* are then drawn from the codes into larger concepts that capture the key findings; quotes are often used to exemplify findings.

Despite qualitative analysis of EHR data being uncommon, there are several studies that have retrospectively examined encounter notes. At an HIV antiretroviral treatment referral program, pharmacists' notes taken during semi-structured interviews with patients were retrospectively analyzed to identify barriers and facilitators of successful treatment (Krummenacher et al., 2014). Also in the HIV medicine area, counseling notes have been qualitatively assessed at a preexposure prophylaxis demonstration site to understand how participants used this medicine and its impact on sexual preferences (Carlo Hojilla et al., 2016). Within the U.S. Department of Veterans Affairs, researchers have qualitatively analyzed "life-sustaining treatments" notes for patients with advanced kidney disease to understand the clinical utility of such notes (Wong, 2022). These studies can serve as prototypical examples for researchers engaging in this type of work.

Researchers should be aware of several controversies with secondary analysis of qualitative data (Ruggiano & Perry, 2019). First, the context of the data collection has been removed when examining clinical notes *post hoc*. That is, the clinician had a specific motivation and intention when documenting and this spirit may be unknown to the researcher, especially if the researcher is not a clinician or otherwise fluent in clinical documentation. As such, this could impact the rigor of the analysis. The three studies mentioned earlier (Carlo Hojilla et al., 2016; Krummenacher et al., 2014; Wong, 2022) involved the local organization and personnel who gathered the original data, minimizing the opportunity for misinterpretation of the notes. Second, informed consent, confidentiality, and anonymity may be compromised with secondary qualitative data. This is especially important given that the frequency of free text in sensitive clinical areas, such as behavioral and mental health. Furthermore, these types of data were never created by the researcher; rather they were created for clinical note-taking with an implicit understanding of privacy. In short, the ethics of qualitative analysis of EHR data should be vetted with the local institutional review board.

Related to the idea of qualitative analysis of encounter notes is the use of bibliometric techniques of encounter notes. *Bibliometrics* is an approach to extract, manipulate, and measure written material, most commonly article citations (Donthu et al., 2021). In its traditional use, bibliometrics may be used to identify patterns and trends in citations, such as by geography, institution, or article performance, to summarize the state of a topic or field.[14] Content analysis is one type of bibliometric technique that can be applied to qualitative EHR data if we view the encounter note as the "text" and the metadata of that note (i.e., recording clinician, date and time, clinical practice, type of note and theme) as the "citation" accompanying the text. By extrapolating bibliometrics to EHR encounter notes citations, these techniques can be used – in an unconventional manner – on assessing relationships between notes, themes of the notes, and temporality of documentation, and their association with patient or provider-level characteristics.

Phenome-wide association studies

The concept of a clinical phenotype, or health state of a patient, was covered in Chapters 2 and 6 of the book (Richesson et al., 2013; Wei & Denny, 2015). A related concept is that of a phenome, or a collection of phenotypes. Phenome-wide association studies (PheWAS) are concerned with identifying how genotypes, or genetic markers frequently defined by single nucleotide polymorphisms, may be correlated with clinical phenotypes. Such studies leverage EHR data – most often International Classification of Diseases codes but could include other clinical data to define the clinical phenotype – as the source population. To do this, genotype data must be available and linkable at the patient level in the EHR. The main goal of a PheWAS is to replicate known gene-disease relationships in the EHR and to search for hidden and unanticipated associations. These studies are similar to genome-wide association studies, which may also use EHR data, except the directionality is reversed: whereas a genome-wide study examines novel genomic associations given a clinical phenotype, a PheWAS examines novel phenotype associations given a genotype.

Denny et al. (2010) described the methodology to conduct a PheWAS in the EHR and provided several didactic examples. Their examples pulled data from a DNA biobank linked to a de-identified EHR at Vanderbilt University, providing genotype and phenotype information for approximately 6,000 study participants. Genotyping was performed for five single nucleotide polymorphisms with previously known disease associations encompassing cardiovascular and autoimmune disease. Phenotyping was performed using International Classification of Diseases codes collapsed into categories by common etiologies. The phenotypes were constructed for all codes deemed useful in a genetic context: in total over 200,000 codes were collapsed into 900 code categories. For each genotype, correlations were examined with the phenotype code categories. For example, for the genotype "rs3135388," which has previously been associated with multiple sclerosis and systemic lupus erythematosus, 8 previously unknown phenotypes were detected in the PheWAS: cancer of the rectum and anus, diabetes mellitus, benign neoplasm of other parts of the digestive system, benign neoplasm of respiratory and intrathoracic organs, conduct disorders, acute renal failure, erythematous conditions, and pulmonary heart disease (Figure 12.10).

PheWAS studies conducted in the EHR must be interpreted with caution due to issues surrounding institutional practices, patient selection into the study, and data

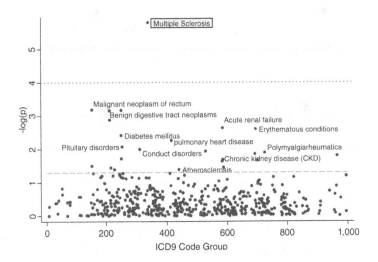

Figure 12.10 Phenome-wide association study results for the association between genotype "rs3135388" and known and unknown clinical phenotypes.

availability and accuracy in the EHR. These issues have been covered extensively in Chapters 6 and 9 of the book. Furthermore, any associations identified should not be viewed as etiologic given the lack of accounting for important confounding factors such as age, sex, and family history. Therefore, these types of studies may best be viewed as hypothesis-generating. Finally, collection of genomic data and linkage with EHR data must be done with care. Given the potentially sensitive and discriminatory nature of the data and to ensure patient safety, security, and privacy, any linked EHR-genomic data should be nonidentifiable.

Notes

1 By high-dimensional data, we mean datasets that have many variables for many observations. Refer to chapter 1 for a definition of "big data."
2 Common unsupervised learning algorithms include K-means, hierarchical clustering, principal components analysis, and Gaussian mixture models.
3 Common supervised learning algorithms include support vector machines, K-nearest neighbors, regularized regression, decision trees, and neural networks. Ensemble models incorporate multiple algorithms, and popular ones include random forest, extreme gradient boosting (XGBoost), and SuperLearner.
4 Tutorials may be found on many websites including https://regex101.com and https://regexone.com, as well as in several dedicated books on regular expressions.
5 https://ctakes.apache.org.
6 https://github.com/stamang/CLEVER.
7 The run chart is the simplest type of chart because it is free from assumptions, but there are many permutations of control charts based on the type of data and assumed distribution. For example, Xbar and S charts examine changes in sample means and standard deviations, respectively, for continuous normally distributed data. The C or U chart may be used to examine events by counts or rates for count data following a Poisson distribution, and the P chart examines event proportions for binomial data. For rare events, the G chart may be used which assumes a geometric distribution.
8 Further information on tokenization may be found here: https://www.clinicalresearch newsonline.com/news/2022/03/29/the-case-for-tokenizing-data-on-clinical-trial-participants.
9 For the US census, these may be obtained from the TIGER/Line Shapefiles website at: https://www.census.gov/geographies/mapping-files/time-series/geo/tiger-line-file.html.
10 Instructions for creating your own shapefiles may be found here: https://www.gold steinepi.com/blog/creatingyourownspatialanalysismapsasshapefileswithqgis/index.html.
11 As with patients' addresses changing over time (see Chapter 6), researchers must keep in mind that patients' rooms may change over time due to transfers or procedures. This can be handled in a variety of ways, such as operationalizing room upon admission, discharge, or procedure; longest length of stay; or as a time-varying measure.
12 One useful resource is BurkeyAcademy: https://spatial.burkeyacademy.com.
13 A credible interval may be interpreted similarly to a confidence interval.
14 Bibliometrics should not be conflated with meta-analyses, where the goal is to summarize empirical evidence of relationships between variables.

References

Abadie A. Semiparametric difference-in-differences estimators. Rev Econ Stud. 2005;72(1):1–19.
Abbe A, Grouin C, Zweigenbaum P, Falissard B. Text mining applications in psychiatry: A systematic literature review. Int J Methods Psychiatr Res. 2016;25(2):86–100.

Alexander N, Alexander DC, Barkhof F, Denaxas S. Identifying and evaluating clinical subtypes of Alzheimer's disease in care electronic health records using unsupervised machine learning. BMC Med Inform Decis Mak. 2021;21(1):343.

Andaur Navarro CL, Damen JAA, Takada T, Nijman SWJ, Dhiman P, Ma J, Collins GS, Bajpai R, Riley RD, Moons KGM, Hooft L. Risk of bias in studies on prediction models developed using supervised machine learning techniques: Systematic review. BMJ. 2021;375:n2281.

Aronson AR. Effective mapping of biomedical text to the UMLS metathesaurus: The MetaMap program. Proc AMIA Symp. 2001:17–21.

Ashby D, Hutton JL, McGee MA. Simple Bayesian analyses for case–control studies in cancer epidemiology. J Royal Statist Soc Ser D (The Statistician). 1993;42(4):385–397.

Bejan CA, Angiolillo J, Conway D, Nash R, Shirey-Rice JK, Lipworth L, Cronin RM, Pulley J, Kripalani S, Barkin S, Johnson KB, Denny JC. Mining 100 million notes to find homelessness and adverse childhood experiences: 2 case studies of rare and severe social determinants of health in electronic health records. J Am Med Inform Assoc. 2018;25(1):61–71.

Bernal JL, Cummins S, Gasparrini A. Difference in difference, controlled interrupted time series and synthetic controls. Int J Epidemiol. 2019;48(6):2062–2063.

Bernal JL, Cummins S, Gasparrini A. Interrupted time series regression for the evaluation of public health interventions: A tutorial. Int J Epidemiol. 2017;46(1):348–355.

Bernal JL, Cummins S, Gasparrini A. The use of controls in interrupted time series studies of public health interventions. Int J Epidemiol. 2018;47(6):2082–2093.

Bhavani SV, Lonjers Z, Carey KA, Afshar M, Gilbert ER, Shah NS, Huang ES, Churpek MM. The development and validation of a machine learning model to predict bacteremia and fungemia in hospitalized patients using electronic health record data. Crit Care Med. 2020;48(11):e1020–e1028.

Bozigar M, Connolly CL, Legler A, Adams WG, Milando CW, Reynolds DB, Carnes F, Jimenez RB, Peer K, Vermeer K, Levy JI, Fabian MP. In-home environmental exposures predicted from geospatial characteristics of the built environment and electronic health records of children with asthma. Ann Epidemiol. 2022;73:38–47.

Bronsert M, Singh AB, Henderson WG, Hammermeister K, Meguid RA, Colborn KL. Identification of postoperative complications using electronic health record data and machine learning. Am J Surg. 2020;220(1):114–119.

Brownson RC, Colditz GA, Proctor EK (Eds). Dissemination and Implementation Research in Health: Translating Science to Practice. 2nd ed. New York, NY: Oxford University Press, 2017.

Carey RG, Lloyd RC. Measuring Quality Improvement in Health Care: A Guide to Statistical Process Control Applications. New York, NY: ASQ Quality Press; 2000.

Carlo Hojilla J, Koester KA, Cohen SE, Buchbinder S, Ladzekpo D, Matheson T, Liu AY. Sexual behavior, risk compensation, and HIV prevention strategies among participants in the San francisco PrEP demonstration project: A qualitative analysis of counseling notes. AIDS Behav. 2016;20(7):1461–9.

Chen B, Alrifai W, Gao C, Jones B, Novak L, Lorenzi N, France D, Malin B, Chen Y. Mining tasks and task characteristics from electronic health record audit logs with unsupervised machine learning. J Am Med Inform Assoc. 2021;28(6):1168–1177.

Cowie MR, Blomster JI, Curtis LH, Duclaux S, Ford I, Fritz F, Goldman S, Janmohamed S, Kreuzer J, Leenay M, Michel A, Ong S, Pell JP, Southworth MR, Stough WG, Thoenes M, Zannad F, Zalewski A. Electronic health records to facilitate clinical research. Clin Res Cardiol. 2017;106(1):1–9.

Cui W, Robins D, Finkelstein J. Unsupervised machine learning for the discovery of latent clusters in COVID-19 patients using electronic health records. Stud Health Technol Inform. 2020;272:1–4.

Danaei G, Rodríguez LA, Cantero OF, Logan R, Hernán MA. Observational data for comparative effectiveness research: An emulation of randomised trials of statins and primary prevention of coronary heart disease. Stat Methods Med Res. 2013;22(1):70–96.

Denny JC, Ritchie MD, Basford MA, Pulley JM, Bastarache L, Brown-Gentry K, Wang D, Masys DR, Roden DM, Crawford DC. PheWAS: Demonstrating the feasibility of a phenome-wide scan to discover Gene-disease associations. Bioinformatics. 2010;26(9):1205–1210.

Desai RJ, Wang SV, Vaduganathan M, Evers T, Schneeweiss S. Comparison of machine learning methods with traditional models for use of administrative claims with electronic medical records to predict heart failure outcomes. JAMA Netw Open. 2020;3(1):e1918962.

Dinh A, Miertschin S, Young A, Mohanty SD. A data-driven approach to predicting diabetes and cardiovascular disease with machine learning. BMC Med Inform Decis Mak. 2019;19(1):211.

Donthu N, Kumar S, Mukherjee D, Pandey N, Lim WM. How to conduct a bibliometric analysis: An overview and guidelines. J Business Res. 2021;133:285–296.

Ehsan K, RWCT–002 Collaborators. Developing and Evaluating Causal Inference Methods for Pragmatic Trials. https://ehsanx.github.io/Causal-Inference-Methods-for-Pragmatic-Trials/ (accessed August 2, 2022), 2021.

Fohner AE, Greene JD, Lawson BL, Chen JH, Kipnis P, Escobar GJ, Liu VX. Assessing clinical heterogeneity in sepsis through treatment patterns and machine learning. J Am Med Inform Assoc. 2019;26(12):1466–1477.

Fong A, Iscoe M, Sinsky CA, Haimovich AD, Williams B, O'Connell RT, Goldstein R, Melnick E. Cluster analysis of primary care physician phenotypes for electronic health record use: Retrospective cohort study. JMIR Med Inform. 2022;10(4):e34954.

Ford E, Carroll JA, Smith HE, Scott D, Cassell JA. Extracting information from the text of electronic medical records to improve case detection: A systematic review. J Am Med Inform Assoc. 2016;23(5):1007–1015.

Fox MP, MacLehose RF, Lash TL. Applying Quantitative Bias Analysis to Epidemiologic Data. 2nd ed. New York, NY: Springer, 2021.

Freitas AA. Data Mining and Knowledge Discovery with Evolutionary Algorithms. Berlin: Springer Science & Business Media; 2002.

Gandrup J, Li J, Izadi Z, Gianfrancesco M, Ellingsen T, Yazdany J, Schmajuk G. Three quality improvement initiatives and performance of rheumatoid arthritis disease activity measures in electronic health records: Results from an interrupted time series study. Arthritis Care Res. 2020 Feb;72(2):283–291.

Gianfrancesco M, Murray S, Evans M, Schmajuk G, Yazdany J. A pragmatic randomized trial to improve safe dosing of hydroxychloroquine [abstract]. Arthritis Rheumatol. 2019; 71 (Suppl. 10). https://acrabstracts.org/abstract/a-pragmatic-randomized-trial-to-improve-safe-dosing-of-hydroxychloroquine/. Accessed August 2, 2022.

Gianfrancesco MA, Tamang S, Yazdany J, Schmajuk G. Potential biases in machine learning algorithms using electronic health record data. JAMA Intern Med. 2018;178(11):1544–1547.

Goldstein ND, Kahal D, Testa K, Burstyn I. Inverse probability weighting for selection bias in a Delaware community health center electronic medical record study of community deprivation and hepatitis c prevalence. Ann Epidemiol. 2021 Aug;60:1–7.

Goldstein ND, LeVasseur MT, McClure LA. On the convergence of epidemiology, bio-statistics, and data science. Harv Data Sci Rev. 2020;2(2). https://doi.org/10.1162/996 08f92.9f0215e6.

Goldstein ND, Tuttle D, Tabb LP, Paul DA, Eppes SC. Spatial and environmental cor-relates of organism colonization and infection in the neonatal intensive care unit. J Perinatol. 2018;38(5):567–573.

Guo CY, Yang YC, Chen YH. The optimal machine learning-based missing data imputa-tion for the cox proportional hazard model. Front Public Health. 2021;9:680054.

Hamilton AJ, Strauss AT, Martinez DA, Hinson JS, Levin S, Lin G, Klein EY. Machine learning and artificial intelligence: Applications in healthcare epidemiology. Antimi-crob Steward Healthc Epidemiol. 2021;1(1):e28.

Harris AD, McGregor JC, Perencevich EN, Furuno JP, Zhu J, Peterson DE, Finkelstein J. The use and interpretation of quasi-experimental studies in medical informatics. J Am Med Inform Assoc. 2006;13(1):16–23.

Hernán MA, Alonso A, Logan R, Grodstein F, Michels KB, Willett WC, Manson JE, Robins JM. Observational studies analyzed like randomized experiments: An applica-tion to postmenopausal hormone therapy and coronary heart disease. Epidemiology. 2008;19(6):766–779.

Hernán MA, Robins JM. Using big data to emulate a target trial when a randomized trial is not available. Am J Epidemiol. 2016;183(8):758–764.

Hirsch AG, Jones JB, Lerch VR, Tang X, Berger A, Clark DN, Stewart WF. The electronic health record audit file: The patient is waiting. J Am Med Inform Assoc. 2017;24(e1):e28–e34.

Hu Z, Melton GB, Moeller ND, Arsoniadis EG, Wang Y, Kwaan MR, Jensen EH, Simon GJ. Accelerating chart review using automated methods on electronic health record data for postoperative complications. AMIA Annu Symp Proc. 2017;2016:1822–1831.

Jäger S, Allhorn A, Bießmann F. A benchmark for data imputation methods. Front Big Data. 2021;4:693674.

James G, Witten D, Hastie T, Tibshirani R. An Introduction to Statistical Learning with Applications in R. 2nd ed. New York, NY: Springer, 2021.

Juhn Y, Liu H. Artificial intelligence approaches using natural language processing to advance EHR-based clinical research. J Allergy Clin Immunol. 2020;145(2):463–469.

Kate RJ, Pearce N, Mazumdar D, Nilakantan V. A continual prediction model for inpa-tient acute kidney injury. Comput Biol Med. 2020;116:103580.

Katsoulis M, Stavola BD, Diaz-Ordaz K, Gomes M, Lai A, Lagiou P, Wannamethee G, Tsilidis K, Lumbers RT, Denaxas S, Banerjee A, Parisinos CA, Batterham R, Patel R, Langenberg C, Hemingway H. Weight change and the onset of cardiovascular diseases: Emulating trials using electronic health records. Epidemiology. 2021;32(5):744–755.

Kirshner J, Cohn K, Dunder S, Donahue K, Richey M, Larson P, Sutton L, Siu E, Don-egan J, Chen Z, Nightingale C, Estévez M, Hamrick HJ. Automated electronic health record-based tool for identification of patients with metastatic disease to facilitate clini-cal trial patient ascertainment. JCO Clin Cancer Inform. 2021;5:719–727.

Koleck TA, Dreisbach C, Bourne PE, Bakken S. Natural language processing of symp-toms documented in free-text narratives of electronic health records: A systematic re-view. J Am Med Inform Assoc. 2019;26(4):364–379.

Köpcke F, Trinczek B, Majeed RW, Schreiweis B, Wenk J, Leusch T, Ganslandt T, Ohm-ann C, Bergh B, Röhrig R, Dugas M, Prokosch HU. Evaluation of data completeness in the electronic health record for the purpose of patient recruitment into clinical trials: A retrospective analysis of element presence. BMC Med Inform Decis Mak. 2013;13:37.

Kreimeyer K, Foster M, Pandey A, Arya N, Halford G, Jones SF, Forshee R, Walderhaug M, Botsis T. Natural language processing systems for capturing and standardizing unstructured clinical information: A systematic review. J Biomed Inform. 2017;73:14–29.

Krummenacher I, Spencer B, Du Pasquier S, Bugnon O, Cavassini M, Schneider MP. Qualitative analysis of barriers and facilitators encountered by HIV patients in an ART adherence programme. Int J Clin Pharm. 2014;36(4):716–724.

Kruschke J. Doing Bayesian Data Analysis: A Tutorial with R, JAGS, and Stan. London: Elsevier, 2014.

Kuan V, Fraser HC, Hingorani M, Denaxas S, Gonzalez-Izquierdo A, Direk K, Nitsch D, Mathur R, Parisinos CA, Lumbers RT, Sofat R, Wong ICK, Casas JP, Thornton JM, Hemingway H, Partridge L, Hingorani AD. Data-driven identification of ageing-related diseases from electronic health records. Sci Rep. 2021;11(1):2938.

Kung B, Chiang M, Perera G, Pritchard M, Stewart R. Identifying subtypes of depression in clinician-annotated text: A retrospective cohort study. Sci Rep. 2021;11(1):22426.

Lechner M. The estimation of causal effects by difference-in-difference methods. Found Trends Econometr. 2011;4(3):165–224.

Meng, XL. Data science: An artificial ecosystem. Harvard Data Science Review, 1(1). 2019.

Mennis JL. Mapping the results of geographically weighted regression. Cartograph J. 2006;43(2):171–179.

Moyé LA. Elementary Bayesian Biostatistics. Boca Raton, FL: CRC Press: 2016.

Murray SG, Yim JWL, Croci R, Rajkomar A, Schmajuk G, Khanna R, Cucina RJ. Using spatial and temporal mapping to identify nosocomial disease transmission of clostridium difficile. JAMA Intern Med. 2017;177(12):1863–1865.

Myers L, Stevens J. Using EHR to Conduct Outcome and Health Services Research. In Secondary Analysis of Electronic Health Records. Cham: Springer, 2016. pp. 61–70.

Naimi AI, Mishler AE, Kennedy EH. Challenges in obtaining valid causal effect estimates with machine learning algorithms. Am J Epidemiol. 2021:kwab201.

Nijman S, Leeuwenberg AM, Beekers I, Verkouter I, Jacobs J, Bots ML, Asselbergs FW, Moons K, Debray T. Missing data is poorly handled and reported in prediction model studies using machine learning: A literature review. J Clin Epidemiol. 2022;142:218–229.

Obermeyer Z, Powers B, Vogeli C, Mullainathan S. Dissecting racial bias in an algorithm used to manage the health of populations. Science. 2019;366(6464):447–453.

Pang X, Forrest CB, Lê-Scherban F, Masino AJ. Prediction of early childhood obesity with machine learning and electronic health record data. Int J Med Inform. 2021;150:104454.

Parikh RB, Takvorian SU, Vader D, Paul Wileyto E, Clark AS, Lee DJ, Goyal G, Rocque GB, Dotan E, Geynisman DM, Phull P, Spiess PE, Kim RY, Davidoff AJ, Gross CP, Neparidze N, Miksad RA, Calip GS, Hearn CM, Ferrell W, Shulman LN, Mamtani R, Hubbard RA. PRACTICE investigators. Impact of the COVID-19 pandemic on treatment patterns for patients with metastatic solid cancer in the United States. J Natl Cancer Inst. 2022;114(4):571–578.

Park JI, Bliss DZ, Chi CL, Delaney CW, Westra BL. Knowledge discovery with machine learning for Hospital-acquired catheter-associated urinary tract infections. Comput Inform Nurs. 2020;38(1):28–35.

Paul DA, Johnson D, Goldstein ND, Pearlman SA. Development of a single-center quality bundle to prevent sudden unexpected postnatal collapse. J Perinatol. 2019;39(7):1008–1013.

Pons E, Braun LM, Hunink MG, Kors JA. Natural language processing in radiology: A systematic review. Radiology. 2016;279(2):329–343.

Rassen JA, Murk W, Schneeweiss S. Real-world evidence of bariatric surgery and cardio-vascular benefits using electronic health records data: A lesson in bias. Diabetes Obes Metab. 2021;23(7):1453–1462.

Reátegui R, Ratté S. Comparison of MetaMap and cTAKES for entity extraction in clinical notes. BMC Med Inform Decis Mak. 2018;18(Suppl. 3):74.

Richesson RL, Hammond WE, Nahm M, Wixted D, Simon GE, Robinson JG, Bauck AE, Cifelli D, Smerek MM, Dickerson J, Laws RL, Madigan RA, Rusincovitch SA, Kluchar C, Califf RM. Electronic health records based phenotyping in next-generation clinical trials: A perspective from the NIH health care systems collaboratory. J Am Med Inform Assoc. 2013;20(e2):e226–e231.

Richesson R, Platt R, Simon G, et al. Using Electronic Health Record Data in Pragmatic Clinical Trials: Specific Uses for EHR Data in PCTs. In: Rethinking Clinical Trials: A Living Textbook of Pragmatic Clinical Trials. Bethesda, MD: NIH Health Care Systems Research Collaboratory. Available at: https://rethinkingclinicaltrials.org/chapters/design/using-electronic-health-record-data-pragmatic-clinical-trials-top/specific-uses-ehr-data-pcts/. Updated December 27, 2021.

Ruggiano N, Perry TE. Conducting secondary analysis of qualitative data: Should we, can we, and how? Qual Soc Work. 2019;18(1):81–97.

Savin NE, White KJ. The Durbin–Watson test for serial correlation with extreme sample sizes or many regressors. Econometrica: J Econ Soc. 1977;45(8):1989–1996.

Savova GK, Masanz JJ, Ogren PV, Zheng J, Sohn S, Kipper-Schuler KC, Chute CG. Mayo Clinical text analysis and knowledge extraction system (cTAKES): Architecture, component evaluation and applications. J Am Med Inform Assoc. 2010;17(5):507–513.

Sheikhalishahi S, Miotto R, Dudley JT, Lavelli A, Rinaldi F, Osmani V. Natural language processing of clinical notes on chronic diseases: Systematic review. JMIR Med Inform. 2019;7(2):e12239.

Shivade C, Raghavan P, Fosler-Lussier E, Embi PJ, Elhadad N, Johnson SB, Lai AM. A review of approaches to identifying patient phenotype cohorts using electronic health records. J Am Med Inform Assoc. 2014;21(2):221–230.

Smith VA, Coffman CJ, Hudgens MG. Interpreting the results of intention-to-treat, per-protocol, and as-treated analyses of clinical trials. JAMA. 2021;326(5):433–434.

Sohn S, Wang Y, Wi CI, Krusemark EA, Ryu E, Ali MH, Juhn YJ, Liu H. Clinical documentation variations and NLP system portability: A case study in asthma birth cohorts across Institutions. J Am Med Inform Assoc. 2018;25(3):353–359.

Spasić I, Livsey J, Keane JA, Nenadić G. Text mining of cancer-related information: Review of current status and future directions. Int J Med Inform. 2014;83(9):605–623.

Spasic I, Nenadic G. Clinical text data in machine learning: Systematic review. JMIR Med Inform. 2020;8(3):e17984.

Szabo L. A reality check on artificial intelligence: Are health care claims overblown? https://khn.org/news/a-reality-check-on-artificial-intelligence-are-health-care-claims-overblown/. Kaiser Health News. 2019.

Tabb LP, McClure LA, Quick H, Purtle J, Roux DAV. Assessing the spatial heterogeneity in overall health across the United States using spatial regression methods: The contribution of health factors and county-level demographics. Health Place. 2018;51:68–77.

Tamang SR, Hernandez-Boussard T, Ross EG, Gaskin G, Patel MI, Shah NH. Enhanced quality measurement event detection: An application to physician reporting. EGEMS (Wash DC). 2017;5(1):5.

Tang S, Davarmanesh P, Song Y, Koutra D, Sjoding MW, Wiens J. Democratizing EHR analyses with FIDDLE: A flexible data-driven preprocessing pipeline for structured clinical data. J Am Med Inform Assoc. 2020;27(12):1921–1934.

Tiwari P, Colborn KL, Smith DE, Xing F, Ghosh D, Rosenberg MA. Assessment of a machine learning model applied to harmonized electronic health record data for the prediction of incident atrial fibrillation. JAMA Netw Open. 2020;3(1):e1919396.

Wang Y, Wang L, Rastegar-Mojarad M, Moon S, Shen F, Afzal N, Liu S, Zeng Y, Mehrabi S, Sohn S, Liu H. Clinical information extraction applications: A literature review. J Biomed Inform. 2018;77:34–49.

Wang Y, Zhao Y, Therneau TM, Atkinson EJ, Tafti AP, Zhang N, Amin S, Limper AH, Khosla S, Liu H. Unsupervised machine learning for the discovery of latent disease clusters and patient subgroups using electronic health records. J Biomed Inform. 2020;102:103364.

Warton EM. Time after time: Difference-in-Differences and interrupted time series models in SAS. SAS Global Forum. 2020;2020.

Watson DP, Weathers T, McGuire A, Cohen A, Huynh P, Bowes C, O'Donnell D, Brucker K, Gupta S. Evaluation of an emergency department-based opioid overdose survivor intervention: Difference-in-difference analysis of electronic health record data to assess key outcomes. Drug Alcohol Depend. 2021;221:108595.

Wei WQ, Denny JC. Extracting research-quality phenotypes from electronic health records to support precision medicine. Genome Med. 2015;7(1):41.

Weinfurt K. What is a Pragmatic Clinical Trial: Why Are We Talking About Pragmatic Trials? In: Rethinking Clinical Trials: A Living Textbook of Pragmatic Clinical Trials. Bethesda, MD: NIH Health Care Systems Research Collaboratory. Available at: https://rethinkingclinicaltrials.org/chapters/pragmatic-clinical-trial/what-is-a-pragmatic-clinical-trial/. Updated September 23, 2021.

Wiemken TL, Kelley RR. Machine learning in epidemiology and health outcomes research. Annu Rev Public Health. 2020;41:21–36.

Williams JB, Ghosh D, Wetzel RC. Applying machine learning to pediatric critical care data. Pediatr Crit Care Med. 2018;19(7):599–608.

Wong SPY, Foglia MB, Cohen J, Oestreich T, O'Hare AM. The VA life-sustaining treatment decisions initiative: A qualitative analysis of veterans with advanced kidney disease. J Am Geriatr Soc. 2022 Sep;70(9):2517–2529.

Wu J, Roy J, Stewart WF. Prediction modeling using EHR data: Challenges, strategies, and a comparison of machine learning approaches. Med Care. 2010;48(Suppl. 6):S106–S113.

Zhang S, Zhang C, Yang Q Data preparation for data mining. Appl Artif Intell 2003;17(5–6): 375–381.

Zhu VJ, Lenert LA, Bunnell BE, Obeid JS, Jefferson M, Halbert CH. Automatically identifying social isolation from clinical narratives for patients with prostate cancer. BMC Med Inform Decis Mak. 2019;19(1):43.

Section III

Interpretation to Application

13 Publication and Presentation

EHR-based research does not occur in a vacuum. Study findings need to be disseminated to the field, whether these results are positive, negative, or equivocal. While the publication process may tend to prefer positive findings – known as the publication bias (Chalmers, 1990) – this should not dissuade the researcher. After all, to move the field forward methodologically, provide transparency and openness of science, and ultimately improve health require full disclosure of all available evidence. Additionally, sometimes the means are as important as the ends, and a study can serve as a prototypical example for researchers working in similar areas. The goal of this chapter is to prepare the research for publication and presentation through a discussion of the peer review process and scientific meeting presentation, as well as promote open and transparent science.

Publication

One of the most common academic ways of disseminating scientific knowledge is through the peer-reviewed publication process. This process is intended to critically evaluate research and share the results with a scientific audience. All clinical and public health journals publish EHR-based studies and deciding which ones to target is largely a subjective choice. Informatics journals tend to focus on studies that are about the EHR as a technology, epidemiology and biostatistics journals tend to focus on studies that are about methods for and validity of EHR research or have broad applications, while substantive and clinical journals tend to focus on studies that are applied in nature. Of course, there are journals that publish articles in all three of these areas. Often researchers look to the journal's *impact factor*, a measure of citations, to decide its merit. This is unfortunate, as many worthwhile articles are published in low-impact journals and the occasional poor article is published in the highest impact journals. Yet a journal's impact factor is so ingrained in the publication mindset, it may be tough to move away from this model. Instead of relying solely on impact factor when targeting a journal for publication, the researcher should also consider:

- The potential impact of the research and ability to move the field forward.
- The appropriateness of the journal to accurately represent the work and have a critical, meaningful editorial and peer review.

DOI: 10.4324/9781003258872-17

- The circulation of the journal, desired audience, and whether it is indexed to allow other scientists to discover the research. Researchers should be aware of the so-called predatory journals and publishers that exist for profit alone.[1]
- The likelihood of the work being accepted for publication. Researchers should balance the journal's prestige with the potential impact of the work.
- Journal policies, including types of manuscripts and word count, article publishing charges if open access, and expediency of the review process.

As mentioned, EHR-based research has appeared in all mainstream journals and the selection of a journal is dependent on many factors. In general, single institution EHR studies from less well-known institutions may be more difficult to place in high-impact national and international journals as compared to multi-institution EHR studies or well-established single institutions at large academic medical centers. There are several strategies for identifying the most appropriate journal to target for submission. The articles cited in the prepared manuscript likely indicate relevant journals for a given research area, as would be gleaned from searching Pub-Med based on the manuscript's title or keywords. Several leading publishers in the biomedical field, including SpringerNature (Springer-Verlag GmbH, Heidelberg, Germany) and Elsevier (Elsevier B.V., Amsterdam, Netherlands), provide journal recommendation engines[2] based on the manuscript's title and abstract, although users should be aware that these are tailored to a given publisher's portfolio of journals and not necessarily journal-agnostic. For a sense of the most common journals for EHR-based research, Figures 13.1 and 13.2 chart the top 15 journals in PubMed with the respective search terms "electronic health record" and "electronic health record epidemiology" for the most recent (as of 2022) 10,000 citations.

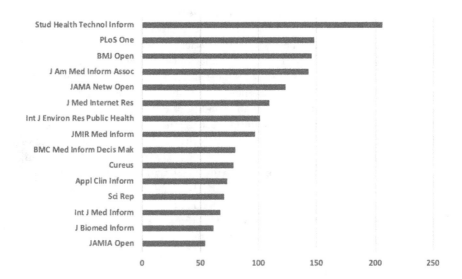

Figure 13.1 Top 15 journals in PubMed for the search term "electronic health record" for the most recent (as of 2022) 10,000 citations. Journal title abbreviations may be decoded here: https://www.ncbi.nlm.nih.gov/nlmcatalog/journals.

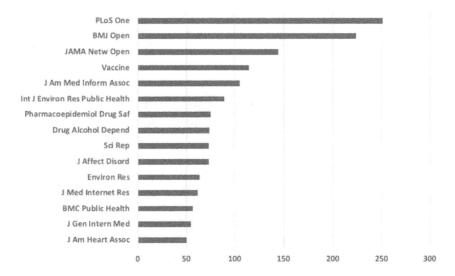

Figure 13.2 Top 15 journals in PubMed for the search term "electronic health record epidemiology" for the most recent (as of 2022) 10,000 citations. Journal title abbreviations may be decoded here: https://www.ncbi.nlm.nih.gov/nlmcatalog/journals.

Aside from publishing in traditional peer-reviewed journals, there is also an increasing use of *preprint servers* such as medRxiv (https://www.medrxiv.org) to host and distribute in-progress manuscripts. The intention of these services is for rapid dissemination and transparency of scientific manuscripts prior to or during the peer review process. As exemplified during the COVID-19 pandemic, preprint articles have entered mainstream use by many authors, publishers, and the media. Unfortunately, the quality of these articles is highly variable, the majority of which never result in a peer-reviewed publication. In fact, a study conducted following the first year of the COVID-19 pandemic observed a publication rate of <6% (Añazco et al., 2021) for articles posted on preprint services. Thus, while posting an article to a preprint service can facilitate its distribution through a self-publication paradigm, these articles require additional scientific scrutiny beyond their peer-reviewed equivalents. Further, posting a manuscript to a preprint server should not be viewed as the end, but rather an intermediate step in the publication process. If a manuscript has been distribution via a preprint service, this should be disclosed upon submission to a peer-reviewed journal.

Formatting research for publication

Regardless of the choice of journal, most observational epidemiology manuscripts are organized as follows.

- *Abstract.* The abstract is a brief synopsis of the work, typically less than 200 words. The abstract may be structured and mirror the sections of the body of the manuscript, or unstructured and presented in a conversational style. The abstract forms the initial impression of an article and therefore it should appropriately motivate the work including the clinical or public health problem, the research goal, and a brief mention of the study design, results, and conclusions as it relates to the field at large.

- *Introduction/Background.* The introduction provides the background of the public health or clinical problem and includes what is known about the topic under inquiry as well as the gaps in scientific knowledge. A well-written introduction culminates in the research question(s), which may be explicitly stated as the final sentence in this section, "In this analysis we sought to..."

- *Methods.* Given that a central theme of this book is the validity of EHR analyses, the methods section should not receive short shrift. The methods define the process by which the research question(s) were answered and should be written in a manner to allow an independent researcher to replicate the work (Goldstein, Hamra & Harper, 2020). Often methods are the primary target for trimming when manuscript word count limits are exceeded; instead of removing them completely, they can be placed in an electronic supplement. For clarity, the methods may be subdivided into sections for the study setting including a description of the institution, catchment area, and EHR; study population including the sampling process to move from the source population to the study population or sample; variable identification including parameterization of the exposure, outcome, and other covariates; and statistical analysis covering the statistical procedures, assumptions, and sensitivity analyses. The methods also commonly include informed consent and institutional review board processes, as well as the statistical software and version used for the analysis.

- *Results.* The results section presents the primary findings and should be clear, concise, and without commentary. When appropriate, results are effectively conveyed as exhibits – tables or figures – with an accompanying description of what each exhibit represents and how to interpret the findings. A typical number of exhibits in the main body of a manuscript is four or five, depending on the journal. Results from secondary endpoints or sensitivity analyses may be included in this section, space permitting, or included in the electronic supplementary material. Many readers will turn to the results section first, and possibly only; thus, the findings need to be able to stand alone.

- *Discussion.* The discussion section forms the commentary that relates the study findings into the greater body of scientific knowledge. A typical discussion section starts by rearticulating the research aims and major findings from the work without being redundant of the results. Then, the results are contextualized with other research in the area, discussing whether the present findings agree or disagree with other studies, along with possible explanations for any deviations. After the primary findings are presented, secondary endpoints or sensitivity analyses can be discussed in a similar fashion. The discussion section also includes an acknowledgement of the study strengths and limitations. This important sub-section demonstrates that the authors have critically reflected upon their work and are transparent in the strengths and weaknesses of the study setting, population, and analyses. Lastly, a concluding paragraph summarizes the value of this work to the field. Optionally, some journals request a paragraph in the discussion section on the clinical or public health implications of the work.

• *Acknowledgements.* This optional and journal-specific section may include funding sources and disclosures, as well as acknowledging individuals who contributed to the work, but did not meet the criteria of authorship. For work that was presented at a scientific conference prior to publication, the authors should acknowledge the meeting including the date and location of the conference.

• *References.* This section includes a listing of all works cited in the manuscript. Journals are particular about the style of references in the manuscript and use of a reference manager can minimize the tediousness of formatting to each journal convention.

STROBE *statement*

Many journals now require prospective authors to report observational epidemiology, including EHR research, according to the STROBE (STrengthening the Reporting of OBservational studies in Epidemiology; http://www.strobe-statement.org) guidelines. These guidelines are the observational epidemiology equivalent to the CONSORT statements for reporting clinical trials (http://www.consort-statement.org). The STROBE statement covers in detail items included in the report of observational studies, and further expands upon the manuscript sections enumerated in the previous section. Readers are encouraged to familiarize themselves with the STROBE requirements (Vandenbroucke et al., 2007); even if the journal does not explicitly request adherence to these guidelines, use of the checklist strengthens the presentation of the work. An extension of STROBE dubbed RECORD for REporting of studies Conducted using Observational Routinely collected Data (http://www.record-statement.org) enhances STROBE for routinely collected health data including EHR data and covers the minimum reporting requirements for methods and results for EHR-based studies (Langan et al., 2013).

Exhibits

Exhibits such as tables and figures are a visual tool to summarize the results and concisely present supporting evidence of study findings. A typical number of exhibits in the main body of a manuscript is four or five, depending on the journal. In almost all observational and experimental research studies, the first table a reader encounters is invariably the characteristics of the study population, with possible stratification by the outcome. Revisiting the *birthwt* analysis from Chapters 10 and 11 on the relationship between maternal smoking during the first trimester of pregnancy and low birthweight infants, a typical "Table 1" is shown in Table 13.1.

Table 13.1 Characteristics of the *birthwt* study population and comparison by low birthweight infants

Characteristic	All infants	Comparison by birthweight outcome		
		Not low birthweight	Low birthweight	P-valuea
Total No. (%)	189 (100)	130 (69)	59 (31)	–
Maternal age, years	23 (5)	24 (5.6)[b]	22 (4.5)	0.08
Maternal weight				0.20
<170 pounds	168 (89%)	113 (87%)	55 (93%)	
≥170 pounds	21 (11%)	17 (13%)	4 (7%)	
Maternal race				0.08
White	96 (51%)	73 (56%)	23 (39%)	
Black	26 (14%)	15 (12%)	11 (19%)	
Other	67 (35%)	42 (32%)	25 (42%)	
Smoking during pregnancy				0.03
No	115 (61%)	86 (66%)	29 (49%)	
Yes	74 (39%)	44 (34%)	30 (51%)	
Previous preterm labor				<0.01
No	159 (84%)	118 (91%)	41 (70%)	
Yes	30 (16%)	12 (9%)	18 (31%)	
Maternal hypertension				0.04
No	177 (94%)	125 (96%)	52 (88%)	
Yes	12 (6%)	5 (4%)	7 (12%)	
Uterine irritability				0.02
No	161 (85%)	116 (89%)	45 (76%)	
Yes	28 (15%)	14 (11%)	14 (24%)	
First trimester doctor visits				0.27
None	100 (53%)	64 (49%)	36 (61%)	
One	47 (25%)	36 (28%)	11 (19%)	
Two	30 (16%)	23 (18%)	7 (12%)	
Three or more	12 (6%)	7 (5%)	5 (9%)	
Gestational age, weeks	39 (2%)	39 (1.7)	38 (1.9)	0.04

[a] Statistical testing using Student's t-test for continuous variables, and chi-squared test for categorical variables, $\alpha = 0.05$.

[b] Estimates are given as mean (standard deviation) for continuous variables, and count (frequency) for categorical variables.

Such study characteristic tables as Table 13.1 provide information germane to the catchment and validity of the EHR population. First, we can assess the overall composition of the study population, including the number of participants (n = 189) and breakdown by outcome (n = 59, or 31% with low birthweight). Further, to aid in the assessment of external validity, we can assess the total distribution of characteristics, and verify if the group is not compositionally overrepresented or underrepresented compared to some target population. Second, we can readily compare characteristics of participants across the outcome of interest. By calculating "column percentages" for each characteristic, we can assess the balance of categorical variables within each of the dichotomous outcome states: low birthweight versus not low birthweight. For example, from Table 13.1, the proportion of women with hypertension is greater among those with low birth-weight infants versus those without low birthweight infants (12% versus 4%, respectively, p = 0.04). Additionally, we can assess whether any categorical cell counts are insufficient for valid statistical inference. Third, potential confounding variables are identifiable based on differences in distributions across the outcome states (a similar table would be required for exposure states to fully evaluate confounding, as discussed in Chapter 11). Finally, the reader gets a general sense of the unadjusted bivariable relationship between the exposure of interest (smoking) and the outcome (low birthweight). There was greater maternal smoking among the low birthweight group (51%) compared to the not low birthweight group (34%); this difference was unlikely due to chance alone (p = 0.03) at an α of 5%.

The body of the results section does not need to repeat this table in its entirety. Rather, we should present in text only the most relevant findings, such as characteristics that are notably different between groups or characteristics that are surprisingly not different. The size of the total population and comparison groups may be presented at the beginning of the results, along with a reminder of the dates and study setting.

Assuming the statistical analysis proceeded from unadjusted analysis as in Table 13.1 to a fully adjusted multivariable regression model, the independent contributions from each covariate can also be depicted in table format. Suppose the *birthwt* dataset was recruited at delivery to include a sample of low birthweight infants along with a random selection of controls, and the data represent an unmatched case–control study. The raw statistical software output from the regression model is shown in Figure 13.3 and the formatted output is shown in Table 13.2. As compared to the raw output, the formatted table readily captures the magnitude of effect of the point estimate (i.e., odds ratio), the precision (i.e., 95% confidence interval), and the result of the hypothesis test (i.e., p-value).

The exact format of Tables 13.1 and 13.2 will vary by convention of the journal, but to facilitate peer review, the tables should be presented to maximize readability using horizontal breaks, borders, and bolded or italicized text. Once accepted for publication, the journal will format the final tables per their stylistic conventions.

Exhibits presented as graphs and figures may depict distributions of variables (Figure 13.4), hypothesized causal diagrams (Figure 13.5), relationships between continuous variables (Figure 13.6), or other findings that cannot be easily replicated in a table. Multi-panel figures, such as Figure 13.4, present related data while not increasing the overall exhibit count. Unless color is a necessity, most figures can be created with grayscale shading and varying line weights (thicknesses) or types, such as dashed lines, dotted lines, or combinations thereof. Grayscale figures will not incur additional charges in print-based journals. If color figures are required and the publication budget allows, researchers should strive to use a color-blind friendly palette. When formatting figures for press, the publisher will require a high-print-resolution figure, typically 300 dots per inch minimum.[3]

```
> summary(glm(low ~ as.factor(smoke) + as.factor(race) + as.factor(ptl_collapsed) +
as.factor(ftv_collapsed) + gestation, data=analytic_dataset, family=binomial(link=logit)))

Call:
glm(formula = low ~ as.factor(smoke) + as.factor(race) + as.factor(ptl_collapsed) +
    as.factor(ftv_collapsed) + gestation, family = binomial(link = logit),
    data = analytic_dataset)

Deviance Residuals:
    Min      1Q   Median      3Q     Max
-1.7248  -0.8425  -0.6108   1.0447  2.1754

Coefficients:
                          Estimate Std. Error z value Pr(>|z|)
(Intercept)                 4.3008     6.5480   0.657  0.51130
as.factor(smoke)1           0.3667     0.6162   0.595  0.55173
as.factor(race)2            1.1103     0.5101   2.176  0.02952 *
as.factor(race)3            0.9095     0.4253   2.138  0.03250 *
as.factor(ptl_collapsed)1   1.4148     0.4522   3.128  0.00176 **
as.factor(ftv_collapsed)1  -0.4916     0.4610  -1.066  0.28626
as.factor(ftv_collapsed)2  -0.3531     0.5083  -0.695  0.48722
as.factor(ftv_collapsed)3   0.2311     0.6591   0.351  0.72588
gestation                  -0.1516     0.1645  -0.922  0.35677
---
Signif. codes:  0 '***' 0.001 '**' 0.01 '*' 0.05 '.' 0.1 ' ' 1

(Dispersion parameter for binomial family taken to be 1)

    Null deviance: 234.67  on 188  degrees of freedom
Residual deviance: 208.06  on 180  degrees of freedom
AIC: 226.06

Number of Fisher Scoring iterations: 4

> exp(0.3667)
[1] 1.442965
```

Figure 13.3 Adjusted unconditional odds ratio of the relationship between maternal smoking during the first trimester and low birthweight infants.

Table 13.2 Results of the multivariable logistic regression and the relationship between maternal smoking during the first trimester and low birthweight infants

Characteristic	Odds ratio	95% Confidence interval	P-value
Smoking during pregnancy			
No	Ref	–	–
Yes	1.44	(0.43, 4.87)	0.55
Maternal race			
White	Ref	–	–
Black	3.04	(1.11, 8.35)	0.03
Other	2.48	(1.09, 5.84)	0.03
Previous preterm labor			
No	Ref	–	–
Yes	4.12	(1.72, 10.27)	<0.01
First trimester doctor visits			
None	Ref	–	–
One	0.61	(0.24, 1.48)	0.29
Two	0.70	(0.25, 1.84)	0.49
Three or more	1.26	(0.33, 4.56)	0.73
Gestational age, weeks	0.86	(0.62, 1.18)	0.36

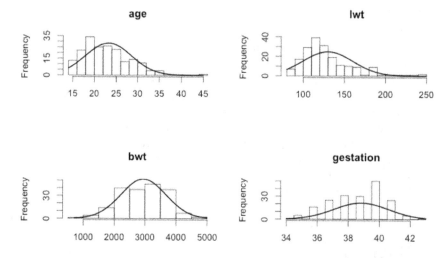

Figure 13.4 Distributions of the continuous variables in the *birthwt* dataset.

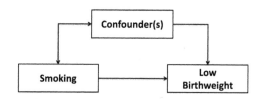

Figure 13.5 Relationship of one or more confounders to the exposure and outcome in the *birthwt* dataset.

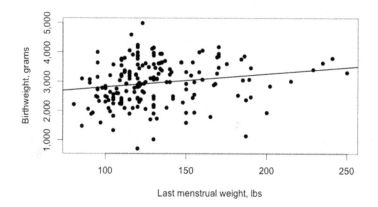

Figure 13.6 A regression model between maternal weight at last menstrual period (the independent predictor) and infant's birthweight (the dependent predictor).

Open access

There has been a trend in scientific publishing to move away from a subscriber-paid publication model to a researcher-paid publication model, termed *open access*. In open access publishing, the researcher or their institution holds the copyright[4] rather than the journal. While open access publishing may be attractive to researchers, there are additional costs in terms of article processing charges that may run several thousand dollars. Investigators from underrepresented institutions or countries may apply for reduced fees, and researchers with grant-funded work may wish to add anticipated publication fees when preparing the grant budget. Dedicated open access publishers, such as PLOS (PLOS, San Francisco, CA), BioMed Central (Springer-Verlag GmbH, Heidelberg, Germany) and Frontiers (Frontiers Media SA, Lausanne, Switzerland), once seen as fringe and low impact, are now common and accepted in the scientific community, publishing high-quality journals. Subscription-based journals offer the option whether the article, if accepted, should be published under the no-cost subscription model or paid open access model. Regardless of whether the journal is open access or not, only peer-reviewed journals should be considered for publication of scientific research. Non-peer-reviewed "gray literature" may still provide valuable information but should be viewed with caution by consumers.

Not to be confused with open access, *public access* is a requirement set forth by the U.S. National Institutes of Health (NIH) stipulating that NIH-funded work must be publicly accessible via PubMed Central. The onus is on the publisher or researcher to submit the NIH-funded article to PubMed Central: further information may be found at https://publicaccess.nih.gov.

Journal submission process

Submitting a manuscript to a journal is a standardized process through publisher use of near ubiquitous submission systems such as EditorialManager (Aries Systems Corporation, North Andover, MA) and ScholarOne (Clarivate, London, United Kingdom). Once a target journal is identified, the "Instructions for Authors" section on the journal or publisher website will contain the necessary information for manuscript submittal, including article types, word and exhibit limits, formatting guidelines, and acceptance rate. When submitting a manuscript, the author needs to pay careful attention to these instructions, lest the manuscript be returned as nonconforming.

In addition to the manuscript, tables, and figures, the researcher should prepare a cover letter and title page. The cover letter is addressed to the editors of the journal, serves to introduce the manuscript and the authors, provides a brief statement about the merit of the work and its importance to the readers of the journal, and states that the work has not been previously published or under consideration for publication elsewhere. While not always required, a cover letter should nonetheless be included, even with revisions. The title page, which may be included in the manuscript text or as a separate file, includes meta-information about the manuscript, such as the title, keywords, funding, conflicts of interest, and the authorship, including affiliations and corresponding author identification.

After the manuscript is submitted, it will first be screened by one of the journal's editors. If the manuscript receives a high enough priority score and is of potential interest to the journal, it will be sent for external peer review. Many journals require nomination of potential peer reviewers among which the editor will select two or three. Even though peer review is often a blinded process, the researcher should avoid nominating individuals at their institution or nominating colleagues who may be familiar with the work. Occasionally, due to the small network of individuals working in a particular area, this may be unavoidable. Potential reviewers can be identified through a literature search or existing citations in the manuscript – especially first and last authors – or from colleague recommendations. During external peer review, experts in the field evaluate the methods and significance of the work, with a recommendation to the editor for disposition and revisions.

Following review, the journal editor will render a decision on the manuscript and inform the corresponding author. The decision may be an outright acceptance, a rejection (with or without peer review), or a revise and resubmit with revisions. If the decision is to reject and there is peer review feedback available, the authors are highly encouraged to consider all comments and revise the manuscript prior to submitting to another journal. If the decision is to revise and resubmit, the authors are requested to address the major and minor concerns raised by the peer reviewers. The authors should be as responsive as reasonably possible to the reviewer critiques, noting the exact changes made in the manuscript in a point-by-point reply (or rebuttal if no changes are made) to the reviewers. After the revised manuscript is resubmitted, it may be sent externally for a subsequent round of peer review or internally evaluated by the editor. Typically, the timeframe from submission to decision ranges from weeks to months, largely depending on bottlenecks in the external review process.

Post-acceptance, the manuscript is transferred to the journal's production and editorial staff. The staff will ensure compliance with journal formatting policies, including text, exhibits, and references, and create article page proofs for review. These page proofs are a final opportunity for the author to confirm author names and affiliations, and correct any typos or grammatical issues in the text. Substantive changes are discouraged unless there is a gross inaccuracy. The proofs may also include "author queries," for example, requests to correct references, clarify ambiguities, provide higher resolution figures, and so on. The proofing process generally has a short window of time – in some cases turnaround is expected within two to three days. Following approval of the proofs, the article will often be published online ahead of print, followed by appearance in the print for subscription-based journals. As part of the post-acceptance process, the journal or publisher sets an *embargo date*, where the author is prohibited from discussing or disseminating the article prior to this date, although this does not preclude scientific presentation based on the abstract. Working with your institution's public relations group can time any media coverage with this embargo date. Lastly, any work that has been funded by an NIH grant will need to be posted in PubMed Central for compliance with the public access policy as detailed on the website: https://publicaccess.nih.gov. Authors should check with the respective journal to confirm whether the author or publisher is responsible for depositing the article.

Presentation

Disseminating research at a scientific meeting provides an opportunity to share recent work with colleagues in an organized setting. Presentation may take the form of a poster or oral platform talk and should occur prior to publication of the corresponding manuscript. In fact, many organizations preclude published work from being presented as a solicited abstract, unless the author is invited to participate in a symposium or panel discussion. Depending on the focus of the research – EHR technology, EHR methods, or applied EHR research – there are many options for conferences both domestic and international.

Submitting work for presentation typically requires an abstract of a few hundred words, an accompanying exhibit (if allowed), and identification of the desired presentation format, whether poster or talk. A platform talk is the more prestigious avenue for presentation, but not specifying a poster or talk upon submission ensures the greatest opportunity for acceptance under either format. Poster presentations are less formal and more of an interactive discussion (often favored by students), while a platform talk is a well-structured ten- to fifteen-minute lecture followed by questions.

Posters can be created using presentation software, such as Microsoft Power-Point (Microsoft Corporation, Redmond, WA). The guidelines for poster formatting typically follow a structured abstract and include background, methods, results, and discussion. A poster is inherently visual, and therefore should heavily rely upon figures and tables, and minimize text. The exact dimensions of the poster will be dictated by the conference and will require the use of a special printer or conference poster-printing services. Slides for a talk are also created using presentation software. The conference or session chair may request a copy of the slides in advance, so they should be created beforehand. As a rule of thumb, a slide deck should have the number of slides approximately equal to the number of minutes in the talk (assuming an average of one minute per slide) and also minimize typed text.

Alternate forms of dissemination

The publication and presentation process discussed thus far was inherently academic and directed toward a scientific audience. However, clinical and public health research impacts more than scientists, and therefore researchers should engage the public via popular press or other means in coordination with their institutions' media relations group. Some general medical journals frequently cited in popular press, for example the *Journal of the American Medical Association* and *Nature*, include talking points or similar summaries that represent clear and concise implications of the work, useful for quoting in popular press. Unfortunately, popular

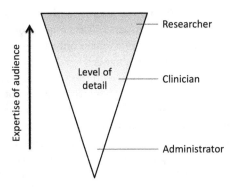

Figure 13.7 Relationship between audience and detail.

press routinely cite select medical journals (Suleski & Ibaraki, 2010), and therefore may be largely unaware of the majority of EHR research. To communicate with a broader audience will take a concerted effort on the part of the researcher and their institution.

For example, many print and online newspapers have health and science sections that could serve as a potential venue for engaging the public. Contacting editors or writers and expressing interest is the first step. Outside of more established channels, writing for health-related websites, blogs, or social media is a straightforward way of reaching a broader, and perhaps younger, audience, and can be undertaken by any researcher (Kapp, Hensel & Schnoring, 2015). The goal of using non-traditional communication channels is to disseminate research to a wider audience.

We all consume data differently. As the target audience broadens and consequently has less expertise, the level of detail correspondingly decreases (Figure 13.7). The researcher will be interested in understanding the study design, analytic methods, statistical results, and potential issues of internal and external validity. The clinician will be focus on the results and their application for treatment and prognosis. Meanwhile decision makers at the executive levels, such as hospital administrators or policymakers, respond to visual representations of the data that are easily digestible, and often require distilled high-level executive summaries of the data instead of the traditional scientific publication. Brownson et al. (2018) provided an overview of approaches for health science communication relevant for clinical and public health researchers. Tables 1 and 2 in Brownson et al. summarize the level of information needed for varied audiences and recommendations and tools for dissemination to nonacademic audiences, respectively.

Other methods of health communication

Presentation of data as figures or tables is commonplace in traditional scientific communications, yet these are static visuals. They do not allow the consumer to interact with the data, such as exploring population stratifications or varying underlying assumptions. By moving toward interactive, non-static representation of the data, consumers will be able to ask real-time questions such as "How does adherence to this quality measure change when only applied toward women?" or "only applied to people in a certain age range?" or "with a certain comorbidity?" without relying on the researchers to update the results and re-run the analyses. The question may no longer be "what is statistically significant?" but rather "what is of biggest interest to your audience?"

These kinds of questions can be addressed with interactive data visualization tools that are becoming commonplace in quality, performance, and process improvement projects, as well as policy and planning activities (Ghazisaeidi et al., 2015). These tools create data visualization dashboards that provide a snapshot or longitudinal view of high-dimensional aggregate data using various types of interactive graphics and plots. While the level of coding and programming necessary to produce these dashboards is a barrier, software is available such as Tableau (Tableau Software, Seattle, WA) or, for R users, Shiny (RStudio, Boston, MA) that will automate the process.

The use of information graphics (a.k.a. "infographic") for summarizing public and clinical health concerns or interventions has advanced over the years with the availability of free software to create the infographic and the ubiquity of social media (Stewart, 2021). Infographics are an effective way to convey complex health-related data through graphic form (Otten, Cheng & Drewnoski, 2015). As the American Planning Association, a collaboration of the U.S. Centers for Disease Control and Prevention and American Public Health Association, states, the strategic use of infographics is of greatest benefit "when the message is more visual in nature and requires more than data or charts to communicate successfully to the target audience" (American Planning Association, 2022). Figure 13.8 is an example infographic created by the Office of the National Coordinator for Health Information Technology that presents the evolution of EHRs and their perceived impact on health and healthcare in the U.S. Ultimately, the researcher needs to consider who their audience is, what the core message is to promote, and how to best achieve it.

Open and transparent EHR research

Improving the quality, rigor, and impact of EHR-based research requires an open and transparent science. This means a full disclosure of research materials, assumptions, and decisions so that others may properly assess the merits and shortcomings of a particular analysis. Science is a self-correcting process: as knowledge accumulates over time, hypotheses are refuted or refined. The speed and ability to do this is related to transparent science. Others have described the so-called replication crisis that exists in epidemiology (Lash, Collin & Van Dyke, 2018). In the context of EHR research, replicability[5] is the ability to arrive at the same results for the same research question using different EHR data. A reproducible finding would hold regardless of the EHR – assuming there is internal and external validity – and thus provide greater evidence of the measure

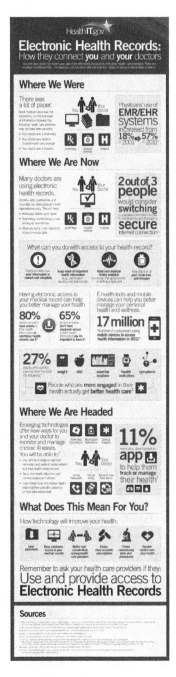

Figure 13.8 Example infographic that presents the evolution of EHRs and how they will impact health and healthcare in the U.S. A full-size version is available at the following website: https://www.Healthit.gov/infographic/electronic-health-records-infographic.

of disease burden or the impact of an exposure or intervention (Reeves et al., 2014). Indeed, reproducible findings are one of the tenets of causal inference (see Chapter 11).

For studies that rely on secondary analysis of healthcare data, including EHRs and claims databases, reproducibility should be viable when the same data are available. In a reproducibility study of 40 studies from 31 publications derived from longitudinal healthcare databases, Wang et al. (2016) largely achieved the goal of reproducing the results with a high degree of accuracy, although this may be more of testament to the ability of the reproducibility team. The authors noted three challenges that are addressable, including reporting of the (1) codes to operationalize the outcomes, covariates, and inclusion/exclusion criteria, (2) decisions made to operationalize covariates that are not dependent on codes, such as calculations or groupings, and (3) timing of cohort entry, inclusion criteria, covariate assessment period, or enrollment period in the original study.

Other studies have had mixed results. Bartlett et al. (2019) evaluated whether 220 clinical trials published in seven leading general medical journals could be replicated using EHR data: in other words, were the "intervention, indication, inclusion and exclusion criteria, and primary end points" available as discrete elements in the EHR or insurance claims data? Optimistically, they calculated that 15% of clinical trials may be replicable using EHR data. Seesaghur et al. (2021) conducted a reproducibility study using EHR data comparing analytic approaches, concluding that transparency in raw data processing, study design and operational decisions, and analytic choices are crucial for reproducible research. Similar conclusions were reached by Goldstein et al. (2020) who noted four challenges in reproducing study findings based on the methods description that accompanies a published scientific article, namely (1) the difficulty in moving from raw data to analytic data, (2) the implicit nature of many methodological assumptions, (3) an overreliance on citations to convey critical information, and (4) lack of a clear definition as to what reproducible should mean.

Despite guidelines such as STROBE and RECORD (described earlier) that help to standardize the process of reporting observational EHR research, some have argued that researchers lack the tools and methods to enact such recommendations (Denaxas et al., 2017), and EHR research has been hampered by lack of adherence to these guidelines (Langan et al., 2013). As such, there are calls for applications of software engineering principles to standardize data creation, develop libraries of analytic approaches, and improve coding and documentation practices to enable reproducible EHR research (Denaxas et al., 2017).

These and other recommendations to improve EHR research largely focus on transparency in data management and analysis as opposed to data sharing, given the private and sensitive nature of EHR data. For examples, researchers have used or created repositories to share clinical codes and phenotypes (Richesson et al., 2021; Springate et al., 2014), data operationalization code for open-source EHRs (Johnson et al., 2018), and computational codes for epidemiologic analysis (Goldstein, 2018). Existing and emerging approaches are available to securely share EHR data via blockchain technology (Dubovitskaya et al., 2020;

Glicksberg et al., 2020) or the Health Insurance Portability and Accountability Act's Privacy Rule (Malin, Benitez & Masys, 2011), as well as decoupling data from analysis (Goldstein & Sarwate, 2016) such as differential privacy (Ficek et al., 2021).

Open-source epidemiology

Many of the underlying questions about methodological, statistical, and data assumptions can be resolved by releasing the original computational codes, known as open-source epidemiology (Goldstein, 2018). There are four main benefits to releasing code: (1) transparency, (2) reproducibility, (3) advancement of methods, and (4) education. The following serves as a how-to guide for researchers interested in releasing their computational codes as part of the publication process using a no-cost solution using two data sharing platforms: GitHub (Microsoft Corporation, Redmond, WA) to store the analytic codes themselves and Zenodo (European Organization for Nuclear Research, Geneve, Switzerland) to obtain a digital object identifier (DOI), which serves as a persistent unique identifier for referencing the code in the manuscript. Free accounts are needed on both GitHub and Zenodo.[6]

Before releasing code, any proprietary or personal information should be redacted and the code prepared according to scientific computing best practices (Wilson et al., 2017). Providing the citation to the published or in-progress manuscript at the top of the source code will link the source code to related publications. Any code released into the public domain should carry an open-source license; the MIT license is the simplest and most permissive, although if the code being released inherits other code, a GPL license may be more appropriate. Researchers may wish to consult with their Institutional Review Board or General Counsel prior to releasing any study materials.

The first step to releasing code is to create a new code repository on GitHub. Having separate repositories per publication allows for a clean mapping from the published work to the underlying analysis. On GitHub, fill in the required information for a new repository, make it publicly accessible, and add an open-source license as appropriate. Within this newly created repository, upload the analytic code source files and any ancillary data to share, such as fitted statistical models, simulated or de-identified datasets, codebooks, survey instruments, etc.

Next, on Zenodo, navigate to the GitHub page under Home > Account and toggle the switch to ON for any repository on GitHub that needs a citable DOI. Back on GitHub, create a release for the repository, which is a snapshot of the files at that point in time. When creating a release, be sure to name the release in a meaningful fashion for example, by using the publication title as the release title or adding the manuscript citation in the description. One may also choose to designate the release a "pre-release" to identify that a manuscript is currently under review and not published. Finally, on Zenodo, click the "Synch now" button toward the top of the GitHub page: your repository will now have a citable DOI associated with it. This DOI can be placed in the methods section of the manuscript, for example, by saying "Analytic codes are available for download from..."

The peer review process creates additional complications for managing publicly released code, as the researcher will need to create a new release for each iteration of the manuscript and corresponding code. On Zenodo, each release creates a new DOI and this identifier needs to be updated in the revised manuscript to correctly associate the code with the performed analysis. However, once the manuscript is accepted for publication, a final release is needed that is not designated a "pre-release." The DOI can be updated one final time during the page-proofing process.

Notes

1 Librarian Jeffrey Beall compiled a list of predatory publishers and journals, available at https://beallslist.net. Researchers are highly encouraged to consult this list prior to publishing. Another good source to consult is the index of journals cited in PubMed: https://www.nlm.nih.gov/bsd/serfile_addedinfo.html. However, this list is not foolproof as researchers may deposit articles in PubMed Central for journals that have not been scrutinized.

2 SpringerNature: https://journalsuggester.springer.com. Elsevier: https://journalfinder.elsevier.com.

3 Users of R may refer to this blog post that details the creation of publication ready graphics: https://www.goldsteinepi.com/blog/publicationreadygraphicsinr/index.html.

4 Work completed by U.S. government employees is usually exempt from this copyright transfer.

5 The terms replication and reproducibility are used interchangeably in this book, although to be true to their original definitions, reproducibility refers to the same data source, whereas replicability refers to different data sources.

6 See this article for configuration instructions for the corresponding Zenodo account: https://docs.github.com/en/repositories/archiving-a-github-repository/referencing-and-citing-content.

References

American Planning Association. Centers for Disease Control and Prevention. https://planning.org (accessed August 15, 2022).

Añazco D, Nicolalde B, Espinosa I, Camacho J, Mushtaq M, Gimenez J, Teran E. Publication rate and citation counts for preprints released during The COVID-19 pandemic: The good, the bad and the ugly. PeerJ. 2021;9:e10927.

Bartlett VL, Dhruva SS, Shah ND, Ryan P, Ross JS. Feasibility of using real-world data to replicate clinical trial evidence. JAMA Netw Open. 2019;2(10):e1912869.

Brownson RC, Eyler AA, Harris JK, Moore JB, Tabak RG. Getting the word out: New approaches for disseminating public health science. J Public Health Manag Pract. 2018;24(2):102–111.

Chalmers I. Underreporting research is scientific misconduct. JAMA. 1990;263(10):1405–1408.

Denaxas S, Direk K, Gonzalez-Izquierdo A, Pikoula M, Cakiroglu A, Moore J, Hemingway H, Smeeth L. Methods for enhancing the reproducibility of biomedical research findings using electronic health records. BioData Min. 2017;10:31.

Dubovitskaya A, Baig F, Xu Z, Shukla R, Zambani PS, Swaminathan A, Jahangir MM, Chowdhry K, Lachhani R, Idnani N, Schumacher M, Aberer K, Stoller SD, Ryu S, Wang F. ACTION-EHR: Patient-centric blockchain-based electronic health record data management for cancer care. J Med Internet Res. 2020;22(8):e13598.

Ficek J, Wang W, Chen H, Dagne G, Daley E. Differential privacy in health research: A scoping review. J Am Med Inform Assoc. 2021;28(10):2269–2276.

Ghazisaeidi M, Safdari R, Torabi M, Mirzaee M, Farzi J, Goodini A. Development of performance dashboards in healthcare sector: Key practical issues. Acta Inform Med. 2015;23(5):317–321.

Glicksberg BS, Burns S, Currie R, Griffin A, Wang ZJ, Haussler D, Goldstein T, Collisson E. Blockchain-authenticated sharing of genomic and clinical outcomes data of patients with cancer: A prospective cohort study. J Med Internet Res. 2020;22(3):e16810.

Goldstein ND. Toward open-source epidemiology. Epidemiology. 2018;29(2):161–164.

Goldstein ND, Hamra GB, Harper S. Are descriptions of methods alone sufficient for study reproducibility? An example from the cardiovascular literature. Epidemiology. 2020;31(2):184–188.

Goldstein ND, Sarwate AD. Privacy, security, and the public health researcher in the era of electronic health record research. Online J Public Health Inform. 2016;8(3):e207.

Johnson AE, Stone DJ, Celi LA, Pollard TJ. The MIMIC code repository: Enabling reproducibility in critical care research. J Am Med Inform Assoc. 2018;25(1):32–39.

Kapp JM, Hensel B, Schnoring KT. Is twitter a forum for disseminating research to health policy makers? Ann Epidemiol. 2015;25(12):883–887.

Langan SM, Benchimol EI, Guttmann A, Moher D, Petersen I, Smeeth L, Sørensen HT, Stanley F, Von Elm E. Setting the RECORD straight: Developing a guideline for the REporting of studies conducted using observational routinely collected data. Clin Epidemiol. 2013;5:29–31.

Lash TL, Collin LJ, Van Dyke ME. The replication crisis in epidemiology: Snowball, snow job, or winter solstice? Curr Epidemiol Rep. 2018;5(2):175–183.

Malin B, Benitez K, Masys D. Never too old for anonymity: A statistical standard for demographic data sharing via the HIPAA privacy rule. J Am Med Inform Assoc. 2011;18(1):3–10.

Otten JJ, Cheng K, Drewnowski A. Infographics and public policy: Using data visualization to convey complex information. Health Aff (Millwood). 2015;34(11):1901–1907.

Reeves D, Springate DA, Ashcroft DM, Ryan R, Doran T, Morris R, Olier I, Kontopantelis E. Can analyses of electronic patient records be independently and externally validated? The effect of statins on the mortality of patients with ischaemic heart disease: A cohort study with nested case-control analysis. BMJ Open. 2014;4(4):e004952.

Richesson RL, Wiley LK, Gold S, Rasmussen L. Finding Existing Phenotype Definitions. In: Rethinking Clinical Trials: A Living Textbook of Pragmatic Clinical Trials. Bethesda, MD: NIH Health Care Systems Research Collaboratory. Available at: https://rethinkingclinicaltrials.org/chapters/conduct/electronic-health-records-based-phenotyping/finding-existing-phenotype-definitions/. Updated September 23, 2021.

Seesaghur A, Petruski-Ivleva N, Banks V, Wang JR, Mattox P, Hoeben E, Maskell J, Neasham D, Reynolds SL, Kafatos G. Real-world reproducibility study characterizing patients newly diagnosed with multiple myeloma using clinical practice research datalink, a UK-based electronic health records database. Pharmacoepidemiol Drug Saf. 2021;30(2):248–256.

Springate DA, Kontopantelis E, Ashcroft DM, Olier I, Parisi R, Chamapiwa E, Reeves D. ClinicalCodes: An online clinical codes repository to improve the validity and reproducibility of research using electronic medical records. PLoS One. 2014;9(6):e99825.

Stewart C. The best infographic maker in 2021. https://www.creativebloq.com/infographic/tools-2131971 (accessed December 2, 2021), 2021.

Suleski J, Ibaraki M. Scientists are talking, but mostly to each other: A quantitative analysis of research represented in mass media. Public Underst Sci 2010;19(1):115e25.

Vandenbroucke JP, von Elm E, Altman DG, Gøtzsche PC, Mulrow CD, Pocock SJ, Poole C, Schlesselman JJ, Egger M, STROBE Initiative. Strengthening the reporting of observational studies in epidemiology (STROBE): Explanation and elaboration. PLoS Med. 2007 Oct 16;4(10):e297.

Wang SV, Verpillat P, Rassen JA, Patrick A, Garry EM, Bartels DB. Transparency and reproducibility of observational cohort studies using large healthcare databases. Clin Pharmacol Ther. 2016;99(3):325–32.

Wilson G, Bryan J, Cranston K, Kitzes J, Nederbragt L, Teal TK. Good enough practices in scientific computing. PLoS Comput Biol. 2017;13(6):e1005510.

14 Applications of Electronic Health Record Research

This penultimate chapter focuses on applications of EHR research. Our goal is not the construction of a research database or analytic dataset, the finding of a significant p-value, or the creation of a publication or scientific presentation. The goal of EHR research is to positively impact, whether directly or indirectly, health and healthcare using the EHR as a source of data. Implicit in this discussion is how results move beyond a single EHR study to inform public health or clinical guidelines. There is an inherent tension between the individual and public, and we must reconcile this in EHR research. What the best answer is for an individual may be different than the public. For example, we could use EHR data to inform estimates about disease prevalence or risk factors for outcomes, which, at a population level, is less critical to "get right": in other words, some error in our research is acceptable. On the other hand, if we use EHR data to predict individual risk, such as the risk of a bad outcome or the prognosis of a good outcome from a given intervention, there is less flexibility for us to arrive at the wrong answer: errors need to be more precise. So, how do we assess health at a population level from the EHR? Surveillance, a core function of public health, utilizes EHRs as one of many data streams to assess population health, and our conversation begins with success stories of using EHR data to improve health and healthcare. Then, we will visit how these surveillance systems work in practice using EHR data. Finally, we will explore the tension in EHR research, understanding the individual role, how clinical and public health does not always benefit the individual, and further, why this is not a prerequisite for successful EHR research.

Success stories using EHR data

Chapter 1 introduced several examples of how EHR data improve public health. The public health value in aggregating EHR data in real-time and large-scale ways has aided in identification of lead poisoning of children in Flint, Michigan (Hanna-Attisha, LaChance & Sadler, 2016), and real-time surveillance for COVID-19 (Burke et al., 2021). Let us explore both successes in more detail.

The lead-contaminated water episode in Flint, Michigan, received national attention in the U.S. By way of a brief background, the city of Flint – an impoverished area with poor health outcomes – switched water supplies from Lake

DOI: 10.4324/9781003258872-18

Huron to the Flint River in 2016 while awaiting a new pipeline to Lake Huron. This was done as a temporary, cost-saving measure. Shortly thereafter, residents noted a change in their tap water's color, taste, and odor, and subsequent tests confirmed presence of bacteria, including *Escherichia coli*, and lead in the water. Using data from their institutional EHR – Epic (Epic Systems Corporation, Verona, WI) – researchers observed a marked difference in the incidence of elevated blood lead levels, from 2.4% to 4.9%, post water source change (Hanna-Attisha et al., 2016). As the lead author, Hanna-Attisha stated in an interview, "If we did not have Epic, if we did not have [the EHR], if we were still on paper, it would have taken forever to get these results" (Walburg, 2016). The study design was a pre–post retrospective analysis of EHR data among 1,473 children less than five years of age who had a blood lead level test between January 1, 2013 to September 15, 2013 (pre-period) and January 1, 2015 to September 15, 2015 (post-period). The EHR data were geocoded and linked to Census data to create neighborhood-level deprivation scores. Spatial interpolation was performed to visualize continuous changes in blood lead levels across the city. Despite the dramatic findings, reflecting on issues of validity and accuracy of EHR data discussed elsewhere in this book, there are some limitations to the analysis. The catchment of this EHR may not reflect a random sample of the population of children in the city, but rather a systematically skewed sampled. Further, the availability of blood lead levels may further skew this sample toward higher-risk children. Importantly, they were able to corroborate their EHR findings with health department programmatic screening.

Capturing worldwide attention was the COVID-19 pandemic. During the early pandemic period in the first half of 2020, testing capacity was scaling up, coupled with issues in the assay itself. Due to mandated shutdown orders, healthcare began to rely on virtual telehealth visits for many non-emergent cases. Researchers from the Cleveland Clinic in Ohio noted this increased demand for virtual visits and posited that documentation in their EHR – Epic (Epic Systems Corporation, Verona, WI) – could be used for COVID-19 surveillance and reporting (Burke et al., 2021). By modifying their clinical note template to capture the clinical and epidemiologic criteria in the Council for State and Territorial Epidemiologists COVID-19 case definition, these data could be extracted in near-real time (within 24 hours) via their data warehouse for public health reporting as probable cases. For a one-week period in April 2020, 526 patients had a virtual visit for COVID-19 of whom 218 (41%) met the criteria for probable COVID-19 and were reported to the health department. For comparison, during the same one-week period, 353 cases of laboratory-confirmed COVID-19 were diagnosed in the Cleveland Clinic system. The authors noted that the EHR "enabled us to easily find and report additional cases [specifically, a 62% increase] to public health authorities for investigation." Such a study demonstrates how EHR data can be used for real-time research and reporting.

There are, of course, many other examples of success stories using EHR data. The U.S. Agency for Healthcare Research and Quality (AHRQ) Digital Healthcare Research Program aims to "produce and disseminate evidence about how the evolving digital healthcare ecosystem can best advance the quality, safety, and effectiveness of healthcare for patients and their families" (Agency for Healthcare Research and Quality, 2022a). AHRQ has touted several EHR-relevant research projects funded under this program that demonstrated a positive impact on healthcare outcomes, including natural language processing for cervical cancer decision support, electronic outcomes-based emergency department triage, postoperative risk assessment clinical decision support, poison control information exchange, and the economics of EHR implementation (Agency for Healthcare Research and Quality, 2022b). The Office of the National Coordinator for Health Information Technology has also compiled a list of success stories, including EHR-based projects that have integrated population health tools, improved reporting tools, identified patients eligible for clinical trials, monitored and optimized performance metrics, sepsis prediction at an earlier and treatable stage, and mining clinical knowledge in pathology reports, among others (Office of the National Coordinator for Health Information Technology, 2022).

EHRs for public health surveillance

Historically, most public health surveillance programs have been conducted passively through state or local notifiable disease reporting systems. Active surveillance has occurred less frequently, typically employed in response to a public health concern, such as influenza monitoring in emergency departments during a severe season, or outbreak investigations for communicable or infectious diseases. Such traditional surveillance systems rely on data obtained from death certificates, epidemic and case reporting, outbreak and field investigations, laboratory reporting, health surveys, environmental monitoring, and registries (Declich & Carter, 1994). Passive surveillance utilizing existing data streams is comparatively easy to perform and has few technical requirements, especially in the case of paper or faxed case reports. On the other hand, this type of surveillance is not real time, suffers from data quality issues, and is incomplete due to missing cases. To supplement traditional reporting systems, newer data sources are being used for disease surveillance. Automated electronic laboratory reporting has been shown to increase the timeliness and completeness of surveillance for notifiable diseases (Overhage, Grannis & McDonald, 2008). The use of healthcare billing and claims records, internet, social media, other digital sources outside of the health domain, veterinary and environmental databases built upon the One Health model, and, of course, EHRs can help improve the timeliness, completeness, and accuracy of disease surveillance (McNabb et al., 2017). For example, compared to traditional surveillance activities, EHR data have improved the assessment of the HIV care continuum (Arey et al., 2019) and COVID-19 vaccination outreach (Bonham-Werling et al., 2021).

Spurred on by "meaningful use" (see Chapter 1), the use of information technology services improves surveillance efforts through several mechanisms (Birkhead, Klompas & Shah, 2015; McNabb et al., 2017). First, data are automatically shared and synchronized with surveillance systems. This data sharing can be bidirectional to also update providers on active public health threats, diagnostic or treatment recommendations, and general guidance. Second, the data are readily analyzable through pre-programmed reports or custom queries. Third and related, the data and analyses occur real time, which is especially important in a public health emergency as exemplified by the COVID-19 pandemic. Lastly, the availability of large-scale electronic data enables advanced approaches to field epidemiology, such as the use of machine learning algorithms and artificial intelligence to flag anomalies or patterns in the data. One such demonstration of this last point is the Centers for Disease Control and Prevention's (CDC) Epidemic Prediction Initiative that extrapolates and predicts disease epidemics for COVID-19, West Nile virus and other vector-borne illnesses, and influenza (Centers for Disease Control and Prevention, 2022a).

Despite these advantages, significant hurdles remain, such as the large capital expenditures and expertise necessary to build and maintain these systems, concerns over data privacy and security, and lack of widespread adoption (McNabb et al., 2017). Kruse et al. (2018) identified 13 facilitator and barriers to the use of EHRs for supporting population health among 55 reviewed articles, summarized in Table 14.1. While the mention of facilitators outweighed barriers 3–2 in the reviewed articles, data quality and integrity were commonly expressed concerns. This finding was corroborated by Aliabadi, Sheikhtaheri and Ansari (2020), who reviewed 49 articles and noted that data quality was the second most common challenge for the development and implementation of EHR-based surveillance, behind investment of finances, time, and resources. Other EHR specific concerns identified in their review include difficulty in using unstructured data and

Table 14.1 Facilitators and barriers of EHR-enabled population health as reported in the biomedical literature

Facilitator[a]	Barrier[a]
1. Productivity/efficiency	1. Missing data/data error
2. Quality	2. No standards
3. Data management	3. Productivity loss
4. Surveillance	4. Technology complex
5. Preventative care	5. Cost
6. Communication	6. Decreased quality
7. Interoperability	7. Limited staff support
8. Decision support	8. Resistance to change
9. Health outcomes	9. Human error
10. Satisfaction	10. Accessibility/utilization
11. Financial assistance	11. Disease management
12. Ease of use	12. Critical thinking/treatment decisions
13. Current technology	13. Privacy concerns

[a] Ordered from most common to least common among 55 reviewed articles.

inadequate population coverage. A summary of all challenges and recommended solutions may be found in Tables 2 and 3 in Aliabadi et al. (2020) – many of these have been covered in detail elsewhere in this book.

EHR-supplemented public health surveillance may be used for syndromic, pharmaco-, and notifiable disease surveillance. *Syndromic surveillance* operates through documented sign and symptoms in the medical record (but may also include diagnoses and other ancillary information); *pharmaco-surveillance* is obtained from prescription and medication data, vaccinations, or device safety monitoring; and *notifiable disease surveillance* is abstracted from diagnoses and discharge reports. For notifiable diseases in the U.S., the CDC's National Electronic Disease Surveillance System enables individual healthcare providers or systems to send reports to local, state, and federal (i.e., CDC) public health authorities via an electronic message using HL7 (National Electronic Disease Surveillance System Working Group, 2001). There are similar calls for national disease-specific – but not traditionally notifiable – surveillance system using EHRs (Williams et al., 2022) with examples underway for chronic diseases (Kraus et al., 2022) including diabetes (DiCAYA, 2022). Also at a national level, syndromic surveillance occurs in the U.S. via the BioSense Platform of the CDC's National Syndromic Surveillance Program (Gould, Walker & Yoon, 2017). BioSense captures EHR data in the form of free text chief complaints, demographics, vital signs, and diagnostic and procedure codes.

There are several applied examples in the literature of syndromic surveillance from EHRs. Based on drug overdose-related emergency department visits in the U.S., researchers have noted that discharge data may provide a more accurate measure of overdose burden while syndromic data may better capture real-time clusters and changes (Vivolo-Kantor, Smith & Scholl, 2021). According to the authors, "syndromic data alone may lead to overestimation of burden in certain communities, and is not the intended purpose of syndromic data, whereas relying on discharge data alone may lead to underestimation of burden," but both data sources play a complementary role. In Ontario, Canada, syndromic surveillance for respiratory diseases using chief complaint data from the emergency department EHR was validated against (1) a discharge-based reporting system using billing codes and (2) a telehealth nurse triage helpline (van-Dijk et al., 2009). The researchers noted considerable overlap between the chief complaint with the two comparison conditions, suggesting that real-time EHR data can be used for syndromic surveillance as compared to the time-lagged data. This surveillance endeavor has expanded into the Acute Care Enhanced Surveillance (ACES) system that covers 95% of Ontario's acute care hospitals and relies on data from both emergency department visits as well as inpatient admissions (KFL&A Public Health, 2022). Real-time communicable and non-communicable data for 84 distinct syndromes are collected via ACES, and respiratory spatial surveillance maps are shared publicly via their website.[1] In the U.S., the CDC's Outpatient Influenza-like Illness Surveillance Network receives data from EHRs across the U.S. to monitor for symptoms of fever, cough, or sore throat (Centers for Disease Control and Prevention, 2022b). As with ACES, data are also publicly available via an interactive website.[2] Advantages to syndromic surveillance from EHRs include early detection of clusters, ability to rapidly characterize outbreaks, and perform quick investigations. Disadvantages may include false alarms (low specificity), failure to detect outbreaks (low sensitivity), and technical expertise required.

In one of the more well-known case studies of EHR-enabled surveillance, the Massachusetts Department of Public Health, in collaboration with Harvard University and the U.S. CDC, has created a surveillance system – MDPHNet – that allows public health to initiate queries against participating practices' EHRs while protecting patient privacy and data security, as the data remain behind the practices' firewalls. There are several components to the overall system. PopMedNet is the controlled access to EHR data for partners via a distributed network, ESP-net is an open-source epidemiological application that automatically queries Pop-MedNet for public health surveillance including notifiable diseases and syndromic surveillance, and RiskScape is the interactive web-based data visualization system (Cocoros et al., 2021; Vogel et al., 2014). MDPHNet provides surveillance data on a variety of infectious and non-infectious diseases, controlled substances and other medication prescriptions, and laboratory testing. Unlike the other examples described earlier, MDPHNet is not publicly available, although the platform's source code is open source.[3] Additional communicable and chronic disease EHR surveillance examples may be found in Birkhead, Klompas, and Shah (2015) and Willis et al. (2019).

As mentioned earlier, the EHR public health surveillance tools described are not necessarily complete for their catchment areas – for example, MDPHNet covers approximately 20% of the state population (Cocoros et al., 2021) – and as such, the representativeness of these data may be skewed to participating practices or sicker patients. These systems can be contrasted to traditional health information exchanges (HIEs; see Chapter 4), that provide a longitudinal patient-level view of patient health regardless of healthcare providers. For example, the Commonwealth of Massachusetts HIE – Mass HIway – provides patient-level data for all healthcare systems in Massachusetts; importantly, the governing regulations exclude nursing homes, dental clinics, behavioral health entities, small medical ambulatory practices, and solo practices (Commonwealth of Massachusetts, 2021). While the HIE may provide a more complete view of a population than the EHR-enabled surveillance systems, it is not perfect, and the data may also not be accessible to researchers. Further, when examining aggregate data, ecological fallacy may occur if inference is applied on an individual level (Greenland, 2001). Catchment is further discussed in Chapter 6.

Concluding salvo

There is an inherent dichotomy between clinical and public health practitioners. The clinician serves as the health advocate for their patients, while public health serves as the health advocate of their populations. Public health speaks in terms of net or average effects from an intervention, while a patient is particularly concerned only with their benefit. Sometimes this can lead to a conflict between the two with a patient questioning why a particular treatment, or behavior modification, did not have an apparent effect. For example, smoking is the leading cause of lung cancer (National Cancer Institute, 2017), yet non-smoking patients can still get carcinomas of the lung, and some lifelong smokers will never get cancers. Therefore, the public's health cannot be examined from a single EHR observation or study.

What is public health?

Before delving further into this tension, let us define key terms. Public health is literally the health of populations of people. Health is not just being free of disease; it is defined by the World Health Organization as a state of complete physical, mental, and social well-being (World Health Organization, 1946). A population may be a town, city, or county (local health departments), an entire state (state health departments), or the entire country (the U.S. CDC). A population may also be defined by subset of people with a shared characteristic in one of these geographies, such as the population of Black women aged 45–50. Healthcare for populations does not occur in a clinical setting, but more often through law, policy, and regulations. Successes through this model include school entry mandatory vaccination, seatbelt laws, recommendations for diet and exercise, smoking cessation interventions, safe sex campaigns, screening for cancers, and social distancing and shelter in place orders during a pandemic (Centers for Disease Control and Prevention, 1999). By having enough people engage in these advised behaviors and lifestyles, the overall population will be healthier. Yet not everyone has agency or desire to adhere to these recommendations or requirements, and some factors may be immutable, such as family history of disease or the aging process.

Population health is measurable through aggregated markers, such as infant mortality and life expectancy. In fact, in the twentieth century life expectancy increased an average of 30 years; a truly remarkable feat of which much of the increase was attributable to public health interventions (Centers for Disease Control and Prevention, 1999). This does not mean that every individual born at the end of the twentieth century lived exactly 30 years longer than previous generations, but this introduces a paradox that arises from the way public health measures are conveyed: what happens at a population level may not be a marker for what happens at an individual level. From an ethics standpoint, public health typically operates under a utilitarianism perspective: the greatest good for the greatest number. Therein lies the well-established tension.

Individual versus public health

Individual health versus public health is not a new concept: a seminal paper discussed sick populations and sick individuals in 1985 (Rose, 1985). When a sick patient seeks guidance and treatment from a physician, often the physician will couch the therapy by saying "In most people, we expect to see..." It is clear from this statement that "most people" implies some population (or EHR) where the therapy was tested, and it may not exactly translate to the individual.

Epidemiologists are trained to be as precise as possible in measuring the risks associated with a behavior or condition, but, when disseminating the results, use imprecise language acknowledging this reality. We may be able to measure the increased risk in lung cancer associated with smoking as 83.4% ($\pm$3.7%) compared to a non-smoker, but we have no way of knowing with complete certainty which public health interventions will benefit which individuals. As implied earlier, there is a notion of altruism at play. If an individual does something that does not directly benefit them, we hope that it benefits someone else.

A lot of public health concerns, particularly infectious disease threats, are well studied and the interventions well known. If an individual chooses not to vaccinate or quarantine to prevent spread of SARS-CoV-2, they may be comfortable with the assumed risk for themselves, but this ignores the risk to others. Epidemiologists provide the evidence at a population level of these interventions. Public health hopes that individuals choose to vaccinate, practice safe sex, quit or never start smoking, and otherwise follow their guidance, but these interventions are not perfect, and the individual, who gets vaccinated, always uses a condom, and never smoked and may come down with COVID-19, has an unintended pregnancy and dies of lung cancer.

There is also a breadth of articles in scholarly literature discussing the tension between public health interventions and the role of individual choice (Gostin, 2005). Public health cannot legislate that having sex without a condom is illegal (although HIV criminalization laws infamously tried this; Harsono et al., 2017), but public health has many policies that are the result of legislation, such as school vaccination requirements. When policy is enacted through legislation, the public's welfare must override the individual's liberty to abstain from these interventions. Court cases that challenge these laws as a violation of Constitutional rights usually fail because these laws do not differentially impact any class or group of individuals. The overriding public interest of keeping the population healthy is paramount.

Challenges faced by public health

As mentioned earlier, individuals do not always have agency, incentive, or desire to adhere to public health recommendations. Perhaps these individuals would like to change but believe the recommendation will not benefit them, or view public health as a threat to their autonomy in decision making. The ability to change is not always an onus placed on individuals. As said in public health, place matters. Quitting smoking is exceedingly difficult when surrounded by other smokers. Living in an impoverished neighborhood or being forced to leave an existing neighborhood due to elevated costs of living associated with gentrification often results from a lack of autonomy and agency, perhaps because of systematic policies of oppression. Again, when turning to the literature, we see that individuals who move frequently or live in a neighborhood below the federal poverty line have worse health than their counterparts who have stable housing or live in a more affluent area (Diez Roux et al., 2017; Oishi & Schimmack, 2010). Public health interventions that improve the neighborhood, such as building playgrounds or a community greenspace, may face challenges if those areas contribute to crime or drug sales and use.

We also must acknowledge the potentially fickle nature of public health. Not only must an area be exceedingly devastated with a health problem, but it also most garner widespread attention before individuals gain agency. Post Hurricane Katrina, the Flint Michigan water crisis, and COVID-19, the initial response was underwhelming, and it was not until local organizations pushed through to the national spotlight that additional relief efforts became available. Many suffered and died during this time and perhaps this failing has led to a further rift and distrust between individuals and public health authorities.

Public health and science are fallible

The reality is public health is not a cure-all to societal ills. It represents the best knowledge about disease and other health conditions at a point in time. This changes as society and the science evolve. As has been said before, the hallmark of a good scientist is one who is willing to change their mind. At one point, science suggested that hormone replacement therapy in postmenopausal women may have been beneficial to reduce risk of heart disease. Then the Women's Health Initiative found it was harmful, increasing risk of certain cancers. Contemporary research seems to think it may be beneficial, but only within a certain segment of the population of women, namely, those perimenopausal and for a short duration of therapy (National Institutes of Health, 2016). As another example, public health messaging has largely shifted from fear-based negative ads to positive ads over the last few decades. Toward the beginning of the HIV/AIDS epidemic, public health ads were often criticized as stigmatizing (Fairchild et al., 2018). It was argued that these ads further exacerbated an already stigmatizing condition, leading to adverse health outcomes. As mentioned in Chapter 13, a host of recent studies have called to question many scientific findings as lacking reproducibility (Baker, 2016). But this does not mean we should abandon progress, defund science, or sow public distrust in scientific findings. Science is self-correcting over time, and we should not discard the advances of the previous century because public health does not always benefit the individual.

How scientific studies can lead to inconsistent evidence

Suppose we conduct a hypothetical study evaluating a COVID-19 vaccine. For the vaccine to be licensed or authorized for emergency use in the U.S., it must undergo thorough and rigorous scientific evaluation, ultimately approved by the Food & Drug Administration. Under the evidence-based medicine paradigm that scientific data are dogma for patient care, a randomized controlled trial must be conducted to establish the efficacy of the vaccine. In this trial, the vaccine will be compared to placebo. This trial is undertaken in a group of participants, the vaccine and placebo are administered at random, and the participants are monitored for incident illness.

Barring a perfect vaccine, we can reasonably expect that a proportion of people within each intervention group will become ill. In advance, we hypothesize the incidence will be greater in the placebo group, but we still expect nominal numbers in the vaccine group. Importantly, as the data are analyzed, the outcome measure becomes an average of each group's effects: the aggregated data trump the individual effect. Consequently, the vaccine may demonstrate efficacy in the majority, but there will be a minority who do not benefit or worse are harmed. This may have to do with individual genetics, social networks and contact with someone who is infected, low level or asymptomatic disease that was not diagnosed, or other myriad factors. Further, in this type of trial, the population recruited to participate may not be representative of the public. It is well known that clinical trials often fail to adequately include minority groups (Food & Drug Administration, 2021).

In contrast to this contrived clinical trial, under a paradigm known as reality-based medicine, we may observationally follow a group of people through the EHR. As investigators we do not manipulate who was vaccinated and who was not, rather we allowed people to naturally select vaccination, as occurs in society outside of the experimental model. This reality-based medicine paradigm may be preferred evidence as to the public health benefits from vaccination, because ideally, we want people to voluntarily choose a public health intervention, not be coerced into it, and we want the participants to be representative of society. Yet as compared to the randomized clinical trial, under this observational study we are likely to see differing performance from the vaccine: the notion of vaccine efficacy versus effectiveness. Individuals who choose to be vaccinated likely engage in other health seeking behaviors and are thus at lower risk of acquiring infectious diseases. The data are aggregated as before to arrive at population-level estimates.

Importantly, under both paradigms, the studies show that vaccination works in some proportion of people (the measure of efficacy or effectiveness), implying that in some *other* proportion of people (one minus the measure of efficacy or effectiveness) the vaccine did not work. If the signal from the vaccinated group is strong enough, that is, if the vaccine appeared to confer adequate protection with minimal risks, the vaccine will be approved for use and promoted as a tool in the public health toolbox.

From the public health perspective, the vaccine works. After real-world data are aggregated, such as from the EHR, there will be demonstrable evidence that among those who chose vaccination, there were fewer cases of COVID-19. Further, for those vaccinated who unfortunately fell ill, the intensity and course of the disease may be minimized. From the individual perspective, the effectiveness of the vaccine depends in part upon on how similar you are to the people under study from the clinical trial and in part how similar you are to the people from the real-world observational study. There may be a preponderance of evidence to suggest you will be protected after vaccination but there is no guarantee.

Who benefits from population health?

Most public health programs are built around the burden of disease at a population level. Surveillance efforts help direct health department allocation of funding; thus, common diseases receive more attention than rare diseases, unless the rare diseases are particularly lethal and contagious, such as Ebola. Public health interventions assume the average population effect and being the average individual will yield direct and tangible benefit. Even for those impacted by a rare disease, being in a healthier community will increase access to resources and availability of care, improve prognosis, and reduce disease sequalae. For example, abstaining from vaccination while living in a community with an overall high proportion of individuals vaccinated may offer protection. Place matters.

More provocatively, as was said in a book of the same name, having less medicine may yield more health (Welch, 2016). Some health interventions, such as population screening for diseases such as breast and colon cancers, have a downside to them: once an individual enters healthcare, they are likely to have a health problem discovered. This may result in unnecessary procedures, with all subsequent risk, monetary expenditure to the healthcare system, and the stress and anxiety of having a false-positive finding on one of these screening tests. As a population, we should not turn away from certain public health services, but we need to recognize they are imperfect.

We are all individuals as well as members of a community

For the EHR researcher, they may find themselves in both camps: clinical health and public health. Mervyn Susser, a professor of epidemiology, sought to bridge the two worlds when he wrote that "[d]espite the epidemiologist's insistence on studying populations, his ultimate concern is with health, disease, and death as it occurs in individuals" (Susser, 1973, p. 59). When discrepancies between the two arise, the interplay between the individual and community may not be immediately apparent. As an example, we can turn to the debate surrounding face masks for prevention of SARS-CoV-2 infection. An individual may be willing to take on a greater risk by not wearing a mask; however, if this individual is in a setting that has a high likelihood of exposure, such as in a healthcare environment, they may place others at risk. As another example we can consider motorcycle helmet laws. While some may maintain this decision only affects themselves, and they are willing to take the risk, there are downstream community implications of this decision. Should this individual be injured while riding, there are potentially substantial costs incurred to the healthcare and insurance systems, where risk is managed through pools of individuals in the community.

Dispassionate scientists or scientist-advocates

This book will not weigh in on the debate of the role of the scientist: researchers may elect to operate under either position. Rather, let us dissect the role of the individual in EHR research. How much can be accomplished by an individual depends on motivation, scope, and funding. Building a research database from a single institutional EHR is possible by an individual, but this book does not necessarily advocate for this approach (see Chapter 1). Rather, the individual's role may be to oversee the entire process as the principal investigator, or to handle discrete components, such as the data management or analysis. Regardless of the role, having the knowledge of data extraction, linkage, and epidemiological modeling will minimize possible errors and maximize research validity.

Researchers who wish to move beyond knowledge generation may engage in *translational epidemiology*. Khoury, Gwinn and Ioannidis (2010) identified four phases of translational epidemiology that occur after the core research has concluded:

Phase 1. *Applications.* Moving from risk factors to identifying potential interventions to mitigate poor health outcomes.

Phase 2. *Guidelines.* Assessing public health interventions with recommendations for practice guidelines.

Phase 3. *Practice.* Once guidelines are created, determining their adherence in practice.

Phase 4. *Outcomes.* Population health changes because of practiced guidelines.

These four phases emphasize the transition of epidemiology from the academic role of knowledge generation into the pragmatic role of knowledge application. Under this perspective, the individual's role does not conclude at knowledge generation. The individual's role is to see that these data are used appropriately and have a meaningful impact. Translational epidemiology requires additional skills beyond study design, measurement, analysis, and causal inference. Dowdy and Pai (2012) suggest the epidemiologist serves as the "accountable health advocate" and focuses on expanding the core research skill of the following:

- *Communication.* Move away from the traditional paradigm of communicating only to a scientific audience. Instead, engage a lay audience through popular press, social media, and novel channels, to convey results of research. This was discussed in Chapter 13.
- *Perspective.* Focus on existing knowledge to improve public or clinical health through translational epidemiology, as much as traditional knowledge generation.
- *Advocacy.* Synthesize previous research to identify trends, incorporate into guidelines, and study the health impact in clinical or public populations.

Some researchers may choose to participate in direct community engagement moving from advocacy to activism. For example, at the dawn of the AIDS epidemic in the U.S., many scientists joined in with grassroots community organizations to fight for discovery of the virus and treatment, and to mitigate stigma in the marginalized groups devastated by the disease. Regardless of the position we ultimately take, the first step in effecting change in health and healthcare is by forming an evidence base, and this book has strived to identify the strengths and weaknesses of using EHR data for this purpose.

Notes

1 https://mapper.kflaphi.ca/respmapper/
2 https://gis.cdc.gov/grasp/fluview/fluportaldashboard.html
3 https://www.esphealth.org

References

Agency for Healthcare Research and Quality. Digital Healthcare Research Home. https://digital.ahrq.gov (accessed August 18, 2022), 2022a.

Agency for Healthcare Research and Quality. Success Stories. https://digital.ahrq.gov/program-overview/success-stories (accessed August 18, 2022), 2022b.

Aliabadi A, Sheikhtaheri A, Ansari H. Electronic health record-based disease surveillance systems: A systematic literature review on challenges and solutions. J Am Med Inform Assoc. 2020;27(12):1977–1986.

Arey AL, Cassidy-Stewart H, Kurowski PL, Hitt JC, Flynn CP. Evaluating HIV surveillance completeness along the continuum of care: Supplementing surveillance with health center data to increase HIV data to care efficiency. J Acquir Immune Defic Syndr. 2019;82(Suppl 1):S26–S32.

Baker M. 1,500 scientists lift the lid on reproducibility. Nature. 2016;533(7604):452–454.

Birkhead GS, Klompas M, Shah NR. Uses of electronic health records for public health surveillance to advance public health. Annu Rev Public Health. 2015;36:345–359.

Bonham-Werling J, DeLonay AJ, Stephenson K, Hendricks KA, Bednarz L, Weiss JM, Gigot M, Smith MA. Using statewide electronic health record and influenza vaccination data to plan and prioritize COVID-19 vaccine outreach and communications in Wisconsin communities. Am J Public Health. 2021;111(12):2111–2114.

Burke PC, Shirley RB, Faiman M, Boose EW, Jones RW, Merlino A, Gordon SM, Fraser TG. Surveillance for probable COVID-19 using structured data in the electronic medical record. Infect Control Hosp Epidemiol. 2021;42(6):781–783.

Centers for Disease Control and Prevention. Ten great public health achievements–United States, 1900-1999. MMWR Morb Mortal Wkly Rep. 1999;48(12):241–243.

Centers for Disease Control and Prevention. About the Epidemic Prediction Initiative. https://predict.cdc.gov/about (accessed August 22, 2022), 2022a.

Centers for Disease Control and Prevention. U.S. Influenza Surveillance: Purpose and Methods. https://www.cdc.gov/flu/weekly/overview.htm (accessed August 22, 2022), 2022b.

Cocoros NM, Kirby C, Zambarano B, Ochoa A, Eberhardt K, Rocchio Sb C, Ursprung WS, Nielsen VM, Durham NN, Menchaca JT, Josephson M, Erani D, Hafer E, Weiss M, Herrick B, Callahan M, Isaac T, Klompas M. RiskScape: A data visualization and aggregation platform for public health surveillance using routine electronic health record data. Am J Public Health. 2021;111(2):269–276.

Commonwealth of Massachusetts. HiWay Regulations FAQS. https://www.masshiway.net/index.php/Regulations/Regulations_FAQs. June 2021.

Declich S, Carter AO. Public health surveillance: Historical origins, methods and evaluation. Bull World Health Organ. 1994;72(2):285–304.

DiCAYA. Assessing the Burden of Diabetes by Type in Children, Adolescents, and Young Adults Network. https://www.dicaya.org/home (accessed November 10, 2022), 2022.

Diez Roux AV, Moore KA, Melly SJ, Wang X, Joshi R. Neighborhood Health and Poverty in Philadelphia. In Urban Collaborative Data Brief Number 2. Philadelphia PA: Dornsife School of Public Health, Drexel University, 2017.

Dowdy DW, Pai M. Bridging the gap between knowledge and health: The epidemiologist as accountable health advocate ("AHA!"). Epidemiology. 2012;23(6):914–918.

Fairchild AL, Bayer R, Green SH, Colgrove J, Kilgore E, Sweeney M, Varma JK. The two faces of fear: A history of hard-hitting public health campaigns against tobacco and AIDS. Am J Public Health. 2018;108(9):1180–1186.

Food & Drug Administration. Clinical Trial Diversity. https://www.fda.gov/consumers/minority-health-and-health-equity-resources/clinical-trial-diversity (accessed August 18, 2022), 2021.

Gostin LO. Jacobson v Massachusetts at 100 years: Police power and civil liberties in tension. Am J Public Health. 2005;95(4):576–581.

Gould DW, Walker D, Yoon PW. The evolution of BioSense: Lessons learned and future directions. Public Health Rep. 2017;132(1_suppl):7S–11S.

Greenland S. Ecologic versus individual-level sources of bias in ecologic estimates of contextual health effects. Int J Epidemiol. 2001;30(6):1343–1350.

Hanna-Attisha M, LaChance J, Sadler RC. Champney schnepp a. Elevated blood lead levels in children associated with the Flint drinking water crisis: A spatial analysis of risk and public health response. Am J Public Health. 2016;106(2):283–290.

Harsono D, Galletly CL, O'Keefe E, Lazzarini Z. Criminalization of HIV exposure: A review of empirical studies in the United States. AIDS Behav. 2017;21(1):27–50.

KFL&A Public Health. Acute Care Enhanced Surveillance. https://www.kflaphi.ca/acute-care-enhanced-surveillance/ (accessed August 22, 2022), 2022.

Khoury MJ, Gwinn M, Ioannidis JP. The emergence of translational epidemiology: From scientific discovery to population health impact. Am J Epidemiol. 2010;172(5):517–524.

Kraus EM, Brand B, Hohman KH, Baker EL. New directions in public health surveillance: Using electronic health records to monitor chronic disease. J Public Health Manag Pract. 2022;28(2):203–206.

Kruse CS, Stein A, Thomas H, Kaur H. The use of electronic health records to support population health: A systematic review of the literature. J Med Syst. 2018;42(11):214.

McNabb S, Ryland P, Sylvester J, Shaikh A. Informatics enables public health surveillance. Journal of Health Specialties. 2017;5(2):55.

National Cancer Institute. Tobacco. http://www.cancer.gov/about-cancer/causes-prevention/risk/tobacco (accessed December 2, 2021), 2017.

National Electronic Disease Surveillance System Working Group. National electronic disease surveillance system (NEDSS): A standards-based approach to connect public health and clinical medicine. J Public Health Manag Pract. 2001;7(6):43–50.

National Institutes of Health. Menopausal Hormone Therapy Information. https://www.nih.gov/health-information/menopausal-hormone-therapy-information (accessed August 18, 2022), 2016.

Office of the National Coordinator for Health Information Technology. Success Stories. https://www.healthit.gov/success-stories (accessed August 18, 2022), 2022.

Oishi S, Schimmack U. Residential mobility, well-being, and mortality. J Pers Soc Psychol. 2010;98(6):980–994.

Applications of Electronic Health Record Research

Overhage JM, Grannis S, McDonald CJ. A comparison of the completeness and timeliness of automated electronic laboratory reporting and spontaneous reporting of notifiable conditions. Am J Public Health. 2008;98(2):344–350.

Rose G. Sick individuals and sick populations. Int J Epidemiol. 1985;14(1):32–38.

Susser M. Causal Thinking in the Health Sciences. New York, NY: Oxford University Press, 1973.

van-Dijk A, Aramini J, Edge G, Moore KM. Real-time surveillance for respiratory disease outbreaks, Ontario, Canada. Emerg Infect Dis. 2009;15(5):799–801.

Vivolo-Kantor AM, Smith H 4th, Scholl L. Differences and similarities between emergency department syndromic surveillance and hospital discharge data for nonfatal drug overdose. Ann Epidemiol. 2021;62:43–50.

Vogel J, Brown JS, Land T, Platt R, Klompas M. MDPHnet: Secure, distributed sharing of electronic health record data for public health surveillance, evaluation, and planning. Am J Public Health. 2014;104(12):2265–2270.

Walburg D. Flint doctor used Epic Systems records to expose lead crisis. Wisconsin State Journal. January 30, 2016. https://madison.com/news/local/health-med-fit/flint-doctor-used-epic-systems-records-to-expose-lead-crisis/article_ef462592-f27b-5ed0-a2ff-33232902ab74.html.

Welch HG. Less Medicine, More Health: 7 Assumptions That Drive Too Much Medical Care. Boston, MA: Beacon Press, 2016.

Williams BA, Voyce S, Sidney S, Roger VL, Plante TB, Larson S, LaMonte MJ, Labarthe DR, DeBarmore BM, Chang AR, Chamberlain AM, Benziger CP. Establishing a national cardiovascular disease surveillance system in the United States using electronic health record data: Key strengths and limitations. J Am Heart Assoc. 2022;11(8):e024409.

Willis SJ, Cocoros NM, Randall LM, Ochoa AM, Haney G, Hsu KK, DeMaria A Jr, Klompas M. Electronic health record use in public health infectious disease surveillance, USA, 2018-2019. Curr Infect Dis Rep. 2019;21(10):32.

World Health Organization. Constitution. https://www.who.int/about/governance/constitution (accessed August 18, 2022), 1946.

15 Case Studies in Electronic Health Record Research

The case studies and case briefs included in this chapter are designed to be used in a classroom discussion setting. Readers may redefine or reshape the cases or the discussion questions to suit their interests. Although the cases are adapted from real-world projects, certain details have been changed to emphasize one or more challenges or limitations of EHR research. Additional case studies using the publicly available Medical Information Mart for Intensive Care (MIMIC) database (described in Johnson et al., 2016) may be found in part III of the open access e-book *Secondary Analysis of Electronic Health Records.*[1]

Case study #1: assessing laboratory testing and diagnosis at an outpatient clinic

This case study is adapted from a project examining the uptake of hepatitis C testing at an outpatient federally qualified health center (Goldstein et al., 2022; Jose et al., 2021; Kahal et al., 2018). The health center was expanding their capacity to diagnose and treat chronic infection with hepatitis C through a universal screening program. To evaluate the success of the program, the researchers required baseline data on historic prevalence of hepatitis C diagnosis and testing patterns at the center, and following the implementation of the universal screening program, post-intervention data on diagnosis rates, and testing uptake. The EHR was queried to provide data on chronic hepatitis C diagnoses – using International Classification of Diseases (ICD) diagnostic codes – and corresponding laboratory orders. These testing orders were captured in the EHR via Current Procedural Terminology (CPT) codes and test results were captured in the EHR via Logical Observation Identifiers Names and Codes (LOINC). The universal screening program was implemented in 2015 via an "alert" if a hepatitis C lab was not found in the EHR. The researchers decided to retrospectively analyze EHR data for a five-year period before and after the intervention, i.e., 2010–2020.

Several notable issues were identified by the researchers during the study. First, the health center switched from ICD-9-CM to ICD-10-CM codes in 2014. Second, healthcare workers and billing personnel may have used various codes for capturing diagnoses and laboratory orders during the 10-year study period. Further, patients may have visited any number of diagnostic laboratories in the study

DOI: 10.4324/9781003258872-19

area, each of which may have reported and interpreted the test result differently. The test results were stored as a free-text note in the EHR as opposed to discrete, coded values. Third, uptake of the program was not instantaneous following the intervention in 2015: there was a ramp-up period of approximately one year while processes were refined, and the healthcare workers became familiar with the workflow changes.

Discussion questions

1 What are the tradeoffs of assessing a diagnosis via ICD codes alone? What are several alternative strategies?
2 What kind of bias could the change in ICD codes during the study period induce? How can the researchers minimize its potential impact?
3 How can researchers form a list of the relevant ICD, CPT, or LOINC codes to be mined from the EHR? How can they verify their assumptions?
4 What options do the researchers have for operationalizing a discrete variable from the free-text reported test result? What are the pros and cons of these approaches?
5 Define how to construct clinic-wide measures of baseline diagnoses and laboratory orders. What data and which patients should comprise the numerator and denominator for these measures? Repeat for measures of post-intervention diagnoses and orders.
6 What study design best describes this case study? What analytic strategies are appropriate for comparing the before and after time periods?

Case study #2: the inpatient hospital setting as a risk factor for disease

This case study is adapted from a project assessing extrinsic risk factors for disease in a neonatal intensive care unit (Goldstein et al., 2016; Goldstein et al., 2017a; Goldstein et al., 2018a). Such extrinsic risk factors included measures of occupancy – that is, the number of patients in the unit – as well as spatial and environmental factors that may influence disease risk. For this project, researchers were interested in assessing whether measures of these extrinsic risk factors correlated with the occurrence of disease. The researchers formed a retrospective cohort of infants admitted to the intensive care unit for a five-year period, from 2015 to 2020 (approximately 5,000 unique admissions). The exposures of primary interest included occupancy, as measured by the average number of other infants in the unit for a given hospitalization, patient room identified by the room number, as well as features of the rooms and intensive care unit, such as size of the room, presence of refrigerators or bathrooms in the room, and nursing care patterns. The primary outcome was incident infection that occurred 72 hours post-admission.

The cohort was identified through the EHR, and pertinent data extracted, including room number, room transfers, intrinsic markers of health among the infants such as gestational age or birthweight, and the study end points of infection or discharge. All other extrinsic factors including the size of the room, features of the room such single or double occupancy, and nursing care patterns were provided to the study team and linked at the patient-level. Missing data were minimal. Given the spatial features of the dataset, special analytic techniques were required to account for the nonindependence of observations (clustering at the room level), and the appropriate regression techniques were employed to estimate incidence of the outcome. Nursing care patterns were used to identify "neighbors" for the determining the presence of spatial dependency in the data.

Discussion questions

1   How can the researchers identify data that exist or do not exist in the EHR as required for this project? How can the researchers determine what data are discrete versus free-text?
2   Compare and contrast the various approaches for abstracting these data from the EHR, assuming the investigators have access to the EHR.
3   Now, assuming that the data are not accessible to the investigators, but rather will be abstracted on their behalf, how can the investigators ensure that the right data are abstracted?
4   What are the limitations of a single-center EHR study for generating generalizable knowledge on the intensive care unit as a risk factor for disease? How do we verify if this intensive care unit is comparable to others?
5   How may assumptions the researchers make about occupancy, room transfers, or nursing assignments impact the analysis? How can these be tested?

Case study #3: catchment of a health center and validity of inference

This case study is adapted from an analysis of community deprivation and diagnosis of chronic hepatitis C infection (Goldstein et al., 2021). The patients forming the study population were derived from an EHR at a federally qualified health center. The researchers were studying whether selection into the health center – and more specifically the EHR – was patterned based on community deprivation and hepatitis C diagnosis. Understanding the catchment area of a health center is a fundamental challenge in EHR research that may impact both internal and external validity. From an internal validity perspective, selection into the study by patterns in the exposure and outcome may lead to selection bias. From an external validity perspective, a nonrepresentative sample may threaten generalizability or transportability. In this study, the target population for inference was the local community.

A cohort of patients for a five-year period (2008–2013) was selected from the EHR, geocoded to their most recent address recorded in the EHR, and mapped to their respective census tracts. After geocoding, census data on education, employment, income and poverty, and household composition were used to form census tract deprivation scores. To model catchment, the researchers explored three distance-based radii from the health center that would capture 75%, 80%, and 90% of the patient population. Then, using the catchment model as an inverse probability weight in the regression model – in other words, patients within the catchment area are likely overrepresented in the data and patients outside the catchment area are likely underrepresented in the data – the authors compared how inference would change between area deprivation and diagnosis of chronic hepatitis C.

Discussion questions

1 What are the general complications of using patients' addresses, and specific complications of using patients' most recent addresses, recorded in the EHR? What are alternative strategies?
2 What are the implications of geocoding into census tracts when the cohort period spans a decennial census? How can this be remediated?
3 Describe the limitations of a distance-based radius from the health center as a proxy for catchment. How else may catchment be assessed?
4 What is the relationship between sampling error, selection bias, and representativeness?
5 Aside from the potential selection bias, discuss how information bias may arise from the EHR data used in this study. How can information bias be addressed in EHR-based studies?
6 Under what conditions would researchers not be concerned with modeling the catchment of an EHR?

Cases study #4: case–control study from the EHR

This case study is adapted from a study of hospital-onset *Clostridioides difficile* infection among patients at an urban safety-net hospital (Vader et al., 2021). The study used case–control sampling of inpatients who were diagnosed with an incident infection 72 hours post-admission, frequency matched on age and length of stay to controls who did not have a documented infection in the EHR. The controls were sampled hospital wide. Eligibility criteria included patients being 18 years and older, not pregnant, and not incarcerated, who were hospitalized between 2010 and 2020. Cases and controls were geocoded to their residential address, and linked to census tract-level indicators of education, employment, income and poverty, and household composition to form census tract deprivation scores. Aside from age, address, and length of stay, other covariates retrieved from the EHR included race, ethnicity, insurance type, referral location, antibiotic use, and proton-pump inhibitor use. The authors noted significant missing data across many variables in the EHR and used multiple imputation to assess the impact. The authors further noted that data were not available on two important factors: recent hospitalizations and prior *Clostridioides difficile* infection. Both descriptive and analytic analyses were used to compare hospital demographics to national surveillance data as well as to isolate the independent contributions of the enumerated covariates.

Discussion questions

1 For each of the variables in the analysis, describe how measurement error may occur in the EHR. Which variables are most likely and least likely to contain measurement error?
2 For each of the variables in the analyses, describe how missing data may occur in the EHR (speculate on the type of missing data mechanism). Which variables are most likely and least likely to contain missing data?
3 How can the EHR be used to identify the eligible participants in this case–control study? How can the EHR be used to identify cases and controls specifically?
4 Name several potential limitations with comparing a single-center EHR to national statistics. What may explain the observed differences?
5 For the two variables not found in the EHR – recent hospitalizations and prior *Clostridioides difficile* infection – how might the researchers obtain these data? If the data are not available, how can the researchers assess the potential impact on the analysis?

Case study #5: simulating a patient care environment using EHR data

This case study is adapted from a simulation model of the neonatal intensive care unit developed to explore the potential for methicillin-resistant *Staphylococcus aureus* (MRSA) transmission in the unit (Goldstein et al., 2017b; Goldstein et al., 2018b). The EHR does not have to be used in a traditional observational analysis: it can be used to inform hypothetical studies as well. Such studies rely on "what-if" simulations that are created and evaluated computationally to compare varying exposures or interventions. They are frequently employed when a real-world study is unfeasible or unethical. In simulation models, the study setting, participants, and modeling parameters may be informed from literature, expert opinion, best guesses, or real-world data, such as the EHR. The advantage of using EHR data as opposed to these other data sources is the ability to ground the work in an actual setting, thereby improving inference and applicability of the study findings to the practice.

In this study, the researchers created a simulation model based on an actual neonatal intensive care unit and the parameters for the number of infants, characteristics of those infants (such as gestational age or birthweight), and healthcare workers interactions with the infants were informed from the local EHR. For example, healthcare worker interactions with infants can be garnered from care documentation events in the EHR, which are then ranked by their capacity to contaminate a healthcare worker with MRSA. Infants can then be linked together by common healthcare providers, and the propensity for MRSA transmission evaluated to inform hand hygiene practices, MRSA surveillance frequency, de-colonization regimens, or other interventions.

Discussion questions

1 What are the tradeoffs in using a single-center EHR to tune the parameters in a simulated setting as opposed to a literature review, expert opinion, best guesses, or other sources of data?
2 Describe common issues with EHR data quality and how those may impact the parameters in this simulation study.
3 How can a simulation model be validated to reflect reality in a patient care?
4 Describe how EHR data may be used to assess factors other than a patient's health in a healthcare setting, such as patient transfers, occupancy, and health-care worker patterns.

Case brief #1: data linkage

Researchers need to link pediatric EHR data to external data sources to inves-tigate how location and environmental factors may affect postnatal outcomes among various racial subgroups. Specifically, the researchers would like to link EHR data to vital statistics (birth records) and retrieve maternal information for each infant in the EHR. There are two overarching challenges: (1) the lack of a clear unique identifier to link data and (2) discrepancies between race as recorded in the EHR and race as recorded on the birth certificate for the infants.

Discussion questions

1 Describe how to link EHR data with other data sources when a unique iden-tifier is not available, along with the advantages and disadvantages to the approaches?
2 How can discrepancies in the data linkage (as described in the case brief) be resolved? In other words, which data are the best to use? Discuss the pros and cons to the approaches.

Case brief #2: data versus analysis

A clinic is interested in assessing the hepatitis C care cascade for a cohort of pa-tients followed in an outpatient EHR. A simplified view of this care cascade is Testing → Disease Staging → Labs → Treatment → Cure. Patients first need to be tested for infection, then have the disease staged (through labs or imaging) for the appropriate treatment, followed by prescribed therapy, and post-treatment labs to determine whether cured. Each step in this cascade can be represented by a percentage metric, yet the EHR does not contain variables corresponding to each of the discrete steps. Rather, the EHR contains data on diagnostic codes, reported lab results, and medication administration for each patient in a time-series fashion.

Discussion questions

1 How can an analytic dataset be constructed to depict the hepatitis C care case based only on the patient-level time-series data found in the EHR? What assumptions are required and what are the implications of those assumptions?
2 For each variable in the care cascade, define the numerator and denominator and how those may be obtained from the EHR.

Case brief #3: data abstraction

Researchers partnering with a community hospital are planning a study of postpartum hemorrhage following labor and delivery among a cohort of 1,000 pregnant women. The cohort will be assembled retrospectively from the EHR, requiring data on the following variables: maternal age, parity, maternal platelet counts by trimester and at delivery, treatment administered for thrombocytopenia, platelet count before and after treatment administered, physician indication for treatment, bleeding events during pregnancy, hospital admissions, gestational age at delivery, mode of delivery, type of anesthesia, birthweight, postpartum hemorrhage, fetal death, and neonatal platelet count. Unfortunately, the informatics group at the hospital is unable to provide an automated extract of these data; therefore, these data must be manually abstract from the EHR.

Discussion questions

1 What resources (e.g., personnel) and technology will be required to perform this manual abstraction?
2 Compare and contrast different approaches for performing this data abstraction. How can the accuracy and integrity of these data be ensured?
3 Design a study to audit the manually abstracted data.

Case brief #4: non-EHR data

Researchers working on a study of surgical outcomes at a large academic medical center require epidemiological data not currently captured in the institutional EHR, including occupation, housing status, income, and employment. A retrospective cohort of 5,000 patients already exists. All other pertinent data have been abstracted from the EHR. This cohort is contemporary, recruited in the past year.

Discussion questions

1 What are several potential approaches to obtaining data that have not been captured in the EHR for the patients in this cohort? Reflect on the pros and cons for each approach, including approaches that require *de novo* data collection and approaches that rely upon existing data.

2 Now suppose that these data were captured in the social history section of a free text note. How might researchers operationalize discrete measures from free text? How can the accuracy of their approach be confirmed?

Case brief #5: surveillance from the EHR

Public health is partnering with a leading health system that provides the majority of inpatient and outpatient obstetrical and pediatric care in an area to participate in their EHR-based surveillance program. These data will be used to inform population health metrics for the entire region, including maternal immunizations, childhood immunizations, infant mortality, and maternal mortality.

Discussion questions

1 Describe how to use an EHR for population health management. Define the setting and the EHR data required.
2 How will the catchment and selection process of this health system impact the population health metrics mentioned in the case brief?
3 How can the accuracy and completeness of the data in the EHR be verified?

Case brief #6: hospital readmissions

A research group is interested in exploring hospital readmission rates in a metropolitan area to predict correlates of readmission for heart disease. The research group is embedded with a single hospital and has access to their institutional EHR, with a catchment of approximately 20% for the geographic area. Other hospitals in this area have similar catchments: there is no one health system that has a monopoly of care. The researchers are relying on discharge codes and death certificates to identify heart disease-related admissions.

Discussion questions

1 What data sources might be used to examine readmissions across catchment areas? What are the pros and cons for each of these data sources?
2 What issues might arise in relying on diagnostic codes to identify heart disease? What issues might arise in relying on death certificates to identify heart disease? What can be done to minimize the impact of these potential biases?
3 How might selection bias impact this study?

Case brief #7: claims versus EHR data

Researchers have access to an EHR-claims linked database covering visits to a women's health clinic that is part of an academic medical center. They are interested in studying diagnosis and treatment of endometriosis over a five-year period.

Given the potential for misdiagnosis of this health condition, the researchers are interested in performing a validation study of the diagnosis before proceeding to other research aims.

Discussion questions

1 What are the differences between claims databases and EHR databases?
2 Which database should the researchers use as the reference "gold standard" for this validation study? How else might the researchers conduct this validation study?

Case brief #8: building a research database

Researchers have been tasked with creating a comprehensive research database of oncology patients that will be used to identify social and environmental drivers of outcomes both within and across multiple locations. Data sources to be linked include a tumor registry, multiple EHRs, claims data, census data, and environmental surveys.

Discussion questions

1 Compare and contrast several approaches for constructing the research database, from a simple spreadsheet to the use of a common data model. What are the tradeoffs inherent in each approach?
2 How can the researchers approach the problem of data linkage with such varied data sources? What are the requirements?

Note

1 The e-book is available at http://dx.crossref.org/10.1007/978-3-319-43742-2.

References

Goldstein ND, Eppes SC, Ingraham BC, Paul DA. Characteristics of late-onset sepsis in the NICU: Does occupancy impact risk of infection? J Perinatol. 2016;36(9):753–757.

Goldstein ND, Eppes SC, Mackley A, Tuttle D, Paul DA. A network model of hand hygiene: How good is good enough to stop the spread of MRSA?. Infect Control Hosp Epidemiol 2017b;38(8):945–952.

Goldstein ND, Ingraham BC, Eppes SC, Drees M, Paul DA. Assessing occupancy and its relation to healthcare-associated infections. Infect Control Hosp Epidemiol. 2017a;38(1):112–114.

Goldstein ND, Jenness SM, Tuttle D, Power M, Paul DA, Eppes SC. Evaluating a neonatal intensive care unit MRSA surveillance programme using agent-based network modelling. J Hosp Infect. 2018b;100(3):337–343.

Goldstein ND, Kahal D, Testa K, Burstyn I. Inverse probability weighting for selection bias in a Delaware community health center electronic medical record study of community deprivation and hepatitis c prevalence. Ann Epidemiol. 2021;60:1–7.

Goldstein ND, Kahal D, Testa K, Gracely EJ, Burstyn I. Data quality in electronic health record research: An approach for validation and quantitative bias analysis for imperfectly ascertained health outcomes via diagnostic codes. Harvard Data Science Review. 2022;4(2). DOI: 10.1162/99608f92.cbe67e91.

Goldstein ND, Tuttle D, Tabb LP, Paul DA, Eppes SC. Spatial and environmental correlates of organism colonization and infection in the neonatal intensive care unit. J Perinatol. 2018a;38(5):567–573.

Johnson AE, Pollard TJ, Shen L, Lehman LW, Feng M, Ghassemi M, Moody B, Szolovits P, Celi LA, Mark RG. MIMIC-III, a freely accessible critical care database. Sci Data. 2016;3:160035.

Jose R, Kahal D, Testa K, Goldstein ND. A qualitative study of implementing universal hepatitis c screening among adults at an urban community-based health provider in Delaware. Dela J Public Health. 2021;7(3):16–23.

Kahal D, Goldstein ND, Bincsik A, Stephens T, Testa K, Szabo S. Expanding care for patients infected with hepatitis c through community partnership in Delaware. Dela J Public Health. 2018;4(5):76–79.

Vader DT, Weldie C, Welles SL, Kutzler MA, Goldstein ND. Hospital-acquired *Clostridioides difficile* infection among patients at an urban safety-net hospital in Philadelphia: Demographics, neighborhood deprivation, and the transferability of national statistics. Infect Control Hosp Epidemiol. 2021;42(8):948–954.

Appendices

Appendix 1

Secondary Data Research Planner

Study aims	*Chapter 3*
Lead researcher (PI):	_____
Co-investigator(s):	_____
	_____
	_____
	_____
Other key personnel:	_____
	_____
Research question(s) or	_____
specific aim(s):	_____
	_____
	_____
	_____
Hypothesis(es):	_____
	_____
	_____
	_____
	_____
IRB needed:	_____ Yes _____ No
IRB review type:	_____ Exempt _____ Expedited _____ Full
IRB (primary):	_____
IRB (secondary):	_____

Funding   *Chapter 3*

Needed: _____ Yes   _____ No

Anticipated budget: $_____

Funding type: _____ Grant/Agreement _____ Contract

                           _____ Other

Potential funders: _____

                           _____

                           _____

                           _____

Competing interests: _____

EHR data source   *Chapter 4*

Data source: _____ Single institution   _____ Multi-institution

                    _____ Claims database   _____ Other

Export method: _____ Chart review   _____ Reporting tool

                    _____ Direct connection   _____ Existing extract

Data location: _____ Internal   _____ External   _____ Other

Data interface: _____ SQL   _____ Data file   _____ Other

Source description: _____

                           _____

                           _____

                           _____

Institution/location(s):   _____

                           _____

EHR data point person: _____

                           _____

Supplementary sources: _____

                           _____

                           _____

                           _____

Data description   *Chapters 4 and 5*

Type of data: _____ Cross-sectional   _____ Longitudinal

Data organization: _____ Wide   _____ Long

Merge/link required: _____ Merging   _____ Linking   _____ Both

Merge/link description: _____

                      _____

                      _____

                      _____

Population description: _____

                      _____

                      _____

                      _____

Years of data: _____

Num. subjects: _____

Num. observations: _____

Additional denominator   _____

  considerations: _____

Variables   *Chapters 4 and 5*

Unique identifier: _____

Primary exposure(s):   _____

Primary outcome(s):   _____

Potential confounder(s):   _____

_____

_____

_____

Potential mediator(s):   _____

_____

Potential modifier(s):   _____

_____

Other core variables: _____

_____

_____

_____

Variables not available: _____

_____

Epidemiology   *Chapters 7 and 8*

Study design: _____ Cross-sectional   _____ Cohort

                           _____ Case-control   _____ Longitudinal

                           _____ Multi-level   _____ Other

Inclusion criteria: _____

                           _____

                           _____

Exclusion criteria: _____

                           _____

                           _____

Power analysis: _____

Matching: _____ Yes   _____ No

Matching factor(s):   _____

Disease measures: _____ Incidence   _____ Prevalence

                           _____ Risk comparison   _____ Survival

Analysis   *Chapters 10 and 11*

Missing data: _____ Yes   _____ No

Missing data type: _____ MCAR   _____ MAR   _____ MNAR

Imputation: _____ Yes   _____ No

Estimate type: _____ Crude   _____ Adjusted

Analytic technique: _____ Descriptive   _____ Other

                           _____ Regression   Specify type: _____

                           _____ ML   Specify type: _____

Regression assumptions: _____ Normality   _____ Independence

                           _____ Linearity   _____ Equal variance

Sensitivity analysis: _____

                           _____

                           _____

Unexpected deviations: _____

                           _____

Publication and Presentation   *Chapter 13*

Dissemination: _____ Publication _____ Presentation

Target journal: _____

Open access: _____ Yes   _____ No

Target conference: _____

Abstract deadline: _____

Abstract type: _____ Talk _____ Poster _____ Either

Other mechanisms: _____

                           _____

                           _____

                           _____

Appendix 2

Example Code Using R

Chapter 3

Code #3.1. Saving the birthwt dataset from the MASS package as a CSV.

```
#load the MASS package
library(MASS)

#load the birthwt dataset into the environment
birthwt=birthwt

#View the dataset in RStudio
View(birthwt)

#save as a CSV
#note that missing values are encoded as empty strings,
#but can be encoded
#in any pattern recognizable by the destination, such as
#"." for SAS
write.csv(birthwt, file="birthwt.csv", na="", row.names=F)
```

Chapter 4

Code #4.1. Using SQL to extract and subset data from a Microsoft SQL Server database.

```
#connect to SQL Server database using the RODBC package
library(RODBC)
```

```
#setup the channel using the ODBC data source
#ImmunizationDB
channel = odbcConnect(dsn="ImmunizationDB",
readOnlyOptimize=T)

#issue the query
immunizations = sqlQuery(channel, paste("SELECT [patient
id], [patient name], [gender], [address], [antigen],
[date administered] FROM [patient demographics] LEFT
JOIN [vaccine administered] ON [patient demographics].
[patient id]=[vaccine administered].[patient id] WHERE
[county]='Philadelphia County';"), stringsAsFactors=F)
close(channel)

#save the output
save(immunizations, file="research_database.Rdata")
```

Chapter 5

Code #5.1. Reshaping data from long to wide.

```
#output showing original long format
#ID: the unique ID per person
#Antigen & Date: the repeated measures
#Vaccine: an index for number of vaccines
```

ID	Name	Gender	Address	Antigen	Date	Vaccine
1	Person #1	F	Address for person #1	MMR	1/1/15	1
1	Person #1	F	Address for person #1	HepB	1/1/15	2
2	Person #2	M	Address for person #2	HepB	3/1/15	1
2	Person #2	M	Address for person #2	HepB	5/1/15	2
3	Person #3	F	Address for person #3	DTaP	6/1/15	1
3	Person #3	F	Address for person #3	IPV	6/1/15	2
4	Person #4	M	Address for person #4	IPV	1/1/15	1
4	Person #4	M	Address for person #4	MMR	2/1/15	2
5	Person #5	F	Address for person #5	MMR	9/1/15	1
5	Person #5	F	Address for person #5	DTaP	9/1/15	2

```
#issue the reshape command
reshape(long_format, v.names=c("Antigen","Date"),
timevar="Vaccine", idvar="ID", direction="wide")

#output showing wide format from the above command
#note the variables Antigen.1, Date.1, Antigen.2, Date.2
#correspond to the four
#vaccine variables necessary after transformation from
#long to wide
```

ID	Name	Gender	Address	Antigen.1	Date.1	Antigen.2	Date.2
1	Person #1	F	Address for person #1	MMR	1/1/15	HepB	1/1/15
2	Person #2	M	Address for person #2	HepB	3/1/15	HepB	5/1/15
3	Person #3	F	Address for person #3	DTaP	6/1/15	IPV	6/1/15
4	Person #4	M	Address for person #4	IPV	1/1/15	MMR	2/1/15
5	Person #5	F	Address for person #5	MMR	9/1/15	DTaP	9/1/15

Code #5.2.   Linkage operation of two datasets with unique identifiers using the integrated merge function.

```
#output showing dataset #1
```

ID	Name	Gender	Address	Antigen	Date
1	Person #1	F	Address for person #1	MMR	1/1/15
2	Person #2	M	Address for person #2	HepB	3/1/15
3	Person #3	F	Address for person #3	DTaP	6/1/15
4	Person #4	M	Address for person #4	IPV	1/1/15
5	Person #5	F	Address for person #5	MMR	9/1/15

```
#output showing dataset #2
```

ID	Name	Gender	Address	Antigen	Date
1	Person #1	F	Address for person #1	HepB	1/1/15
2	Person #2	M	Address for person #2	HepB	5/1/15
3	Person #3	F	Address for person #3	IPV	6/1/15
4	Person #4	M	Address for person #4	MMR	2/1/15
5	Person #5	F	Address for person #5	DTaP	9/1/15

```
#link the two vaccine variables from the second dataset
#into the first dataset
#join by ID, and keep all observations from the first
#dataset
```

```
merge(x=dataset1, y=dataset2[,c("ID","Antigen","Date")],
by="ID", all.x=T)

#output showing the linked datasets

ID Name    Gender Address       Antigen.x Date.x Antigen.y Date.y
1  Person F        Address for MMR       1/1/15 HepB      1/1/15
   #1              person #1
2  Person M        Address for HepB      3/1/15 HepB      5/1/15
   #2              person #2
3  Person F        Address for DTaP      6/1/15 IPV       6/1/15
   #3              person #3
4  Person M        Address for IPV       1/1/15 MMR       2/1/15
   #4              person #4
5  Person F        Address for MMR       9/1/15 DTaP      9/1/15
   #5              person #5
```

**Code #5.3.   Linkage operation of two datasets with
unique identifiers using a coded algorithm.**

```
#initialize two new vaccine variables in the first dataset
dataset1$Antigen.2 = NA
dataset1$Date.2 = NA

#initialize a variable to keep track of matches
dataset2$Matched = F

#loop through each observation in the first dataset
for (i in 1:nrow(dataset1))
{
    #look for a match by ID
    matched = which(dataset2$ID==dataset1$ID[i])

    if (length(matched) > 0)
    {
        #found a match, copy over vaccine variables
        dataset1$Antigen.2[i] = dataset2$Antigen[matched]
        dataset1$Date.2[i] = dataset2$Date[matched]

        #indicate a match occurred
        dataset2$Matched[matched] = T
    }
}

#the above code can also be accomplished with the
#integrated merge function by
#specifying the argument all.y=T
```

Code #5.4. Fuzzy matching and linkage approach using the Levenshtein distance.

```
library(vwr) #for levenshtein.distance

#create matching variables in each dataset
#a combination of last name, gender, and date of birth
#upper case with non-alphanumeric characters removed
dataset1$NewID = gsub("[^A-Z0-9]","", toupper(paste
(dataset1$Last_name,dataset1$Gender,dataset1$Date_
of_birth)))
dataset2$NewID = gsub("[^A-Z0-9]","", toupper(paste
(dataset2$Last_name,dataset2$Gender,dataset2$Date_
of_birth)))

#initialize two new vaccine variables in the first
#dataset
dataset1$Antigen.2 = NA
dataset1$Date.2 = NA

#initialize a variable to keep track of matches
dataset2$Matched = F

#loop through each observation in the first dataset
for (i in 1:nrow(dataset1))
{
    #get a list of potential matches
    distance = levenshtein.distance(dataset1$NewID[i],
    dataset2$NewID);

    #check for a match using a distance of 3 as the
    #initial criteria
    if (min(distance)<=3)
    {
        #find the match, note there may be more than one
        #match,
        #but we'll just take the first
        matched = which(distance == min(distance))[1]

        #and copy the vaccine variables
        dataset1$Antigen.2[i] = dataset2$Antigen[matched]
        dataset1$Date.2[i] = dataset2$Date[matched]

        #indicate a match occurred
        dataset2$Matched[matched] = T
    }
}
```

Code #5.5.   Common data type casting operations.

```
#check the data types
str(dataset)

#cast to numeric
dataset$dose_numeric = as.numeric(dataset$dose)

#cast to date, the format argument specifies the format
#of the date
dataset$antigen_date = as.Date(dataset$date,
format="%m/%d/%Y")

#cast to text
dataset$name_text = as.character(dataset$name)

#make categorical
dataset$gender_category = as.factor(dataset$gender)
```

Code #5.6.   Recoding examples.

```
#scenario 1
dataset$gender_mf = ifelse(dataset$gender=="Male" |
dataset$gender=="M", "M", ifelse(dataset$gender=="Female"
| dataset$gender=="F", "F", NA))

#scenario 2
dataset$yesno_10 = ifelse(dataset$yesno_21==2, 1,
ifelse(dataset$yesno_21==1, 0, NA))

#scenario 3
dataset$married_category = ifelse(dataset$married==
"Married", 0, ifelse(dataset$married=="Not Married", 1, NA))

#scenario 4
dataset$weight_kgs = ifelse(is.numeric(dataset$weight_
lbs), (dataset$weight_lbs / 2.2), NA)

#scenario 5
dataset$race_category = ifelse(dataset$race_ethnicity==
"non-Hispanic Caucasian" | dataset$race_ethnicity==
"Hispanic Caucasian", 0, ifelse(dataset$race_ethnicity==
"non-Hispanic African American" | dataset$race_
ethnicity=="Hispanic African American", 1,
```

```
ifelse(dataset$race_ethnicity=="non-Hispanic Asian" |
dataset$race_ethnicity=="Hispanic Asian", 2, NA)))

dataset$ethnicity_category = ifelse(dataset$race_
ethnicity=="non-Hispanic Caucasian" | dataset$race_
ethnicity=="non-Hispanic African American" |
dataset$race_ethnicity=="non-Hispanic Asian", 0,
ifelse(dataset$race_ethnicity=="Hispanic Caucasian" |
dataset$race_ethnicity=="Hispanic African American" |
dataset$race_ethnicity=="Hispanic Asian", 1, NA))

#scenario 6
dataset$education_category = ifelse(dataset$education==
"grade school or below" | dataset$education=="middle
school" | dataset$education=="high school no diploma",
0, ifelse(dataset$education=="high school diploma or
equivalent" | dataset$education=="college without
degree", 1, ifelse(dataset$education=="associates
degree" | dataset$education=="bachelors degree" |
dataset$education=="masters degree" | dataset$education==
"doctoral degree", 2, NA)))

# scenario 7
dataset$region_category = ifelse(dataset$northeast==1,
"Northeast", ifelse(dataset$south==1, "South",
ifelse(dataset$midwest==1, "Midwest",
ifelse(dataset$west==1, "West", NA))))

#scenario 8
dataset$bmi_calculated = ifelse(is.
numeric(dataset$weight_kgs) &
is.numeric(dataset$height_m), (dataset$weight_kgs /
(dataset$height_m^2)), NA)

#scenario 9
dataset$ibuprofen = ifelse(length(grep("ibuprofen",
dataset$medications, ignore.case=T))>0, 1, 0)
```

Code #5.7.   Splitting one observation into two observations.

```
#create a linking variable placeholder in original
#dataset
dataset$split_record = NA
```

```
#copy the observation in position i to a temporary
#dataset to split
split_observations = dataset[i, ]

#duplicate the observation for a total of two new
#records
split_observations = rbind(split_observations,
split_observations[1,])

#create a linking variable that is based on position i
#with the suffix of the
#number of new records, separated by a period
split_observations$split_record = paste(i, "2", sep=".")

#perform any other variable manipulations here, such as
#to remove any data
#related to the second offspring from split_
#observations[1, ] and likewise to
#remove any data related to the first offspring from
#split_observations[2, ]

#merge the two new observations back to the original
#dataset
dataset = rbind[dataset, split_observations]

#drop the original observation
dataset = dataset[-i, ]
```

**Code #5.8.   Proposed fuzzy matching approach for
duplicate observation detection.**

```
library(vwr) #for levenshtein.distance

#create a matching variables in the dataset
#a combination of last name, gender, and date of birth
#upper case with non-alphanumeric characters removed
dataset$NewID = gsub("[^A-Z0-9]","", toupper(paste
(dataset$Last_name,dataset$Gender,dataset$Date_
of_birth)))

#initialize a variable to keep track of potential duplicates
dataset$Duplicate = NA
```

```
#loop through each observation in the dataset
for (i in 1:nrow(dataset))
{
    #get a list of potential matches, but will self match
    distance = levenshtein.distance(dataset$NewID[i],
    dataset$NewID);

    #set the self match above the distance threshold
    distance[i] = 99

    #check for a match using a distance of 3 as the
    #initial criteria
    if (min(distance)<=3)
    {
        #find the match, note there may be more than one
        #match
        matched = which(distance<=3)

        #record the potential duplicate(s)
        dataset$Duplicate[i] = paste(matched, collapse=",")
    }
}

#review list of potential duplicates
dataset[!is.na(dataset$Duplicate), ]
```

Chapter 7

Code #7.1.   Assembling a cross-section from the research database.

```
#subset by inclusion/exclusion criteria
analytic_dataset = subset(research_database, year>=2001
& year<=2020 & born_at_hospital==1)

#keep only core variables
analytic_dataset = analytic_dataset[, c("ID", "birth_
weight", "staph_infection", "delivery_method", "sex",
"race", "ethnicity", "mom_marital_status", "mom_age",
"+other variables")]
```

Code #7.2. Assembling a cohort from the research database.

```
#subset by inclusion/exclusion criteria
working_dataset = subset(research_database, year>=2001 &
year<=2020 & born_at_hospital==1)

#keep only core variables
working_dataset = working_dataset[, c("ID", "birth_
weight", "staph_infection", "delivery_method", "sex",
"race", "ethnicity", "mom_marital_status", "mom_age",
"+other variables")]

## OPTION1: entire cohort
analytic_dataset = working_dataset

## OPTION2: randomly select unexposed 1:1 with exposed
#sample on exposure, all VLBW<1500g
analytic_dataset = subset(working_dataset, VLBW<1500)

#seed ensures consistency if need to reproduce
set.seed(777)

#randomly select unexposed, without replacement
analytic_dataset = rbind(analytic_dataset, working_
dataset[sample(which(working_dataset$VLBW>=1500),
nrow(analytic_dataset), replace=F), ])
```

Code #7.3. Assembling a case-control sample from the research database.

```
#subset by inclusion/exclusion criteria
working_dataset = subset(research_database, year>=2001 &
year<=2020 & born_at_hospital==1)

#keep only core variables
working_dataset = working_dataset[, c("ID", "birth_
weight", "staph_infection", "delivery_method", "sex",
"race", "ethnicity", "mom_marital_status", "mom_age",
"+other variables")]
```

```
#create a placeholder for matched case and control
working_dataset$matched = NA

#sample all cases (assume case = 1 and control = 0)
analytic_dataset = subset(working_dataset, case==1)

#list of eligible controls by unique identifier
eligible = working_dataset$MRN[working_dataset$case==0]

#seed ensures consistency if need to reproduce
set.seed(777)

#iterate over all cases to select one control per case
for (i in 1:nrow(analytic_dataset))
{
  #sample a control
  potential = sample(eligible, 1)

  need_control = TRUE
  while (need_control)
  {
    #check for matching characteristics, if any
    #when match, set need_control to FALSE, otherwise
    #sample a new potential
    #control using: potential = sample(eligible, 1)
  }

  #add as a control for this case
  analytic_dataset = rbind(analytic_dataset, working_
  dataset[which(working_dataset$MRN==potential), ])

  #track match using the case ID
  analytic_dataset$matched[i] = analytic_dataset$ID[i]
  analytic_dataset$matched[nrow(analytic_dataset)] =
  analytic_dataset$ID[i]

  #remove from control eligible list
  eligible = eligible[-which(eligible==potential)]
}
```

**Code #7.4.   Transforming the analytic dataset from wide
to long format.**

```
#output showing wide format of analytic_dataset

ID Name   Gender Address      Antigen.1 Date.1 Antigen.2 Date.2
1  Person F      Address for  MMR       1/1/15 HepB      1/1/15
   #1            person #1
2  Person M      Address for  HepB      3/1/15 HepB      5/1/15
   #2            person #2
3  Person F      Address for  DTaP      6/1/15 IPV       6/1/15
   #3            person #3
4  Person M      Address for  IPV       1/1/15 MMR       2/1/15
   #4            person #4
5  Person F      Address for  MMR       9/1/15 DTaP      9/1/15
   #5            person #5


#issue the reshape command
#Vaccine will define the vaccine number for each
#individual
#drop removes the original identifier to be replaced with
#a new identifier
reshape(analytic_dataset, varying=c("Antigen.1",
"Date.1","Antigen.2","Date.2"), direction="long",
timevar="Vaccine", drop="ID")


#output showing long format

Name       Gender Address      Vaccine Antigen Date   ID
Person #1  F      Address for  1       MMR     1/1/15 1
                  person #1
Person #2  M      Address for  1       HepB    3/1/15 2
                  person #2
Person #3  F      Address for  1       DTaP    6/1/15 3
                  person #3
Person #4  M      Address for  1       IPV     1/1/15 4
                  person #4
Person #5  F      Address for  1       MMR     9/1/15 5
                  person #5
Person #1  F      Address for  2       HepB    1/1/15 1
                  person #1
Person #2  M      Address for  2       HepB    5/1/15 2
                  person #2
Person #3  F      Address for  2       IPV     6/1/15 3
                  person #3
Person #4  M      Address for  2       MMR     2/1/15 4
                  person #4
Person #5  F      Address for  2       DTaP    9/1/15 5
                  person #5
```

Chapter 10

Code #10.1.   Loading the birthwt dataset and creating the follow-up time variable, gestation.

```
#load the birthwt dataset from the MASS package
library(MASS)
analytic_dataset = birthwt

#seed ensures consistency if need to reproduce
set.seed(777)

#simulate a gestational age variable, where
#smoking increases likelihood of preterm birth
analytic_dataset$gestation = ifelse(analytic_
dataset$smoke==0, round(rnorm(n=nrow(analytic_dataset),
mean=40, sd=1),0), round(rnorm(n=nrow(analytic_dataset),
mean=37, sd=1),0))
```

Code #10.2.   A descriptive analysis of the birthwt analytic dataset.

```
library(gmodels) #CrossTable function
library(psych) #describe function

CrossTable(analytic_dataset$low)
describe(analytic_dataset$age)

#dichotomize maternal weight
analytic_dataset$lwt_170 = ifelse(analytic_
dataset$lwt<170, 0, 1)
CrossTable(analytic_dataset$lwt_170)

CrossTable(analytic_dataset$race)
CrossTable(analytic_dataset$smoke)

#collapse preterm labors
analytic_dataset$ptl_collapsed = ifelse(analytic_
dataset$ptl>1, 1, analytic_dataset$ptl)
CrossTable(analytic_dataset$ptl_collapsed)

CrossTable(analytic_dataset$ht)
CrossTable(analytic_dataset$ui)
```

```
#collapse doctor visits
analytic_dataset$ftv_collapsed = ifelse(analytic_
dataset$ftv>3, 3, analytic_dataset$ftv)
CrossTable(analytic_dataset$ftv_collapsed)

describe(analytic_dataset$bwt)
describe(analytic_dataset$gestation)
```

Code #10.3. Example regression code predicting infant birthweight from maternal weight (two parameterizations).

```
#linear regression, continuous predictor
summary(lm(bwt ~ lwt, data=analytic_dataset))

#linear regression, categorical predictor
summary(lm(bwt ~ as.factor(lwt_170), data=
analytic_dataset))

#logistic regression, categorical predictor
summary(glm(low ~ as.factor(lwt_170), data=analytic_
dataset, family=binomial(link=logit)))
```

Chapter 11

Code #11.1. Estimating the relationship of the potential confounders with the exposure and outcome.

```
library(gmodels) #CrossTable function
library(psych) #describe function

#exposure
describeBy(analytic_dataset$age, analytic_dataset$smoke);
t.test(analytic_dataset$age ~ analytic_dataset$smoke)
CrossTable(analytic_dataset$lwt_170, analytic_dataset$smoke,
prop.r=F, prop.t=F, prop.chisq=F, chisq=T)
CrossTable(analytic_dataset$race, analytic_
dataset$smoke, prop.r=F, prop.t=F, prop.chisq=F, chisq=T)
CrossTable(analytic_dataset$ptl_collapsed, analytic_
dataset$smoke, prop.r=F, prop.t=F, prop.chisq=F, chisq=T)
```

```
CrossTable(analytic_dataset$ht, analytic_dataset$smoke,
prop.r=F, prop.t=F, prop.chisq=F, chisq=T)
CrossTable(analytic_dataset$ui, analytic_dataset$smoke,
prop.r=F, prop.t=F, prop.chisq=F, chisq=T)
CrossTable(analytic_dataset$ftv_collapsed, analytic_
dataset$smoke, prop.r=F, prop.t=F, prop.chisq=F, chisq=T)
describeBy(analytic_dataset$gestation, analytic_
dataset$smoke); t.test(analytic_dataset$gestation ~
analytic_dataset$smoke)

#outcome
describeBy(analytic_dataset$age, analytic_dataset$low);
t.test(analytic_dataset$age ~ analytic_dataset$low)
CrossTable(analytic_dataset$lwt_170, analytic_
dataset$low, prop.r=F, prop.t=F, prop.chisq=F, chisq=T)
CrossTable(analytic_dataset$race, analytic_dataset$low,
prop.r=F, prop.t=F, prop.chisq=F, chisq=T)
CrossTable(analytic_dataset$ptl_collapsed, analytic_
dataset$low, prop.r=F, prop.t=F, prop.chisq=F, chisq=T)
CrossTable(analytic_dataset$ht, analytic_dataset$low,
prop.r=F, prop.t=F, prop.chisq=F, chisq=T)
CrossTable(analytic_dataset$ui, analytic_dataset$low,
prop.r=F, prop.t=F, prop.chisq=F, chisq=T)
CrossTable(analytic_dataset$ftv_collapsed, analytic_
dataset$low, prop.r=F, prop.t=F, prop.chisq=F, chisq=T)
describeBy(analytic_dataset$gestation, analytic_
dataset$low); t.test(analytic_dataset$gestation ~
analytic_dataset$low)
```

Code #11.2.   Estimating the change in effect of the potential confounders with the exposure and outcome.

```
#change in estimates, without confounder
summary(glm(low ~ as.factor(smoke), data=analytic_dataset,
family=binomial(link=logit)))

#with confounder
summary(glm(low ~ as.factor(smoke) + age, data=analytic_
dataset, family=binomial(link=logit)))
summary(glm(low ~ as.factor(smoke) + as.factor(lwt_170),
data=analytic_dataset, family=binomial(link=logit)))
summary(glm(low ~ as.factor(smoke) + as.factor(race),
data=analytic_dataset, family=binomial(logit)))
```

```
summary(glm(low ~ as.factor(smoke) + as.factor
(ptl_collapsed), data=analytic_dataset, family=
binomial(link=logit)))
summary(glm(low ~ as.factor(smoke) + as.factor(ht),
data=analytic_dataset, family=binomial(link=logit)))
summary(glm(low ~ as.factor(smoke) + as.factor(ui),
data=analytic_dataset, family=binomial(link=logit)))
summary(glm(low ~ as.factor(smoke) + as.factor
(ftv_collapsed), data=analytic_dataset, family=
binomial(link=logit)))
summary(glm(low ~ as.factor(smoke) + gestation,
data=analytic_dataset, family=binomial(link=logit)))
```

Code #11.3. Creating a matched case-control study from the birthwt analytic dataset.

```
#create a unique identifier
analytic_dataset$id = 1:nrow(analytic_dataset)

#create a placeholder for matched case and control
analytic_dataset$matched = NA

#sample all cases
matched_dataset = subset(analytic_dataset, low==1)

#list of eligible controls by unique identifier
eligible = analytic_dataset$id[analytic_dataset$low==0]

#seed ensures consistency if need to reproduce
set.seed(776)

#iterate over all cases to select one control per case
for (i in 1:nrow(matched_dataset))
{
  #sample a control
  potential = sample(eligible, 1)

  need_control = TRUE
  while (need_control)
  {
    #match on age +/- 2 years
    if (abs(analytic_dataset$age[potential] - matched_
    dataset$age[i]) <=2) {
      need_control = FALSE
    } else {
```

```
        potential = sample(eligible, 1)
    }
  }

  #add as a control for this case
  matched_dataset = rbind(matched_dataset, analytic_
  dataset[which(analytic_dataset$id==potential), ])

  #track match using the case id
  matched_dataset$matched[i] = matched_dataset$id[i]
  matched_dataset$matched[nrow(matched_dataset)] =
  matched_dataset$id[i]

  #remove from control eligible list
  eligible = eligible[-which(eligible==potential)]
}
```

**Code #11.4. Example analytic models to estimate the
association between smoking and low birthweight in the
birthwt analytic dataset assuming various study designs.**

```
#unadjusted prevalance odds ratio via logistic regression
summary(glm(low ~ as.factor(smoke), data=analytic_dataset,
family=binomial(link=logit)))
exp(0.7041)

#unadjusted prevalance rate ratio via log-binomial
#regression
summary(glm(low ~ as.factor(smoke), data=analytic_dataset,
family=binomial(link=log)))
exp(0.4748)

#adjusted prevalance odds ratio via logistic regression
summary(glm(low ~ as.factor(smoke) + as.factor(race) +
as.factor(ptl_collapsed) + as.factor(ftv_collapsed) +
gestation, data=analytic_dataset, family=binomial
(link=logit)))
exp(0.3667)

#unadjusted cumulative incidence relative risk
library(epitools)
no_outcome_unexposed = sum(!analytic_dataset$low
[analytic_dataset$smoke==0])
outcome_unexposed = sum(analytic_dataset$low
[analytic_dataset$smoke==0])
```

```
no_outcome_exposed = sum(!analytic_dataset$low
[analytic_dataset$smoke==1])
outcome_exposed = sum(analytic_dataset$low
[analytic_dataset$smoke==1])
riskratio(c(no_outcome_unexposed,outcome_unexposed,
no_outcome_exposed,outcome_exposed))

#unadjusted incidence rate ratio
outcome_unexposed = sum(analytic_dataset$low[analytic_
dataset$smoke==0])
outcome_exposed = sum(analytic_dataset$low[analytic_
dataset$smoke==1])
persontime_unexposed = sum(analytic_dataset$gestation
[analytic_dataset$smoke==0])
persontime_exposed = sum(analytic_dataset$gestation
[analytic_dataset$smoke==1])
rateratio(c(outcome_unexposed,outcome_exposed,
persontime_unexposed,persontime_exposed))

#adjusted cumulative incidence relative risk estimated
#via logistic regression
summary(glm(low ~ as.factor(smoke) + as.factor(race) +
as.factor(ptl_collapsed) + as.factor(ftv_collapsed),
data=analytic_dataset, family=binomial(link=logit)))
exp(0.8031)

#adjusted cumulative incidence relative risk estimated
#via modified poisson regression
library(sandwich) #robust standard errors
poissonmod = glm(low ~ as.factor(smoke) + as.factor(race) +
as.factor(ptl_collapsed) + as.factor(ftv_collapsed),
data=analytic_dataset, family=poisson())
poissonmod.cov.matrix = vcovHC(poissonmod, type="HC0")
poissonmod.std.err = sqrt(diag(poissonmod.cov.matrix))
poissonmod.r.est = cbind(Estimate= coef(poissonmod),
"Robust SE" = poissonmod.std.err, "Pr(>|z|)" = 2 *
pnorm(abs(coef(poissonmod)/poissonmod.std.err), lower.
tail=FALSE), LL = coef(poissonmod) - 1.96 * poissonmod.
std.err, UL = coef(poissonmod) + 1.96 * poissonmod.std.
err)
exp(poissonmod.r.est[, c(1,4,5)])

#adjusted cumulative incidence relative risk estimated
#via cox proportional hazards regression
library(survival)
summary(coxph(Surv(gestation, low)~as.factor(smoke) +
as.factor(race) + as.factor(ptl_collapsed) + as.
factor(ftv_collapsed), data=analytic_dataset))
```

```
#adjusted incidence rate ratio estimated via poisson
#regression
summary(glm(low ~ as.factor(smoke) + as.factor(race) +
as.factor(ptl_collapsed) + as.factor(ftv_collapsed),
offset=log(gestation), data=analytic_dataset, family=
poisson()))
exp(0.5540)

#unadjusted survival plot
plot(survfit(Surv(gestation, low) ~ as.factor(smoke),
data=analytic_dataset), lty=c(1,2), xlim=c(30,45),
xlab="Gestation in weeks", ylab="1 - Risk of low
birthweight")
legend(31,0.3,lty=c(1,2),c("Nonsmoker","Smoker"))
summary(coxph(Surv(gestation, low) ~ as.factor(smoke),
data=analytic_dataset))

#unadjusted odds ratio
control_unexposed = sum(!analytic_dataset$low[analytic_
dataset$smoke==0])
case_unexposed = sum(analytic_dataset$low[analytic_
dataset$smoke==0])
control_exposed = sum(!analytic_dataset$low[analytic_
dataset$smoke==1])
case_exposed = sum(analytic_dataset$low[analytic_
dataset$smoke==1])
oddsratio(c(control_unexposed,case_unexposed,control_
exposed,case_exposed))

#adjusted odds ratio estimated via logistic regression
summary(glm(low ~ as.factor(smoke) + as.factor(race) +
as.factor(ptl_collapsed) + as.factor(ftv_collapsed) +
gestation, data=analytic_dataset, family=binomial(link=
logit)))
exp(0.3667)

#adjusted odds ratio estimated via conditional logistic
#regression
summary(clogit(low ~ as.factor(smoke) + as.factor(race) +
as.factor(ptl_collapsed) + as.factor(ftv_collapsed) +
gestation + age + strata(matched), data=matched_dataset))
```

Index

Note: Page references in *italics* denote figures, in **bold** tables and with "n" endnotes.